Practical Guide to

Moderate Sedation/Analgesia

Practical Guide to

Moderate
Sedation/Analgesia

Second Edition

Jan Odom-Forren, RN, BSN, MS, CPAN, FAAN
Perianesthesia/Perioperative Consultant;
Co-editor, Journal of PeriAnesthesia Nursing
Louisville, Kentucky

Donna Watson, RN, MSN, CNOR, ARNP, FNP-C
IV Moderate Sedation Consultant and Educator
Fox Island, Washington

With 22 illustrations

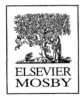

ELSEVIER
MOSBY

ELSEVIER
MOSBY

11830 Westline Industrial Drive
St. Louis, Missouri 63146

Practical Guide to Moderate Sedation/Analgesia
Copyright © 2005, Mosby, Inc.

Previous edition copyrighted 1998.

ISBN-13: 978-0-323-02024-4
ISBN-10: 0-323-02024-0

Executive Editor: Michael S. Ledbetter
Senior Developmental Editor: Lisa P. Newton
Publishing Services Manager: Pat Joiner
Project Manager: Rachel E. Dowell
Senior Designer: Amy Buxton

Transferred to Digital Printing 2010

Contents

1 HISTORY OF MODERATE SEDATION

2 PRESEDATION ASSESSMENT, MONITORING PARAMETERS, AND EQUIPMENT

3 PHARMACOLOGY

4 MANAGEMENT OF COMPLICATIONS

5 PATIENT DISCHARGE

6 INSTITUTION POLICY AND GUIDELINE DEVELOPMENT: STANDARD OF CARE

7 COMPETENCE IN PATIENT MANAGEMENT

8 PEDIATRIC SEDATION

9 GERIATRIC SEDATION

10 SEDATION IN THE MECHANICALLY VENTILATED PATIENT

11 RISK MANAGEMENT/LEGAL ISSUES

APPENDICES

A   ASA Standards for Basic Anesthetic Monitoring

B   State Boards of Nursing Positions on Moderate Sedation and Administration of Anesthetic Agents

C   Position Statement on the Role of the RN in the Management of Patients Receiving IV Moderate Sedation for Short-Term Therapeutic, Diagnostic, or Surgical Procedures

D   ASA Practice Guidelines for Sedation and Analgesia by Non-Anesthesiologists

E   American Association of Nurse Anesthetists' Position Statement: Qualified Providers of Sedation and Analgesia; Considerations for Policy Guidelines for Registered Nurses Engaged in the Administration of Sedation and Analgesia

F   AORN Recommended Practices for Managing the Patient Receiving Moderate Sedation/Analgesia

G   Pediatric Sedation Standards 2002-2004

Contributors

MARCIA BIXBY, RN, MS, CS, CCRN
Clinical Nurse Specialist—Surgical
  Critical Care
Beth Israel Deaconess Medical Center
Boston, Massachusetts

**CHARLOTTE L. GUGLIELMI, RN, BSN,
  CNOR**
Clinical Nurse Specialist
Perioperative Services
Beth Israel Deaconess Medical Center
Boston, Massachusetts

LISA HEARD, RN, CGRN
Clinical Coordinator, Endoscopy
  Program
Children's Hospital Boston
Division of Gastroenterology and
  Nutrition
Boston, Massachusetts

**VALLIRE D. HOOPER, MSN, RN,
  CPAN**
Clinical Assistant Professor
School of Nursing
Medical College of Georgia
Augusta, Georgia;
Clinical Nurse Specialist, Surgical
  Services
St. Joseph Hospital
Augusta, Georgia

**MICHAEL J. KREMER, DNSC, CRNA,
  FAAN**
Associate Professor, Adult Health
  Nursing
Co-Director, Rush University
  Simulation Labs
Assistant Director, Nurse Anesthesia
  Program
Rush University College of Nursing
Chicago, Illinois

KATHY PICARD, RN, MS, CCRN
Clinical Nurse Specialist—Medical
  Critical Care
Beth Israel Deaconess Medical Center
Boston, Massachusetts

NANCY RAYHORN, BSN, CGRN
Clinical Scientist-Medical Science
  Liaison
Centocor, Inc
Malvern, Pennsylvania;
Pediatric Gastroenterology Nurse
  Clinician
Formerly with Phoenix Children's
  Hospital
Phoenix, Arizona

**NANCY M. SAUFL, MS, RN, CPAN,
  CAPA**
Coordinator
Preadmission Testing
Florida Hospital Memorial Division
Ormond Beach, Florida

Reviewers

JOANNE D. CIMORELLI, RN, BS, CNOR, CRNFA
President
First Assistant Services
Havertown, Pennsylvania;
Staff RN and RN First Assistant
Presbyterian Medical Center of University of Pennsylvania Health System
Philadelphia, Pennsylvania

THERESA L. CLIFFORD, MSN, RN, CPAN
PACU Resource Nurse
Mercy Hospital
Portland, Maine

RANDALL C. CORK, MD, PhD
Professor and Chair
Louisiana State University Health Sciences Center
Department of Anesthesiology
Shreveport, Louisiana

DONNA DeFAZIO QUINN, BSN, MBA, RN, CPAN, CAPA
Director
Orthopaedic Surgery Center
Concord, New Hampshire

BEVERLY GEORGE-GAY, MSN, RN, CCRN
Assistant Professor, Coordinator of Distance Education
Department of Nurse Anesthesia
Virginia Commonwealth University, School of Allied Health
Richmond, Virginia

JULIE GOLEMBIEWSKI, PharmD
Clinical Associate Professor
University of Illinois at Chicago
Department of Pharmacy Practice & Anesthesiology
Chicago, Illinois

MYRNA E. MAMARIL, MS, RN, CPAN, CAPA
Clinical Nurse; Nurse Specialist
Weinberg/Carnegie Prep/PACU
Johns Hopkins Hospital
Baltimore, Maryland

DENISE O'BRIEN, MSN, APRN, BC, CPAN, CAPA, FAAN
Clinical Nurse Specialist
UMH-Postanesthesia Care Unit
Department of Operating Rooms/PACU
University of Michigan Health System
Ann Arbor, Michigan

STEPHEN D. PRATT, MD
Director of Quality Improvement
Anesthesia and Critical Care
Beth Israel Deaconess Medical Center
Harvard Medical School
Boston, Massachusetts

LOIS SCHICK, MN, MBA, RN, CPAN, CAPA
Entrepreneur and Staff Nurse
PACU, Ambulatory Surgery
Denver, Colorado

MARTIN YATES, BSN, CRNA
Director of Anesthesia Services
Presbyterian Hospital of Dallas
Dallas, Texas

To

my husband, Gary, for his patience and understanding,
Andrew, Patrick, Kelsey, and Brittany for their support and encouragement.

JAN ODOM-FORREN

my family—Bob, Chris, and Danny.

DONNA WATSON

Preface

The second edition of this book builds on the first edition. Our wish is for this edition to continue as a guide for a safe standard of care for the patient receiving moderate sedation/analgesia. The information included is based on updated national recommended practices, guidelines, and position statements from various nursing and medical organizations. This book is intended for any health care worker who is interested in the safe administration and monitoring of patients undergoing moderate sedation/analgesia during a short-term therapeutic, diagnostic, or surgical procedure in any department or setting. The book is especially tailored as a guide for the RN managing the care of those patients. Our only departure is in Chapter 10 where we discuss all areas of sedation in the mechanically ventilated patient, including long-term ventilation.

Chapter 1 provides vital information for the RN who is managing the patient receiving moderate sedation/analgesia. It gives the reader a short history of the process that helped to define safety standards for the patient undergoing moderate sedation/analgesia as well as the first and only national position statement written by specialty organizations and disseminated by the American Nurses Association. It also highlights recommended practices from various specialty organizations. There is a discussion of the controversial practice of RNs administering anesthetic agents to patients for the purpose of moderate sedation. This chapter also discusses the impact of position statements or other various statements issued from state boards of nursing regarding the role and responsibilities of RNs in their respective states. The chapter goes on to define sedation and discuss the objectives of sedation.

Chapter 2 focuses on guidelines and expectations concerning presedation assessment, patient monitoring, and necessary equipment. Chapter 3 discusses the medications commonly used for moderate sedation/analgesia and provides a quick reference of those medications. Chapter 4 is dedicated to the complications that can occur in the patient undergoing moderate sedation/analgesia, and includes information about the high-risk patients. Chapter 5 is directed to benefit those patients who are discharged home after the procedure or intervention. Chapter 6 discusses institutional policy and guideline development to assist in obtaining a facility-wide standard of care for all patients that access the health care organization. Chapter 7 focuses on the required competence of any RN who will be managing the care of patients who receive moderate sedation/analgesia. Chapter 8 discusses the special population of pediatric patients. Chapter 9 is an addition to this second edition to discuss the special needs of the geriatric population. Chapter 10 is directed to those RNs who care for the mechanically ventilated patient. Chapter 11 was added to this edition to focus on methods of preventing liability for the nurse who takes on the added responsibilities of administering and monitoring moderate sedation/analgesia.

A proliferation of published information discussing the role of the RN in appropriate management of the sedated patient is available. The goal of this book is to provide a guidebook of expected roles and responsibilities for those RNs based on national guidelines and state board of nursing statements. The focus of this book is the patient. The emphasis of every chapter is on safe patient care with a positive outcome for the patient. Through adherence to the guidelines recommended throughout the book and implementation of appropriate monitoring parameters, the RN can significantly lower the risk of an untoward patient event and achieve a high quality of patient care with a positive outcome for the patient. Our desire is to give to the RN a guidebook that can be easily read and referenced and that will facilitate a good outcome for the patient.

JAN ODOM-FORREN
DONNA WATSON

Acknowledgments

We would like to thank the contributors to this edition of *Practical Guide to Moderate Sedation/Analgesia*. This book is even better because of the contributions of knowledgeable experts who share their wisdom with others. Many thanks to Vallire Hooper who contributed chapters on managing complications and competence in patient management; Charlotte Guglielmi who contributed the chapter on institutional policy and guideline development; Lisa Heard and Nancy Rayhorn who contributed the chapter on pediatric sedation; Marcia Bixby and Kathy Picard who added their expertise in the area of sedation in the mechanically ventilated patient; and Nancy Saufl who added a new chapter on sedation in the geriatric population.

The production of this book would not be possible without the dedication and hard work of many individuals. We would like to thank those reviewers who spent time reading and making suggestions for better ways to impart our message: Denise O'Brien, Theresa Clifford, Dr. Randall Cork, Beverly George-Gay, Julie Golembiewski, Myrna Mamaril, Lois Schick, Donna DeFazio Quinn, Martin Yates, and Joanne Cimorelli. A special thanks goes to Lisa Newton, Senior Developmental Editor, who provided us with support and expertise, gave a push when necessary, and answered countless questions; to Michael Ledbetter, Executive Editor, who was instrumental in publishing the first edition of the book and seeing the need for this second edition; and Rachel E. Dowell, Project Manager, for her tireless work with the details of words.

Finally, we would like to thank our colleagues, friends, and families who have tirelessly supported our careers and efforts. Thank you Gary, for watching football games alone while I worked on the book, Andrew and Patrick for always telling me that I could do it, and Brittny and Kelsey for caring.

JAN ODOM-FORREN

Contents

1 HISTORY OF MODERATE SEDATION 1

History—Nursing Perspective 3
Scope of Practice Issues 4
    State Boards of Nursing 5
    Standards of Practice 5
    Position Statements 8
    Practice Guidelines 8
    Recommended Practices 10
    Controversial Issue: Nurse Administered Propofol Sedation 11
    Development of a Standard of Care 12
Levels of Sedation 13
Objectives of Conscious Sedation 16
Patient Selection 17
Conclusion 18

2 PRESEDATION ASSESSMENT, MONITORING PARAMETERS, AND EQUIPMENT 20

Preprocedure Assessment 20
    Nursing History and Physical Evaluation 21
    Patient Selection 29
    Psychosocial Assessment 35
    Diagnostic Assessment 36
    Patient Education 36
    Informed Consent 37
Intraprocedural Monitoring 37
    Patient Monitoring 37
    Circulation 42
    Electrocardiogram 45
    Level of Consciousness 46
    Emergency Equipment 48
Postprocedure Assessment 48
Documentation 49
Conclusion 50

3 PHARMACOLOGY 53

    Michael J. Kremer

Intravenous Administration 53
    IV Push 54

IV Titration 55
IV Continuous Infusion 55
Benzodiazepines 56
    General Pharmacology 56
    Mechanism of Action 56
    Pharmacokinetics 56
    Clinical Uses 57
        Diazepam 57
        Lorazepam 59
        Midazolam 61
Benzodiazepine Antagonist 63
        Flumazenil 63
        Opioid Agonists 65
    General Pharmacology 65
    Mechanism of Action 65
        Morphine Sulfate 67
        Meperidine 70
        Fentanyl 71
Opioid Agonist-Antagonists 73
        Nalbuphine 73
        Butorphanol 74
Opioid Antagonist 76
        Naloxone 76
Other Drugs 77
        Propofol 77
Phencyclidine Derivative 79
        Ketamine 79
Conclusion 80

4 MANAGEMENT OF COMPLICATIONS 82

Vallire Hooper

Complication Trends 82
Patient Risk Factors 84
    NPO Status 84
    Neck and Airway Assessment 84
    ASA Patient Classification Status 85
    High-Risk Patients 86
Complications and Their Management 89
    Emergency Equipment 89
    Respiratory Complications 90
    Cardiovascular Complications 98
    Allergic Reactions and/or Anaphylaxis 102
Conclusion 103

5 PATIENT DISCHARGE 107

The Report 107
Postprocedure Assessment 109
Patient Discharge 111
Discharge Teaching and Instructions 115
Postprocedure Phone Call 116
Conclusion 118

6 INSTITUTION POLICY AND GUIDELINE DEVELOPMENT: STANDARD OF CARE 120

Charlotte L. Guglielmi

Process for Developing a Single Standard of Care 121
    Step 1: Selection of Team Members 121
    Step 2: Evaluation of Nationally Endorsed Position Statements,
        Recommended Practices, and Guidelines 122
    Step 3: Determining Policy Format 123
    Step 4: Communication 141
    Step 5: Outcome Evaluation 141
Conclusion 144

7 COMPETENCE IN PATIENT MANAGEMENT 146

Vallire Hooper

An Overview of Competence 146
Determining Appropriate Competencies 147
Sedation-Specific Competencies 148
    Medication Administration and Interaction 149
    Airway Management 151
    Basic Dysrhythmia Recognition and Management 151
    Emergency Management 152
Program Implementation 152
Conclusion 152

8 PEDIATRIC SEDATION 155

Lisa Heard and Nancy Rayhorn

Guidelines 157
    Goals 158
    Patient Selection 159
    Personnel and Facility 159

Preprocedure Assessment   160
Intraprocedure Assessment   165
Postprocedure Assessment   166
    Developmental Approaches to the Care of the Child Undergoing Sedation
      and Analgesia   167
Medication Administration   169
    Determination of Dosage   170
    Route of Administration   170
    Commonly Administered Medications   172
Conclusion   172

9 GERIATRIC SEDATION   179

Nancy M. Saufl

Physiologic Changes of Aging   180
    Cardiovascular   180
    Respiratory   181
    Central Nervous System   181
    Renal/Genitourinary   182
    Gastrointestinal   182
    Integumentary   182
    Sensory   182
Patient Selection   183
Care of the Patient   184
Age-Specific Competency   184
Conclusion   185

10 SEDATION IN THE MECHANICALLY VENTILATED PATIENT   187

Marcia Bixby and Kathy Picard

Pathophysiologic Mechanisms of Agitation and Delirium   189
    Agitation   190
    Delirium   190
    Brain Function   193
    Metabolic Disturbances   193
    Withdrawal—Alcohol and Substance   195
Pharmacologic Measures   196
    Analgesics   199
    Anxiolytics and Hypnotics   205
Antagonists   208
    Narcan   208
    Flumazenil   208

Neuroleptics and Sympathetic Inhibiting Agents 209
  Haloperidol 209
Combination Therapy 211
  Tolerance and Extended Elimination Half-Lives 212
Nonpharmacologic Measures 213
Sedation Scale and Other Measures of Sedation 214
Daily Wake Up 219
Sedation and Weaning Protocol 221
Drug Tolerance and Weaning from Ventilator 221
Conclusion 225

11 RISK MANAGEMENT/LEGAL ISSUES 227

Legal Concepts 228
  Duty 228
  Breach of Duty 228
  Causation 228
  Damages or Injuries 229
Management of Risks and Liability in the Patient Receiving Moderate
  Sedation 229
  Practice Issues 229
  Policies and Procedures 230
  Education and Competence 230
  Preprocedure Care 231
  Medication Administration 231
  Monitoring of Patient 232
  Communication 232
  Emergencies 232
  Documentation 233
  Wrong Site Surgery 233
  Administration of Anesthetic Agents 234
Conclusion 236

APPENDICES

A   ASA Standards for Basic Anesthetic Monitoring 238

B   State Boards of Nursing Positions on Moderate Sedation and
    Administration of Anesthetic Agents 242

C   Position Statement on the Role of the RN in the Management of Patients
    Receiving IV Moderate Sedation for Short-Term Therapeutic, Diagnostic, or
    Surgical Procedures 258

D   ASA Practice Guidelines for Sedation and Analgesia by Non-
    Anesthesiologists 261

E   American Association of Nurse Anesthetists' Position Statement: Qualified Providers of Sedation and Analgesia; Considerations for Policy Guidelines for Registered Nurses Engaged in the Administration of Sedation and Analgesia   *290*

F   AORN Recommended Practices for Managing the Patient Receiving Moderate Sedation/Analgesia   *295*

G   Pediatric Sedation Standards 2002-2004   *309*

Practical Guide to

Moderate Sedation/Analgesia

1

History of Moderate Sedation

I n recent years outpatient surgery has drastically increased because of advances in technology, pharmacology, and anesthesia technique. In 1995 close to 4 million procedures were performed at outpatient surgery centers in the United States. By 2004, nearly 6 million surgeries were performed in more than 3300 Ambulatory Surgery Centers (FASA, 2004). Today the anesthesia technique of choice for a significant portion of outpatient surgery is intravenous moderate sedation and analgesia. Many physicians, nurses, and patients prefer the administration of moderate sedation and analgesia as opposed to a general anesthesia for patients who meet appropriate selection criteria. In the future an increase in the administration of moderate sedation and analgesia over a general anesthesia can be expected for specific short-term therapeutic, diagnostic, and surgical procedures.

One of the main advantages of moderate sedation and analgesia is the patient's rapid return to presedation levels. Such patients generally experience a shorter recovery period, ambulate earlier, and more readily participate in the discharge process than do patients receiving a general anesthesia. Side effects from the medications are minimal and complications are few.

At issue is determining the most appropriate provider to administer and monitor the patient receiving moderate sedation and analgesia. The demand for such anesthesia providers is greater than the supply, resulting in an increased use of nonanesthesia providers to administer moderate sedation and analgesia. The nonanesthesia provider is generally a professional registered nurse (RN) who receives additional training in administering moderate sedation and analgesia medications and monitoring the patient. In some instances the nonanesthesia provider is a technician and not an RN. Issues concerning the role and use of the nonanesthesia provider include appropriateness of allowing health care providers who are not specifically trained and educated in the techniques of delivering anesthesia to administer moderate sedation and analgesia medications; determining the competency of the health care provider; selecting patients based on identified criteria; identifying types of medications that may be administered safely by the nonanesthesia provider; and identifying appropriate levels of sedation and types of procedures with few predicted complications (Box 1-1).

Box 1-1 PROCEDURES PERFORMED WITH PATIENT UNDER MODERATE SEDATION AND ANALGESIA AND MONITORED BY NONANESTHESIA RNs*

Head and Neck Procedures

Molar extractions
Blepharoplasty
Rhytidoplasty
Rhinoplasty
Laceration repair
Cataract extraction

Superficial Thoracic Procedures

Breast augmentation
Breast biopsy
Bronchoscopy
Chest tube insertion

Extremity Procedures

Carpal tunnel release
Trigger finger release
Removal of pins/wires/screws
Closed reduction

Gastrointestinal Abdominal Procedures

Endoscopic retrograde cholangiopancreatography
Colonoscopy
Endoscopic ultrasonography
Gastroscopy

Vascular Procedures

Hemodialysis access placement
Pacemaker insertion
Angiography
Cardiac catheterization
Radiofrequency ablation
Electrophysiologic testing

Gynecologic/Urologic Procedures

Dilation and curettage
Fulguration vaginal lesions
Fulguration anal lesions
Cystoscopy
Incision and drainage of Bartholin's cyst
Vasectomy

Emergency Department Procedures

Reduction of dislocation, simple fracture, e.g., dislocated shoulder
Complex suturing, especially for pediatric patient
Insertion of elective chest tube

Radiology Procedures

Magnetic resonance imaging (MRI)
Arteriograms
Liver biopsy

*This list of examples is not intended to be all-inclusive.

HISTORY—NURSING PERSPECTIVE

Moderate sedation is a technique that originated in the practices of oral surgery and dentistry. The American Dental Association published one of the first definitions of conscious sedation as "a minimally depressed level of consciousness that retains the patient's ability to independently and continuously maintain an airway and respond appropriately to physical stimulation and verbal command, produced by a pharmacologic or nonpharmacologic method, or combination" (McCarthy 1984). It is popular and widely used to supplement local or regional anesthesia during a variety of short-term, therapeutic, and diagnostic procedures. Many patients prefer the lighter sleep of moderate sedation and analgesia versus a general anesthesia and like the added amnesic benefit that many of the medications provide. The goals of patient care are to provide adequate analgesia and sedation safely, while allaying patient fears and anxiety.

When moderate sedation first began in the 1980s, the RN's primary technique of moderate sedation and analgesia included administering a benzodiazepine (i.e., diazepam) and/or a narcotic (i.e., meperidine) for the adequate control and management of pain versus sedation. Procedures were relatively low risk, and patients were usually young and healthy with no other preexisting illness. The parameters monitored during the procedure varied and generally included blood pressure, heart rate, and respiration. Patient assessment findings and monitoring parameters were documented at 15- to 30-minute intervals. One RN was assigned to the patient and had circulating and monitoring responsibilities. The patient was transported for recovery to the postanesthesia care unit (PACU) and monitored in the same way as a patient receiving a general anesthesia. The patient was then discharged home or transferred to a nursing unit.

Today's very different scenario can be attributed to the continual increase in ambulatory surgery, reimbursement regulations, and consumer demand. Patients are demanding painless surgery with the latest technology, and they expect only minimal disruption in their daily lives during the recovery phase. Many surgical inpatient procedures that formerly required several days of hospitalization have been replaced by minimally invasive outpatient procedures performed in units outside the traditional operating room.

Third-party payers, private insurers, and Medicare closely monitor billing submitted for monitored anesthesia care (MAC). Each carrier determines the types of procedures and patient criteria allowable for reimbursement of services rendered by anesthesia personnel. The result is a change in business as usual.

Significant changes have occurred in the provision and definition of MAC. The American Society of Anesthesiologists (ASA) updated its position on MAC in 1998. According to the ASA Newsletter (Novak, 1998), MAC now includes the following elements:

- It is a clinical anesthesia service
- Involvement of an anesthesiologist is requested by another physician

- Personnel performing the service possess training and skills usually found only in qualified anesthesia personnel
- Usual preprocedure, intraprocedure, and postprocedure anesthesia services are required
- Level of sedation, short of general anesthesia, may vary widely during a single case and from case to case
- Since MAC is a complete anesthesia service, billing and reimbursement levels should be the same as other anesthesia services

MAC is also distinguished from moderate sedation by the ASA as specifically involving a second independently functioning physician.

This situation raises many questions and issues regarding the nonanesthesia provider's responsibility for monitoring and/or administering medications for moderate sedation and analgesia. The newer medications are close to ideal: they are of short duration, are rapid acting, can be administered through a variety of routes, and have greater predictability and fewer side effects. However, the one significant disadvantage of the newer medications is the increasing difficulty of determining if the patient is approaching the outer boundaries of moderate sedation and analgesia (i.e., unconsciousness). The patient may be responsive and talking while the monitoring parameters indicate that the patient is experiencing mild hypoxemia. Some nonanesthesia providers administer anesthesia medications that are manufactured for use in general anesthesia. This improper administration of these medications can rapidly induce the patient to a level of deep sedation or general anesthesia, a state clearly beyond the scope of practice for the nonanesthesia provider.

One area that has been difficult to define is the acceptable standard of care to be provided by the nonanesthesia provider. The growing expectation is that the nonanesthesia provider should be held to the same standard of care as are anesthesia personnel (i.e., the American Society of Anesthesiology "Standards for Basic Anesthetic Monitoring" [see Appendix A). The patient should not receive a lesser standard of care when moderate sedation and analgesia is administered and/or monitored by a nonanesthesia provider under the direction of a physician with little training and experience in the practice of anesthesia. As nonanesthesia providers participate in the monitoring and/or administration of medications that produce a state of sedation and analgesia, it is imperative that they demonstrate competence and provide services within an accepted scope of practice—one that does not extend to the practice of anesthesia.

SCOPE OF PRACTICE ISSUES

As RNs continue to define and refine their role as providers of moderate sedation and analgesia, state boards of nursing have been consulted regarding patient care. Consequently, several state nursing boards have developed advisory opinions, position statements, declaratory rulings, or guidelines to ensure that the RN is capable, experienced, and competent to provide safe patient care. The responses issued by state boards of nursing assist in preventing inappropriate use of nursing staff who are not trained in anesthesia practice or with little experience in the administration of agents of moderate sedation and analgesia. The movement toward the involvement of each state will focus concern on the safety and welfare of the patient.

State Boards of Nursing

Many RNs managing the care of a patient receiving moderate sedation and analgesia rely on administrative authorities to develop a standard of care (i.e., policy and procedures) to guide their daily practice. To have all the necessary information to make practice decisions, many RNs have requested assistance from individual state boards of nursing to define acceptable practices for the nonanesthesia RN administering moderate sedation and analgesia. Every RN managing the care of patients receiving moderate sedation and analgesia should remain current on information about this subject issued by his or her state board of nursing.

Appendix B presents survey information from each state about the status of the nonanesthesia RN administering moderate sedation (Odom-Forren, 2004). The survey results are summarized as follows:

- Overall consensus on the definition of moderate sedation to include the fact that the patient must "respond purposefully to verbal commands, either alone or accompanied by light tactile stimulation."
- State boards of nursing that have formalized rulings issue them as declaratory rulings, position statements, advisory opinions, guidelines, policy statements, or frequently asked questions (FAQs) on the website.
- All states responding to the survey agreed that the administration and monitoring of moderate sedation and analgesia were within the scope of practice for the educated and competent nonanesthesia RN.
- A few states have ruled that it is within the scope of practice for the competent and educated RN to administer propofol for sedation; other states have ruled that it is not within the scope of practice for the RN who is not a Certified Registered Nurse Anesthetist (CRNA). Many states have not addressed the issue. (See further discussion in this chapter.)

The RN managing the care of a patient receiving moderate sedation and analgesia should periodically consult the state board of nursing for any recent and relevant information. Institution policies and procedures should be consistent with the state board of nursing's recommendations, which reflect current practice. Appendix B shows a summary of the study results.

Standards of Practice

Several resources can be used to develop the standards of practice for the RN who manages the care of a patient receiving moderate sedation and analgesia.

These resources include state board of nursing statutes; professional organiza-tion position statements, guidelines, and recommended practices; literature review; and actual practices occurring in an institution. Often the practices fol-lowed in an institution fall below the national standards set by professional organizations. It is important for institutions and the RN managing the care of a patient receiving moderate sedation and analgesia to be knowledgeable about national standards and recommendations, which are used in courts of law to determine malpractice or negligence.

The American Nurses Association (ANA) recognized the need for nursing standards in the 1960s. In 1965 the ANA Committee on Nursing Services devel-oped the first nursing standards for organized nursing services (Flanagan, 1976). In 1973 the ANA published the first standards for nursing practice. These generic nursing standards were specific to the practice of nursing, based on the nursing process, and intended to apply to every RN. After those standards were developed, many specialty organizations promulgated their own nursing stan-dards, resulting in confusion caused by the lack of consistency in definitions, intent, and format.

In 1991, nearly two decades after issuing its first standards, the ANA pub-lished revised standards for nursing practice. The 1991 standards were revised in 1998 and again in 2004 (ANA, 2004). These generic standards are intended to apply to every practicing RN. The ANA collaborated with specialty nursing organizations in making these revisions and in devising a framework for these organizations to use to develop criteria for specialty nursing standards (e.g., oper-ating room, emergency department, postanesthesia care unit). This collaboration between specialty nursing organizations and the ANA ensures more consistent interpretation of nursing standards.

The RN managing the care of the patient receiving moderate sedation and analgesia should clearly understand nursing standards and how they are used to define the RN's scope of practice. A standard describes an expected level of nursing care; there is little room for variation in practice. Under similar cir-cumstances all RNs are expected to exercise the same sound judgment reflected in the standards of care. For example, every RN is expected to provide a plan of care for the patient based on assessment, diagnosis, outcome identification, plan-ning, implementation, and evaluation. Simply stated, standards are "authorita-tive statements by which the nursing profession describes the responsibilities for which its practitioners are accountable" (ANA, 2004). The ANA's Nursing: Scope & Standards of Practice includes "Standards of Practice" and "Standards of Professional Performance" (Box 1-2), which outline expected knowledge, skills, and professional behavior for the RN.

Professional nursing organizations are responsible for the development and dissemination of acceptable standards of practice. The RN administering mod-erate sedation and analgesia during short-term therapeutic, diagnostic, or sur-gical procedures should be conversant with pertinent research published in

Box 1-2   AMERICAN NURSES ASSOCIATION NURSING: SCOPE & STANDARDS OF PRACTICE

Standards of Practice

Assessment
Diagnosis
Outcomes identification
Planning
Implementation
    Coordination of care
    Health teaching and health promotion
    Consultation
    Prescriptive authority and treatment
Evaluation

Standards of Professional Performance

Quality of practice
Education
Professional practice evaluation
Collegiality
Collaboration
Ethics
Research
Resource use
Leadership

Data from American Nurses Association: Nursing: Scope & standards of practice, Washington, DC, 2004, American Nurses Association.

professional nursing and medical journals. These publications reflect current trends in practice that institutions use to develop policy and procedures for the RN's care of patients receiving moderate sedation and analgesia. The memberships of several associations consist of RNs who manage the care of patients receiving moderate sedation and analgesia on a routine basis (e.g., Association of Operating Room Nurses, American Association of Nurse Anesthetists (AANA), Society for Gastrointestinal Nurses and Associates, American Society of PeriAnesthesia Nurses, Emergency Nurses Association, and American Association of Critical Care Nurses). Each of these nursing associations has published relevant recommended practices, position statements, guidelines, and articles that reflect the latest trends and techniques for safe administration of moderate sedation and analgesia.

In addition, many other nursing and medical associations have been active in the development or endorsement of practice guidelines, position statements, or recommended practices for managing the care of a patient receiving moderate sedation and analgesia. Each professional association contributes to the development of acceptable practice standards. However, some confusion still persists despite the increase in the number of practice standards. Much of this confusion is due to the inconsistent interpretation of position statements, practice guidelines, and recommended practices regarding who should monitor the patient and minimal monitoring standards along with appropriate drugs to be administered by the RN.

Position Statements

Position statements are issued by specialty nursing organizations, state boards of nursing, or other professional associations on actual or emerging practice trends (e.g., moderate sedation and analgesia, patient and health care workers with human immunodeficiency virus, and unlicensed assistive personnel). Position statements are developed by a panel of experts. Generally a position statement is based on a professional consensus of the developing group. Research is used as available for an evidence-based position statement. Because practice is an emerging trend, little scientific research is usually available. Instead, recommendations are based on current practice trends and safe implementation. The position statement may be brief or may outline suggested implementation criteria. Position statements are generally developed because of concern for an area of practice that may be detrimental to patient safety.

In January 1991 the first discussion group was convened by the ANA at the National Federation for Specialty Nursing Organizations in response to concerns expressed by the AANA. The goal was to develop a position statement describing specific recommendations for the safe administration of "conscious" sedation and analgesia by the RN. The final position statement was made available in the fall of 1991 and included the endorsement of 23 specialty nursing organizations. The "Position Statement on the Role of the Registered Nurse (RN) in the Management of Patients Receiving IV Conscious Sedation for Short-Term Therapeutic, Diagnostic, or Surgical Procedures" is significant to all RNs managing the care of patients receiving moderate sedation and analgesia.

This position statement has had tremendous impact on the implementation and delivery of nursing care provided to the patient receiving moderate sedation and analgesia. Today many state boards of nursing, state nursing associations, and specialty nursing associations endorse the position statement or reference it when nursing practice opinions on moderate (conscious) sedation and analgesia are requested (see Appendix C).

Practice Guidelines

Practice guidelines are "systematically developed recommendations that assist the practitioner and patient in making decisions about health care" (ASA, 2002). The basic criteria for development of guidelines include that they be "science-based, documented, unbiased, and clear" (Lohr, 1995). The National Guideline Clearinghouse (NGC), an initiative of the Agency for Healthcare Research and

Quality (AHRQ), is a comprehensive database of evidence-based clinical practice guidelines and related documents. The mission of the NGC is to provide objective, detailed information on clinical practice guidelines to health care professionals and to further their dissemination, implementation, and use. Criteria for inclusion of Clinical Practice Guidelines in the NGC are included in Box 1-3.

One example of practice guidelines is the ASA's "Practice Guidelines for Preoperative Fasting and the Use of Pharmacologic Agents to Reduce the Risk of Pulmonary Aspiration: Application to Healthy Patients Undergoing Elective Procedures" (ASA, 1999). Guidelines such as these are advisory in nature and are not intended to be the only approach to patient management of the clinical problem. The intent is to guide practice while allowing for deviation when necessary. Implementation of practice guidelines is optional and may include full or partial implementation, or none at all. Practice guidelines are recommended options; they are considered as emerging standards of practice that may eventually become mandated. Guidelines may be used in a legal suit to determine acceptable practice.

Practice guidelines were first taken seriously at the federal level through the approval of the Omnibus Budget Reconciliation Act of 1989, which provided funding for the development of national guidelines through the Agency for Health Care Policy and Research (AHCPR). The Healthcare Research and Quality Act of 1999 reauthorized AHCPR until the end of 2005 and changed its name to the AHRQ. The AHCPR guideline "Acute Pain Management: Operative or Medical Procedures and Trauma" (1992) applies to the RN administering moderate sedation and analgesia, and it details suggested management of pain.

Box 1-3   CLINICAL PRACTICE GUIDELINE CRITERIA FOR INCLUSION IN THE NGC

Guidelines contain systematically developed statements that include recommendations, strategies, or information that assists physicians and/or other health care practitioners and patients to make decisions about appropriate health care for specific clinical circumstances.

Guidelines produced under auspices of medical specialty associations; relevant professional societies, public or private organizations, government agencies at the federal, state, or local level, or health care organizations or plans.

Corroborating documentation can be produced and verified that a systematic literature search and review of existing scientific evidence published in peer reviewed journals was performed during the guideline development.

Guideline is English language, current, and most recent version produced. Guideline developed, reviewed, or revised within the last five years.

Data from National Guideline Clearinghouse: Inclusion criteria, 2004, retrieved May 19, 2004, from http://www.guideline.gov/about/inclusion.aspx.

The agency ended its clinical guidelines program in 1996 and now supports the development of evidence reports through its 12 evidence-based practice centers and dissemination of those guidelines through the NGC (AHRQ, 1999).

The American Dental Society of Anesthesiology and the American Association of Oral and Maxillofacial Surgeons have published guidelines on the administration of moderate sedation and analgesia that are similar to the American Academy of Pediatrics "Guidelines for Monitoring and Management of Pediatric Patients During and After Sedation for Diagnostic and Therapeutic Procedures" described in Chapter 8. The ASA (2002) revised "Guidelines for Sedation and Analgesia by Non-anesthesiologists" (see Appendix D). More recently the AANA (2003) has revised "Qualified Providers of Conscious Sedation" and "Considerations for Policy Guidelines for Registered Nurses Engaged in the Administration of Sedation and Analgesia" (see Appendix E).

These recommended guidelines for the administration of moderate sedation and analgesia were developed by medical and nursing organizations that represent professionals involved in the administration of moderate sedation and analgesia. Each guideline includes a recommended set of criteria and should be viewed as clinically flexible. The strength of each guideline is verified by supporting evidence. This gives the guidelines a great deal of credibility. Many associations maintain extensive lists of pertinent literature for their members. It is up to the individual practitioner and institution to choose the most appropriate implementation from interventions and monitoring parameters suggested by the guideline.

Recommended Practices

Recommended practices such as those available from the Association of periOperative Registered Nurses (AORN) represent the association's official position on questions of aseptic and procedural practice performed by perioperative nurses (see Appendix F). Recommended practices are "statements of optimum performance criteria on the various aspects of technical and professional perioperative nursing practices" (AORN, 2002). They are based on current nursing practice, available scientific data, and standards and regulations from agencies such as the Joint Commission on Accreditation of Healthcare Organizations (JCAHO), the Centers for Disease Control and Prevention, and the Occupational Safety and Health Administration (OSHA). Recommended practices serve as guidelines for nursing practice. In making such recommendations, these nursing organizations seek achievable, optimal care, and compliance with practices are not mandated.

Typically, during a malpractice proceeding related to sedation and analgesia, the previously mentioned guidelines, position statements, recommended practices from national organizations, and recommendations from pharmaceutical companies are presented as an expected and acceptable standard of care. If the standard of care in the case did not meet the recommendations, the defendant (i.e., RN, technician, physician, or other) would have to justify and explain exactly how the standard of care delivered was determined. This would include the defendant's attempt to justify why national guidelines, position statements, and recommended practices were not implemented and why the care failed to yield to the best interest of the patient.

Controversial Issue: Nurse-Administered Propofol Sedation

As the practice of nurse-administered moderate sedation has evolved, there have been concerns voiced over the categories of medications that are administered. Of particular interest is the present controversy over nurse-administered propofol sedation (NAPS). Those in favor of nurses administering propofol for sedation cite advantages such as the short action of propofol, the faster recovery and better postoperative function of patients, the lower postoperative nausea and vomiting (PONV) rates, and the faster discharge of patients. Those opposed to the practice of NAPS discuss the disadvantages of the practice, such as unpredictability of propofol leading to unwarranted deep sedation, demanding airway management requirements, no known reversal drugs, and its classification by the package insert as an anesthesia agent to be used only by individuals trained in the administration of general anesthesia (AstraZeneca, 2004; Byrne & Baillie, 2002; Meltzer, 2003).

Several state boards of nursing have looked at the issue of NAPS and rendered a decision that it is not within the scope of practice for RNs to administer propofol. Other state boards of nursing have discussed the issue and decided that it is within the scope of practice for an appropriately educated and competent RN to administer propofol for sedation. Many state boards of nursing either have decision trees that assist RNs to make their own decisions or do not specifically address the issue at all (see Appendix B).

To illustrate the controversy, the American Gastroenterological Association (AGA) issued a press release on March 4, 2004, stating that three gastroenterology specialty groups (the AGA, the American College of Gastroenterology [ACG], and the American Society for Gastrointestinal Endoscopy [ASGE]) had issued a joint statement on sedation in endoscopy supporting nurse-administered propofol sedation by adequately trained nonanesthesiologists (AGA, 2004). On April 14, 2004, the ASA and AANA issued a joint statement regarding propofol administration that declares propofol should be administered only by persons trained in the administration of general anesthesia (Box 1-4) (ASA & AANA, 2004). In addition, the American Association for Accreditation of Ambulatory Surgery Facilities (AAAASF) changed its standards and requires that only anesthesiologists or nurse anesthetists administer propofol after March 1, 2004 (AAAASF, 2004).

The RN who is asked to administer propofol for sedation should check with state boards of nursing regarding any pertinent decisions and any guidelines, position statements, or recommended practices issued by medical or nursing organizations. Institutional policy and state laws and regulations should allow for the practice before the RN agrees. The RN must also understand that if sued

> **Box 1-4**   AANA-ANA Joint Position Statement Regarding
> Propofol Administration
>
> **AANA-ASA Joint Statement Regarding Propofol Administration***
> April 14, 2004
>   Because sedation is a continuum, it is not always possible to predict how an individual patient will respond. Due to the potential for rapid, profound changes in sedative and/or anesthesia depth and the lack of antagonistic medications, agents such as propofol require special attention.
>   Whenever propofol is used for sedation/anesthesia, it should be administered only by persons trained in the administration of general anesthesia, who are not simultaneously involved in these surgical or diagnostic procedures. This restriction is concordant with specific language in the propofol package insert, and failure to follow these recommendations could put patients at increased risk of significant injury or death.
>   Similar concerns apply when other intravenous induction agents are used for sedation, such as thiopental, methohexital or etomidate.
>
> | American Society of | American Association of Nurse |
> |---|---|
> | Anesthesiologists | Anesthetists |
> | 520 N. Northwest Highway | 222 South Prospect Avenue |
> | Park Ridge, IL 60068-2573 | Park Ridge, IL 60068-4001 |
> | Ph: (847) 825-5586 | Ph: (847) 692-7050 |
> | Fax: (847) 825-1692 | Fax: (847) 692-6968 |
> | www.asahq.org | www.aana.com |
> | www.anesthesiasafety.info | www.anesthesiapatientsafety.com |
>
> *AANA & ASA: AANA-ASA joint statement regarding propofol administration, 2004, retrieved 5/19/04 from www.aana.com/news/2004/news050504_joint.asp and www.asahq.org/news/propofolstatement.htm.*
> *This statement is not intended to apply when propofol is given to intubated, ventilated patients in a critical care setting.*

in the event of a dire patient outcome, it would be difficult at this time to defend the practice of NAPS. Reasons for the difficulty with defense are the classification of propofol as an anesthesia agent, disapproval by the expert bodies of the ASA and AANA, and the fact that it is not widely accepted or approved by a majority of boards of nursing.

Development of a Standard of Care

Guidelines, position statements, and recommended practices all contribute to the development of a standard of care (i.e., what the RN is expected to do for the patient). The following suggestions may be helpful in defining a standard of care for the RN who is not trained and educated as an anesthesia provider but is responsible for managing the care of a patient receiving moderate sedation and analgesia.

1. Contact state board of nursing. Determine if the administration of moderate sedation and analgesia is within the legal scope of nursing practice for a nonanesthesia RN. Are there specific medications that should not be administered by the nonanesthesia RN for purposes of moderate sedation and analgesia in that specific state? Are there any special conditions or criteria that must be in place (e.g., monitoring parameters, required equipment that must be present, or continuing education requirements)?
2. Obtain position statements, guidelines, and recommended practices on the role of the nonanesthesia provider for managing the care of a patient receiving moderate sedation and analgesia from professional associations. Determine commonalities and differences among the professional associations on issues related to standards of care (e.g., monitoring parameters). Assess and determine which recommendations the institution is willing to implement. Be able to provide a rationale based on continuous quality improvement documentation and scientific data from the literature.
3. Determine if insurance carriers have specific criteria that must be in place. Insurance carriers generally do not issue guidelines related to patient care. However, some have issued guidelines in the past. Determine if the carrier has such guidelines and implement accordingly.
4. Assess the standard of care provided to the patient receiving moderate sedation and analgesia. Does this standard meet the recommendations presented in the national position statements, guidelines, and recommended practices? If not, determine why and evaluate overall patient safety and potential for harm.
5. Evaluate the different departments administering moderate sedation and analgesia. Determine if there is a consistent standard of care provided to all patients under similar conditions. If the answer is no, evaluate why the differences exist and correct them according to information found. See Chapter 6 for institutional policy and guideline development.

LEVELS OF SEDATION

The nonanesthesia provider managing the care of the patient receiving moderate sedation and analgesia should be able to define the different levels of sedation. Sedation occurs on a continuum, with minimal sedation at one end and general anesthesia at the other (Figure 1-1). The nonanesthesia provider should be knowledgeable about the differences in the sedation levels and able to determine when the patient is approaching deep sedation or general anesthesia.

No sedation   Light sedation   Moderate sedation   Deep sedation   General anesthesia

Figure 1-1 Sedation continuum.

The continuum of sedation allows for the patient to progress from one degree to another, based on the medications administered, route, and dosages. "Minimal sedation" is the administration of oral medications for the reduction of anxiety (e.g., premedication). The patient is technically awake, but under the influence of the medication administered. The following statements are applicable to a patient under "minimal sedation."

1. Protective reflexes are intact (e.g., normal respirations, eye movement, and ability to communicate).
2. The patient does not experience amnesia.
3. The patient's anxiety level and fear are lowered.

The widely accepted definition of moderate sedation and/or analgesia is a "drug-induced depression of consciousness during which patients respond purposefully to verbal commands, either alone or accompanied by light tactile stimulation. No interventions are required to maintain a patent airway, and spontaneous ventilation is adequate. Cardiovascular function is usually maintained" (ASA, 2002; JCAHO, 2004). The clinical characteristics of a patient under moderate sedation and analgesia include the following:

1. Maintenance of protective reflexes (e.g., ability to control secretions, avoid aspiration, and breathe without assistance)
2. Independent and continuous maintenance of a patent airway
3. Appropriate response to physical stimulation and/or verbal command
4. Easy arousal—responds to verbal or light tactile stimulation
5. Cardiovascular status is usually maintained

The ASA (2002) defines deep sedation and/or analgesia as "a drug-induced depression of consciousness during which patients cannot be easily aroused but respond purposefully following repeated or painful stimulation. The ability to independently maintain ventilatory function may be impaired. Patients may require assistance in maintaining a patent airway, and spontaneous ventilation may be inadequate. Cardiovascular function is usually maintained."

The following clinical conditions are indicative of a deeply sedated patient:

1. Not easily aroused
2. May require repeated or painful stimulation to elicit a response
3. Partial or complete loss of protective reflexes
4. Loss of ability to maintain a patent airway independently
5. Cardiovascular function usually maintained

Deep sedation is similar to general anesthesia in that the protective reflexes are lost and the patient is unable to maintain a patent airway. Monitoring parameters for deep sedation should be the same as for general anesthesia. The ASA (2002) and JCAHO (2004) define general anesthesia as "a drug-induced loss of consciousness during which patients are not arousable, even by painful stimulation." The other characteristics described are:

1. Ability to maintain ventilatory function often impaired
2. Assistance in maintaining a patent airway required
3. Positive pressure ventilation is often required
4. Cardiovascular function may be impaired

It is not always possible to predict an individual patient's reaction to sedation. See Table 1-1. Therefore, practitioners should be able to rescue patients who move to the next level of sedation beyond that intended. The ASA (2002) and JCAHO (2004) state that persons administering moderate sedation and/or analgesia should be capable of rescuing patients who enter a state of deep sedation and/or analgesia and those administering deep sedation and/or analgesia should be capable of rescuing patients who move into a state of general anesthesia. The potential for complications increases with deep sedation, and the nonanesthesia provider should avoid managing the care of a patient with clinical indications of deep sedation. Exceptions to this would occur in areas such as the critical care

Table 1-1 | Continuum of Depth of Sedation

	Minimal Sedation (Anxiolysis)	Moderate Sedation/ Analgesia	Deep Sedation/ Analgesia	General Anesthesia
Responsiveness	Normal response to verbal stimulation	Purposeful response to verbal or tactile stimulation	Purposeful response following repeated or painful stimulation	Unarousable even with painful stimulus
Airway	Unaffected	No intervention required	Intervention may be required	Intervention often required
Spontaneous ventilation	Unaffected	Adequate	May be inadequate	Frequently inadequate
Cardiovascular function	Unaffected	Usually maintained	Usually maintained	May be impaired

From ASA. (1999). *Continuum of depth of sedation.* Accessed 1/29/04 from www.asahq.org/publicationsAndServices/standards/20.htm.

unit, where the patient is mechanically ventilated and compromised respiratory status rendered by deep sedation is not an issue.

OBJECTIVES OF CONSCIOUS SEDATION

Under the direction of a physician, the RN may be responsible for titrating medications to the patient's response and monitoring the patient under moderate sedation and analgesia. For proper titration, the RN should be knowledgeable of the goals and objectives of moderate sedation and analgesia. The primary goal of moderate sedation and/or analgesia is to reduce the patient's anxiety and discomfort (AORN, 2002). Other objectives for the patient are (Kost, 2004):

1. Altered mood. Many patients fear general anesthesia and will avoid being "put to sleep" if at all possible. These patients have a high level of fear and apprehension. Many medications alter the patient's mood, allowing for greater acceptance of the procedure about to be performed.
2. Enhanced patient cooperation. If a patient is uncooperative, it may be impossible to complete the procedure. An anesthesia provider may be requested to place the patient under deep sedation or general anesthesia. If administering moderate sedation and analgesia in conjunction with regional anesthesia, the RN should allow sufficient time for the local anesthesia to take effect after injection (i.e., blockage of nerve impulse).
3. Elevation of pain threshold and controlled pain. As mentioned previously, a regional anesthesia may be administered to manage procedural or operative pain. However, opioids may also be administered to elevate the pain threshold. Proper patient education is essential. Because it is unlikely that the diagnostic or operative procedure will be pain free, the patient should be aware that tugging, pulling, and discomfort may ensue. The medications simply elevate the pain threshold. Because the technique of moderate sedation and analgesia does not render the patient unconscious, total absence of pain is unlikely. Opioids, however, are administered to control any pain the patient may encounter.
4. Intact protective reflexes. A patient with intact protective reflexes should be able to respond to physical and verbal commands. The patient should also be capable of communicating any discomfort or other relevant information to the monitoring RN. Eye movements should be normal. Pharyngeal and laryngeal reflexes (e.g., swallowing, retching, or vomiting) should be intact. Respirations should be regular and normal, ventilatory function normal, and the patient should be able to maintain a patent airway without assistance.
5. Stable vital signs. Only little variation in physiologic monitoring parameters from the baseline should be noted. Depending on the method of administration and injection technique (i.e., bolus versus slow titration), there may be some variation in vital signs; however, these are usually only transient and vital signs should return rapidly to the baseline.

6. A degree of amnesia. The amnesic effect varies with the type of medication and the dosage administered. Certain procedures and diagnostic studies may be recalled as unpleasant experiences for the postprocedure patient. From this standpoint the amnesic effects rendered by agents such as the benzodiazepines are desirable—especially for the patient who can expect repeated exposures to certain short-term therapeutic, diagnostic, or surgical procedures (e.g., colonoscopy and cardioversion).
7. Rapid recovery. The time required for recovery from moderate sedation and analgesia is individualized and dose-dependent. Medications are titrated until anxiety is decreased and pain is controlled. However, the medications used for moderate sedation and/or analgesia require a quicker recovery time than those medications typically used for general anesthesia.

The nurse responsible for managing the care of the patient should be knowledgeable about every objective and apply them in daily practice. The RN is responsible for monitoring and assessing the patient throughout the procedure or diagnostic study. Continuous patient assessment is important to determine if the objectives of moderate sedation and analgesia are being met (i.e., relaxed and cooperative, easily aroused, or patent airway).

PATIENT SELECTION

The ideal patient for moderate sedation and analgesia is one who has received proper education about the procedure and is cooperative. Not all patients are amenable to the techniques of moderate sedation and analgesia; some patients may be more appropriately managed by an anesthesia provider. Patients who have a high level of anxiety, pediatric patients, a previous or current history of drug abuse or alcoholism, or posttraumatic stress syndrome may pose difficulties to the nonanesthesia provider who is administering moderate sedation and analgesia.

Patients should be selected on an individual basis, with consideration given to the existing medical diagnosis, past medical history, age, type of procedure and current history, physical examination, and medical condition. Any of these considerations may increase the risk for an undesirable outcome for the patient under moderate sedation and analgesia. The objective is to avoid any patient with an existing complication that may increase the likelihood of a poor outcome. The RN who for any reason does not feel comfortable managing the care of a patient should consult with an anesthesia provider and the attending physician. A joint decision should be made concerning who is the most appropriate person to monitor the patient and the appropriate medications and monitoring parameters to use.

Moderate sedation and analgesia is administered in a variety of settings within an institution. These include, but are not limited to, surgery, PACU, cardiac catheterization laboratory, radiology, emergency department, intensive and/or coronary care units, cardiac nursing units, electrophysiology department, gastroenterology department, and pain management center. It is not uncommon for a specialty unit to receive a patient who is considered at risk because of a high acuity level (e.g., cardiac insufficiency). If the RN who will be responsible for managing the care of the patient receiving moderate sedation and analgesia does not have the proper training and education to manage the basic care of the patient, it is inappropriate to place the patient under the full management of this RN, even in the immediate presence of a physician. The most appropriate care for such a patient may be provided by an anesthesia provider or an additional RN with the necessary competency to assist in management of the patient's care. The bottom line is safe patient care and the best possible patient outcome.

CONCLUSION

The nonanesthesia provider responsible for managing the care of the patient receiving moderate sedation and analgesia should be knowledgeable about national position statements, guidelines, recommended practices, and state board of nursing recommendations. These should be carefully evaluated and integrated into written policies and procedures relating the accepted standard of practice for the given institution. The policies and procedures should be reviewed annually and revised to reflect current practices and scientific principles as available.

REFERENCES

Agency for Health Care Policy and Research, Public Health Services, U.S. Department of Health and Human Services. (February 1992). Acute pain management: Operative or medical procedures and trauma. Clinical practice guideline (AHCPR Pub. No. 92-0032). Rockville, MD: Acute Pain Management Guideline Panel.

Agency for Healthcare Research and Quality. (1999). Reauthorization fact sheet. Retrieved 5/19/04 from www.ahrq.gov.about/ahrqfact.htm.

American Association for Accreditation of Ambulatory Facilities, Inc. (February 17, 2004). 2004 revised standards memo. Accessed 5/19/04 from www.aaaasf.org/standards/.

American Association of Nurse Anesthetists. (2004). In the news: AANA-ASA joint statement regarding propofol administration. Retrieved 5/19/04 from www.aana.com/news/2004/news050504_joint.asp.

American Gastroenterological Association. (March 8, 2004). AGA News Release: Three gastroenterology specialty groups issue joint statement on sedation in endoscopy. Accessed   5/19/04   from   www.gastro.org/media/newsRelease04/statement-SedationEndoscopy.html.

American Nurses Association. (2004). Nursing: Scope & standards of practice. Washington, D.C.: Author.

American Society of Anesthesiologists. (1999). Continuum of depth of sedation. Retrieved 1/29/04 from www.asahq.org/publicationsAndServices/standards/20.htm.

American Society of Anesthesiologists. (1999). Practice guidelines for preoperative fasting and the use of pharmacologic agents to reduce the risk of pulmonary aspiration: Application to healthy patients undergoing elective procedures. Retrieved 5/19/04 from http://www.asahq.org/publicationsAndServices/npoguide.html.

American Society of Anesthesiologists. (2002). Practice guidelines for sedation and analgesia by non-anesthesiologists. Anesthesiology, 96, 1004-1017.

American Society of Anesthesiologists. (2004). AANA-ASA joint statement regarding propofol administration. Retrieved 5/19/04 from www.asahq.org/news/propofolstatement.htm.

Association of periOperative Registered Nurses. (2002). Recommended practices for managing the patient receiving moderate sedation/analgesia. AORN Journal, 75, 642-652.

Association of periOperative Registered Nurses. (2002). Standards, recommended practices, and guidelines. Denver, CO: Author.

AstraZeneca. (2004). Diprivan® prescribing information. Retrieved 5/19/04 from www.astrazeneca-us.com/pi/202014Diprivan.pdf.

Byrne, M.F., & Baillie, J. (2002). Editorials: Propofol for conscious sedation? Gastroenterology, 123, 373-375.

Federated Ambulatory Surgery Association (2004). The history of ASCs. Retrieved 5/15/04 from http://www.fasa.org/aschistory.html.

Flanagan, L. (1976). One strong voice. Kansas City: American Nurses Association.

Joint Commission on Accreditation of Healthcare Organizations. (2004). Hospital accreditation standards. Oakbrook Terrace, IL: Author.

Kost, M. (2004). Moderate sedation/analgesia. In L. Schick & D.M.D. Quinn (Eds.). PeriAnesthesia nursing core curriculum. St. Louis: Saunders, pp. 432-443.

Lohr, K.N. (1995). Guidelines for clinical practice: What they are and why they count. Journal of Law, Medicine & Ethics, 23, 49-56.

McCarthy, F.M. (1984). Conscious sedation: Benefits and risks. JADA, 109, 546-557.

Meltzer, B. (2003). RNs pushing propofol. Outpatient Surgery Magazine, 4(7), 24-37.

National Guideline Clearinghouse. (2004). Inclusion criteria. Retrieved 5/19/04 from www.guideline.gov/about/inclusion.aspx.

Novak L.C. (1998). ASA updates its position on monitored anesthesia care. ASA Newsletter, 62(12) Retrieved 5/4/04 from www.asahq.org/Newsletters/1998/12_98?ASAupdates_1298.html.

Odom-Forren, J. (2004). Moderate sedation survey. Unpublished research.

2

Presedation Assessment, Monitoring Parameters, and Equipment

Because there is ongoing controversy regarding the monitoring of patients receiving medications for moderate sedation and analgesia, many state boards of nursing are defining specific parameters that must be in place for the registered nurse (RN) managing the care of such patients. Professional organizations such as those described in Chapter 1 periodically update existing position statements, guidelines, and recommended practices that identify specific monitoring parameters. Such parameters are important because they aid the RN in preventing and detecting complications that can have serious consequences for patients.

The RN managing the care of a patient receiving moderate sedation and analgesia is responsible for collecting qualitative and quantitative data. Qualitative data include observations of parameters such as the patient's skin color, depth and character of respirations, movement, pupil size, and sedation level. Quantitative data include physiologic measurements, such as blood pressure, respiration rate, heart rate and rhythm, and oxygen saturation. Continuous monitoring of both qualitative and quantitative parameters ensures early detection of complications that may result from the administration of medications or from the procedure. The patient should be thoroughly assessed to determine any contraindications or risks that may interfere with a predictable positive patient outcome before the RN administers any medication for moderate sedation and analgesia.

PREPROCEDURE ASSESSMENT

The primary purpose of the preprocedure nursing assessment is to obtain baseline health information and determine preexisting illnesses and conditions that might render nurse-monitored sedation inappropriate. Procedures performed with the patient under nurse-monitored sedation are becoming increasingly complex, with deeper sedative levels and a higher patient acuity level. Every RN responsible for the continuous monitoring of a patient receiving moderate sedation and analgesia should be aware of the instances for which care is more appropriately managed by an anesthesia provider. An appropriate preprocedure assessment decreases the risk of adverse outcomes for the patient receiving moderate sedation (ASA, 2002). If the RN determines that it is not in the patient's best interest to be monitored by a nonanesthesia provider, the RN, the physician, and the anesthesia provider should consult to determine the most appropriate person to monitor the patient and the appropriate monitoring parameters.

The RN monitoring the patient throughout the short-term diagnostic, therapeutic, or surgical procedure is responsible for the preprocedure assessment. The preprocedure assessment consists of data collection from a variety of sources, such as chart review, patient assessment and interview, and consultation with other health care providers as appropriate. The assessment includes patient identification and site identification.

Nursing History and Physical Evaluation

If a medical history and physical are included in the patient's chart, the RN may obtain information as appropriate. Obtaining a thorough nursing history is important to the care of the patient. This history should include current medications (prescription or over-the-counter) and herbal use, adverse drug reactions, especially pertaining to previous sedation and/or analgesia or anesthesia, allergies (including medications, latex), medical illnesses, prior procedures, tobacco or alcohol use, family history of diseases or disorders, social history, fasting status, present psychologic status, communication ability, pain assessment, current laboratory values, and understanding of the procedure and of moderate sedation and analgesia.

Physical evaluation by the monitoring RN should include assessment of the heart and lungs, and an evaluation of the airway. Physical assessment should include baseline vital signs, height, weight, age, oxygen saturation, and a review of systems. This information is necessary to determine any indication of circulation impairment and/or difficulties in breathing. The physician should be notified of any abnormalities, and a 12-lead electrocardiogram should be considered. The skin should be assessed for general appearance and color and to determine if the skin is intact, diaphoretic, cold, warm, jaundiced, pale, or cyanotic. Any bruises or lacerations present should be noted and documented. Information that could be included in a presedation assessment is included in Table 2-1. The monitoring RN should develop an individual nursing care plan based on the data collected.

With patient safety at the forefront, it is essential that the patient is identified correctly. The Joint Commission on Accreditation of Healthcare Organizations requires two separate patient identifiers that do not include the patient's location (JCAHO, 2004a). Site identification is also an essential patient safety issue. Any procedures with right and/or left distinction, multiple structures (fingers and toes), or levels (spine) should be marked by the practitioner performing the procedure (JCAHO, 2003).

The administration of sedation and analgesia medications may interfere with the patient's ability to maintain a patent airway; therefore preprocedure evalua-

Table 2-1 | **Presedation History and Physical Evaluation by RN**

General health	Height and weight
	Obesity or recent weight loss
	Current infection
	Current medications (prescription or over-the-counter)
	Current herbal use
	Last food intake (fasting history)
	Physical handicaps and level of mobility
	Baseline vital signs and temperature
	History of tobacco or alcohol use
	Pain assessment (chronic or acute)
Cardiovascular	History of cardiovascular disease
	Recent cardiac surgery or myocardial infarction
	Angina, aortic stenosis, congestive heart failure
	Presence of a pacemaker or implantable cardioverter defibrillator
Respiratory	Smoking history
	Chronic cough
	History of lung surgery or emphysema
	Shortness of breath
	History of tuberculosis, pneumonia, asthma, or bronchitis
	Baseline oximetry reading
	Airway assessment
	Mallampati assessment or other, such as having patient open mouth, stick out tongue, and flex neck
	Craniofacial abnormalities
	History of sleep apnea
Neurologic	General affect including behavior, speech patterns, gait
	Level of consciousness and orientation
	History of seizures, headaches
	Motor abilities
	Preexisting neurologic deficit
Musculoskeletal	Muscle strength, mobility, range of motion
	Use of orthopedic devices or prostheses
	History of arthritis, scoliosis, fractures
Integumentary	Color (cyanosis or jaundice)
	Temperature and texture
	Skin turgor
	Integrity of skin
	Piercings

Table 2-1 | **Presedation History and Physical Evaluation by RN—cont'd**

Gastrointestinal	Chronic diarrhea or constipation Predisposition to nausea and vomiting Time of last oral intake Previous surgery or procedures
Renal/Hepatic	Kidney function, e.g., end stage renal disease for revision of arteriovenous fistula Liver disease including cirrhosis, hepatitis, anemia
Endocrine	Diabetes most common abnormality

Data from Odom, J. (2002). Conscious sedation/analgesia. In N. Burden, D.M.D. Quinn, D. O'Brien, & B.S.G. Dawes (Eds.). Ambulatory surgical nursing, (2nd Ed.). Philadelphia: Saunders, pp. 313-315; American Society of PeriAnesthesia Nurses. (2002). Standards of perianesthesia nursing practice, Cherry Hill, NJ: ASPAN, pp. 27-28; Ferrara-Love, R. (2004). History and physical examinations. In D.M.D. Quinn & L. Schick (Eds.). PeriAnesthesia nursing core curriculum. St. Louis: Saunders, pp.235-251; Association of periOperative Registered Nurses. (2002). Recommended practices for managing the patient receiving moderate sedation/analgesia. AORN Journal, 75, 642-652.

tion of the lungs and airway is essential. The lungs should be assessed for any abnormal breath sounds, such as rales or wheezing. The airway may be assessed using the Mallampati technique, which is used by anesthesia providers to determine possible intubation difficulty, information of potential value to the monitoring RN. The Mallampati technique categorizes the airway into one of three classes (Mallampati, Gatt, Gugino, Desai, Waraksa, Freiberger et al, 1985):

Class 1: Visualization of the faucial pillars, soft palate, and uvula.
Class 2: Visualization of the faucial pillars and soft palate. The uvula is masked by the tongue.
Class 3: Visualization of only the soft palate.

If possible, the patient should be assessed in a sitting position. The patient is directed to open his or her mouth as wide as possible and protrude the tongue, exposing the faucial pillars and uvula at the tongue base. If the classification exceeds class 1, the physician should be notified regarding the appropriate plan of action (Figure 2-1). This simple precautionary measure alerts the monitoring RN and physician to anticipate difficulty in the event of respiratory depression requiring intubation. Some facilities use a simple technique of observing for craniofacial abnormalities, asking the patient to stick out the tongue, open the mouth, and flex the neck. The RN is observing for any craniofacial abnormalities that would cause difficulties with the fit of a positive pressure bag-mask device. If the patient opens the mouth without problem, the RN would be able to easily insert an oral airway. If the patient flexes the neck, the RN would be able to extend the neck in the event of a respiratory problem.

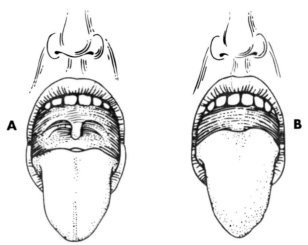

Figure 2-1 Mallampati class 1 airway **(A)** and class 3 airway **(B)**. *(From Dierdorf, S.F. [1995]. ASA practice guidelines for management of the difficult airway. Current Reviews for Nurse Anesthetists, 17, 170.)*

In addition to assessing the heart, lungs, and airway, the following questions are pertinent and helpful in the management of the care for the patient receiving moderate sedation and analgesia.

Question 1

Is there any history of seizure disorder?

Long-term benzodiazepine administration (e.g., diazepam) is often prescribed for patients with convulsive disorders and status epilepticus. Flumazenil, a benzodiazepine antagonist, may be administered to reverse the sedative effects of benzodiazepines. If the patient is undergoing long-term benzodiazepine therapy (e.g., control of intracranial pressure or status epilepticus) the administration of flumazenil is contraindicated because of the risk of seizures. Research is ongoing in this area, and the practitioner should refer to the scientific literature for further guidance. The potential benefits of the drug should be weighed against the potential risk for these patients.

Question 2

Is there any history of cardiovascular problems?

The RN should evaluate any current or past cardiovascular problem(s) to determine if the patient is at increased risk for developing complications during the procedure while under the effects of moderate sedation and analgesia. Consultation between the monitoring nurse, physician, and anesthesia provider is necessary to determine the most appropriate provider to monitor the patient.

Question 3

Is there any history of respiratory problems, such as emphysema or asthma?
Because many of the medications administered for moderate sedation and analgesia may result in respiratory depression, the patient with an existing respiratory problem is at greater risk for developing complications.

Emphysema is common in patients with bronchitis and asthma. The patient may have a distended barrel-shaped chest and a lower respiratory reserve. A state of chronic hypercarbia exists for patients with chronic obstructive pulmonary disease (e.g., emphysema). The low hypoxic level provides the stimulus for the patient to breathe. Large concentrations of oxygen block the patient's stimulus to breathe. To allow for better control of inspired oxygen fractions and to avoid compromising the drive to breathe in the patient with chronic obstructive pulmonary disease, the RN should consider delivering oxygen via a Venturi mask, which allows for a more precise titration of fixed amounts of oxygen in concentrations between 24% and 55% (O'Brien, 2003).

The asthmatic patient suffers from attacks of wheezing and dyspnea caused by partial obstruction of the bronchi and bronchioles. The RN should be aware of any causative factors, how the patient manages an episode, and current medications and should have immediately accessible the aerosol inhalant the patient takes to prevent attacks.

Question 4

Is there any history of liver disease?
Most of the sedation and analgesia medications administered are metabolized in the liver. The sedative effects may be exaggerated and prolonged because of delayed biotransformation. The extent of liver impairment and the appropriateness of nurse management should be determined by the physician.

Question 5

Is there any history of renal disease?
Benzodiazepines and opioid metabolites are excreted in the urine and may be administered with caution to the patient diagnosed with renal insufficiency. The attending physician should be consulted as appropriate.

Question 6

Is there any history of thyroid disorder?
Hyperthyroidism is not contraindication of the administration of moderate sedation and analgesia. However, medications such as atropine and local agents

administered with epinephrine may further increase the heart rate and precipitate a thyroid crisis. Patients with hyperthyroidism may be difficult to sedate within normal recommended dosages because of hypermetabolism related to the disorder. Hypothyroidism may exaggerate the effects of intravenous moderate sedation and analgesia medications. The IV medications should be slowly titrated to the desired effects while the patient is closely monitored. With any thyroid disorder that is medically managed and controlled, the patient should be treated in the same manner as any other patient receiving moderate sedation and analgesia (Monette, 2004).

Question 7

Is there any history of substance abuse?

The administration of sedative and analgesia medications may have little or no effect on known substance abusers. Inform the physician and determine a plan of action that includes an anesthesia provider back-up in the event that the patient becomes uncooperative or combative or the medications have little effect on the patient.

Question 8

Are there any known allergies to medications?

Although a true allergic reaction to a medication is infrequent, the RN should investigate any adverse reaction that a patient describes as an allergy (e.g., rash, pruritus, nausea, vomiting, dizziness, or headache). Verify that allergies are clearly documented. For each medication administered, the RN should be knowledgeable about the effects, contraindications, recommended dosage, potential complications, and populations at increased risk for reactions.

Question 9

Are there any current medications?

The current medication therapy can be reviewed to determine possible drug interactions when these drugs are administered with sedative agents or an invasive procedure is performed (Table 2-2). The patient's use of herbal products and other alternative therapies should also be reviewed for possible interactions (Table 2-3). One study that explored complementary and alternative medication (CAM) use in ambulatory surgical patients found that during the 2 weeks before surgery, 42.7% of 208 patients consumed CAMs. Of those patients, 19.8% (92) took CAMs that inhibit coagulation, 14.4% (70) consumed CAMs with cardiac effects, and 8% (39) of patients consumed CAMs with sedative effects (Wren, Kimbrall, Norred, 2002).

Table 2-2 | Potential Drug Interactions

Category/Drug	Intraoperative Concern	Management	Discontinuation Issues
Cardiovascular			
Angiotensin-converting enzyme	Hypotension with/without bradycardia, intolerance to hypovolemia	Hydration, moderate doses of vasopressor	Brief interruption tolerated; continuation may improve regional blood flow and oxygen delivery, and preserve renal function; consider withholding in patients taking amiodarone, multiantihypertensives
Diuretics	Hypokalemia, hypovolemia	Maintain hydration, check potassium level	May hold morning dose; might be desirable to continue for chronic renal failure
Antiarrhythmics	Cardiac depression; prolonged neuromuscular blockade	Monitor serum levels	Discontinuation rarely recommended
Amiodarone	Hypotension and atropine-resistant bradycardia—may need pacer		
Hemostasis			
Nonsteroidal anti-inflammatory agents	Impaired platelet function, altered renal function, gastrointestinal bleeding		Unless patient is at particular risk for bleeding or impaired renal function, may continue up to morning of surgery
Anticoagulants (heparin, warfarin sodium)	Increased hemorrhage	Reverse heparin with intravenous protamine, reverse warfarin sodium with vitamin K or fresh frozen plasma	Heparin—stop intravenously 4-5 hr and check PTT; warfarin sodium—stop 3-5 days and check PT

*In Ziolkowski, L., & Strzyzewski, N. (2001). Perianesthesia assessment: Foundation of care. Journal of PeriAnesthesia Nursing, 16, 363. From Dunn, D. (1998). Preoperative assessment criteria and patient teaching for ambulatory surgery patients. Journal of PeriAnesthesia Nursing, 13, 274-291.
PTT, Partial thromboplastin time; PT, protime.*

Continued.

Table 2-2 | Potential Drug Interactions—cont'd

Category/Drug	Intraoperative Concern	Management	Discontinuation Issues
Fibrinolytic drugs (streptokinase, urokinase, TPA)	Hemorrhage	Antifibrinolytic agent may be indicated	Discontinuation not an option when administered for life-threatening conditions (eg, MI)
Hypoglycemic agents Insulin	Hyperglycemia, hypoglycemia	Monitor glucose, use of insulin sliding scale	Morning dose withheld or reduced, dose dependent on glucose value
Oral hypoglycemic agents	Hyperglycemia, hypoglycemia	Monitor serum glucose, maintain hydration	Withhold oral hypoglycemic agents beginning on day of surgery
Central nervous system MAO inhibitors	Hypertension secondary to indirect-acting sympathomimetic drugs causes release of norepinephrine; excitatory state (from meperidine) or depressive reaction secondary to opioid	Avoid known triggering agents such as meperidine and indirect-acting sympathomimetic agents (eg, ephedrine)	Older, nonselective MAO inhibitors—discontinue 2-3 wk with risk of psychiatric consequence; new MAO inhabitors have shorter half-life and may stop on morning of surgery

MI, *Myocardial infarction*; MAO, *monoamine oxidase.*

Question 10

What is the patient's fasting status?

The American Society of Anesthesiologists (ASA) recommends (2002) that clear liquids can be taken up to 2 hours before the procedure and that a light meal can be consumed up to 6 hours before the procedure (Table 2-4). There should be sufficient time for gastric emptying to occur. When the patient does not meet established fasting requirements, the potential harm must be weighed against proceeding with the procedure.

Question 11

Is there any history of pain?

It is important to assess the patient for any pain that may be present. A discussion of presence, location, quality, and intensity of the pain should occur. A plan should be formulated to meet the patient's needs before, during, and after the procedure. Not every procedure is painful, although most produce anxiety. (Pasero, 1999). Even if the patient presents with no pain before the procedure, it is vital that the RN plan for any pain that may be experienced during or after the procedure. The patient should be taught how to use the appropriate pain scale. See Figure 3-2.

Question 12

Are there any piercings?

Care of the patient with piercings requires that the nurse responsible for moderate sedation identify whether the piercings can stay in or must be removed. Institutional protocols or guidelines can give clear instructions. The nurse's main concern is to assure the patient's safety. Piercings have the potential to become a foreign body (e.g., tongue piercing), source of infection (close to site of procedure), metal conductor (electrosurgery burn), and a possible snag (drapes or EKG leads with accidental tearing.) The nurse must support and educate the patient with piercings to the health and safety factors in the decision to ensure a positive and safe experience (Marenzi, 2004).

Patient Selection

The patient should be assessed as an appropriate candidate for nurse-monitored sedation based on selection criteria adopted by the facility or outpatient setting. The ASA ranks patient physical status on a scale of 1 to 6 (Table 2-5). Although used most often by anesthesia personnel, many institutions also use this classification system to determine patient selection for nurse-monitored sedation. It is common for patients who are healthy or have a mild systemic disease (e.g., P1 and P2) to be monitored by an RN. In patients with a disease process,

Table 2-3 | Commonly Used Herbs and Implications for Moderate Sedation

Herb	Actions	Common Usage
Black Cohosh	Estrogenic activity; sedative, antiinflammatory and antispasmodic effects	Approved by German Commission E for treatment of PMS, dysmenorrhea, and menopausal symptoms
Echinacea	Has antiinflammatory, immunostimulating effects; causes activation of cell mediated immunity	Used as immune stimulant and for immune support; prophylaxis for colds, influenza, and other viral, fungal, and bacterial infections; more effective when taken at onset of illness
Ephedra	Causes vasoconstriction of blood vessels, resulting in increased blood pressure; amphetamine effects cause bronchodilation, decreased gastrointestinal motility, and CNS stimulation	Used to treat asthma, bronchitis, headache, pulmonary congestion, and joint inflammation; recently used as appetite suppressant
Feverfew	Antimigraine, anti-inflammatory; prostaglandin inhibitor	Used to treat migraines, fever, and arthritis
Garlic	Antimicrobial, cholesterol- and triglyceride-lowering actions, antiplatelet action	Used to treat hypertension, hypercholesterolemia, arteriosclerosis, and infection

Data from Flanagan, K. (2001). Preoperative assessment: Safety considerations for patients taking herbal products. Journal of PeriAnesthesia Nursing, 16, 10-26; Goodwin, S.A., & Dierenfield, J.C. (2004). Complementary and alternative therapies. In D.M.D. Quinn & L. Schick (Eds.). PeriAnesthesia nursing core curriculum. St. Louis: Saunders; Skidmore-Roth, L. (2004). Mosby's handbook of herbs & natural supplements. St. Louis: Mosby.
PMS, Premenstrual syndrome; CNS, central nervous system; BP, blood pressure; HR, heart rate; NSAIDs, nonsteroidal antiinflammatory drugs.

Side Effects/ Complications	Moderate Sedation Implications	Preprocedure Discontinuation
Hypotension, slow heart rate, uterine stimulation, nausea, vomiting, anorexia, miscarriage	May cause hypotension and bradycardia; can potentiate action of antihypertensives	2 wk
Immunosuppression can occur after extended therapy; do not use more than 8 wk without a 3 wk rest period; do not give concomitantly with immunosuppressants; can cause transplant rejection; hypersensitivity reactions can occur; use caution with asthma, allergic rhinitis	Causes inhibition of hepatic enzymes; can affect many anesthetic agents	2 wk
Nervousness, dizziness, headache; increases in BP and HR; severe hypertension, cardiac arrest, seizures, stroke	May cause hypertension or dysrhythmias	7 days
Interferes with blood clotting; mouth ulcers; muscle and joint pain	Anticoagulant effects caused by platelet inhibition (prolonged bleeding time)	2 wk Discontinuation after prolonged use can cause a rebound effect, resulting in symptoms of migraine, insomnia, and anxiety; a slow withdrawal may reduce these effects
Nausea, stomach irritation; inhibits platelet function and fibrinogen; not recommended for concomitant use with aspirin, NSAIDs, or anticoagulants	Anticoagulant effects caused by platelet inhibition; can cause hypotension	2 wk

Continued.

Table 2-3 | Commonly Used Herbs and Implications for Moderate Sedation—cont'd

Herb	Actions	Common Usage
Ginger	Antiemetic, antinausea, antiinflammatory	Used to prevent nausea caused by motion sickness, chemotherapy, pregnancy, anesthesia
Ginkgo biloba	Cognitive enhancement, vasoprotective and tissue-protective actions; antioxidant and antiarthritic actions	Improves memory and mental function, increases blood circulation; used to decrease intermittent claudication
Ginseng	Decreased fatigue, increased physical performance, improved mental function, hypoglycemic action	Increases energy, decreases stress; improves concentration and overall well-being
Kava	Sedative, analgesic, and anxiolytic actions	Alleviates stress, anxiety, tension, and nervousness; used as anxiolytic and sedative; relieves tension headaches and muscle spasms
Saw Palmetto	Decreases symptoms of BPH and swelling of prostate	Used to treat BPH; used as mild diuretic to treat chronic cystitis
St. John's Wort	Antidepressant, antiretroviral/ antimicrobial	Used to treat anxiety, mild to moderate depression, sleep disorders; used topically as antiinflammatory to relieve hemorrhoids

PONV, Postoperative nausea and vomiting; *BPH,* benign prostatic hypertrophy; *GI,* gastrointestinal; *MAOIs,* monoamine oxidase inhibitors; *SSRIs,* selective serotonin reuptake inhibitors.

Side Effects/ Complications	Moderate Sedation Implications	Preprocedure Discontinuation
Nausea, vomiting, especially when taken on empty stomach; may inhibit platelet function	Prolonged bleeding time	2 wk Some studies found that when ginger was given just before surgery to reduce PONV, no increased bleeding was seen
Headache, anxiety, nausea, vomiting, abnormal bleeding; concomitant use with aspirin, NSAIDs, or anticoagulants not recommended	Prolonged bleeding time caused by platelet inhibition	2 wk
Hypertension, tachycardia, anxiety, insomnia; may lower blood glucose levels; should not use with insulin; may decrease action of anticoagulants	Hypoglycemic; can cause hypertension and tachycardia during surgery	2 wk
Blurred vision, red eyes, nausea, vomiting, liver damage, decreased platelets, yellowing skin, and scaling with high doses	Should not be used concomitantly with barbiturates or benzodiazepines; causes excessive sedation; anticoagulant effect caused by platelet inhibition	24 hr
Headache, mild GI distress	Avoid concurrent use with anticoagulants, NSAIDS, antiplatelets	Not necessary
Dizziness, insomnia, fatigue, restlessness, photosensitivity, serotonergic crisis— avoid concomitant use with MAOIs and SSRIs; decreases antiretroviral action of indinavir	Prolongs sedative effects of anesthetic medications	7 days

Continued.

Table 2-3 | Commonly Used Herbs and Implications for Moderate Sedation—cont'd

Herb	Actions	Common Usage
Valerian	Antianxiety, antinsomnia	Used to treat nervous disorders, such as anxiety, restlessness, and insomnia

Table 2-4 | Summary of American Society of Anesthesiologists Preprocedure Fasting Guidelines

Ingested Material	Minimum Fasting Period*
Clear liquids[†]	2h
Breast milk	4h
Infant formula	6h
Nonhuman milk[‡]	6h
Light meal[§]	6h

From American Society of Anesthesiologists. (2002). Practice guidelines for sedation and analgesia by non-anesthesiologists. Anesthesiology, 96, 1004-1017.

These recommendations apply to healthy patients who are undergoing elective procedures. They are not intended for women in labor. Following the guidelines does not guarantee a complete gastric emptying has occurred.

*The fasting periods apply to all ages.

[†]Examples of clear liquids include water, fruit juices without pulp, carbonated beverages, clear tea, and black coffee.

[‡]Since nonhuman milk is similar to solids in gastric emptying time, the amount ingested must be considered when determining an appropriate fasting period.

[§]A light meal typically consists of toast and clear liquids. Meals that include fried or fatty foods or meat may prolong gastric emptying time. Both the amount and type of foods ingested must be considered when determining an appropriate fasting period.

the condition must be medically controlled and no contraindications to the sedation and/or analgesia medications should be present. Patients in the P1 and P2 categories are less likely to develop complications related to the administration of medications for moderate sedation and analgesia or to the procedure itself. Any patient with a systemic disease process (e.g., P3 or higher) should be individually assessed to determine that the systemic disease is medically controlled

Side Effects/ Complications	Moderate Sedation Implications	Preprocedure Discontinuation
Headache, nausea; avoid concomitant use with barbiturates, alcohol, and benzodiazepines because excessive sedation can occur	May potentiate sedation caused by anesthesia/ sedation	7 days Abrupt discontinuation in patients who are physically dependent may cause withdrawal; taper over several weeks

and stable. There should be no contraindication to the administration of moderate sedation and analgesia medications.

Psychosocial Assessment

The course of the diagnostic, therapeutic, or surgical procedure produces stress and anxiety in most patients. The emotional state of the patient should be assessed. Assessment should include identification of any underlying medical problems (e.g., angina pectoris and sickle cell disease) that may exacerbate during stress. Also, a patient undergoing psychiatric care may take medications that interact with most central nervous system depressants commonly administered for moderate sedation and analgesia. Many patients who undergo diagnostic or surgical procedures are anxious and fearful. They may be concerned about the outcome of the test or other family members. They may be fearful of the procedure itself, possibility of pain, or of the unknown. The nurse can provide the support necessary to help the patient cope with the situation.

The cognitive ability of the patient should also be assessed. The patient needs to understand the procedure and any instructions for postprocedure care. This is especially important if the patient is having the procedure as an outpatient. The patient must understand the home care instructions to ensure compliance once discharged.

The social environment and home support for outpatients should also be assessed. This includes proximity to facility or physician's office, presence of telephone in the home, and availability of support from friends or family.

Consultation among the monitoring RN, surgeon, and anesthesia provider may be necessary to determine the most appropriate plan of care.

Table 2-5	Physical (P) Status Classification of the American Society of Anesthesiologists	
Status* (Symbol)†	**Definition**	**Description and Examples**
P1	A normal healthy patient	No physiologic, psychologic, biochemical, or organic disturbance
P2	A patient with mild systemic disease	Cardiovascular disease with minimal rest, asthma, chronic bronchitis, obesity, or diabetes mellitus
P3	A patient with severe systemic disease that limits activity but is not incapacitating	Cardiovascular or pulmonary disease that limits activity; severe diabetes with systemic complications; history of myocardial infarction, angina pectoris, or poorly controlled hypertension
P4	A patient with severe systemic disease that is a constant threat to life	Severe cardiac, pulmonary, renal, hepatic, or endocrine dysfunction
P5	A moribund patient who is not expected to survive 24 hours with or without the operation	Surgery is done as last resort or resuscitative effort; major multisystem or cerebral trauma, ruptured aneurysm, or large pulmonary embolus
P6	A patient declared brain dead, whose organs are being removed for donor purposes	

From the American Society of Anesthesiologists, 520 N Northwest Parkway, Park Ridge, Ill 60068-2573.

*In status 2, 3, and 4, the systemic disease may or may not be related to the reason for surgery.
†For any patient (P1 through P5) requiring emergency surgery, an E is added to the physical status; for example, P1E, P2E.
ASA 1 through ASA 6 is often used for physical status.

Diagnostic Assessment

A thorough evaluation of any preprocedure tests ordered for the patient should be completed. Any abnormal results should be brought to the attention of the physician.

Patient Education

The patient should be assessed for any learning needs before the procedure. Any information about the procedure and sedation should be given at this time. This is also an appropriate time to begin discharge teaching for the outpatient. Some of the medications given during moderate sedation produce amnesia, particularly the benzodiazepines. However, that amnesic effect is not retroactive, so the patient remembers information given preprocedure. It is important to offer as much information as possible before the procedure to the patient. This will increase the compliance with the postprocedure regimen and decrease anxiety and fear before the procedure (Odom, 2000).

Informed Consent

Patients or legal guardians should be informed of risks, benefits, limitations, and alternative treatments of sedation. The informed consent is the responsibility of the physician or other licensed independent practitioner. However, the RN must assure that consent was obtained. Many facilities have a separate consent form for sedation and for the procedure. The consent for sedation can be part of the procedural consent as long as the risks of sedation are specifically outlined. Another benefit of the informed consent is that it seems to increase patient satisfaction with the process (ASA, 2002; Odom, 2000).

INTRAPROCEDURAL MONITORING

Controversy about universal versus selective monitoring is ongoing. Some of the ongoing issues have included the following: Should a patient undergoing an endoscopic procedure be monitored differently than a patient undergoing a surgical procedure or a patient in the emergency department? Should a history and physical examination be required for every patient who will receive moderate sedative and analgesia medications? What is minimal laboratory work that should be done? What are minimal documentation intervals? Should the RN and the physician be certified in advanced cardiac life support? What is the minimal fasting status for the patient undergoing moderate sedation and analgesia? Should the patient be monitored with an electrocardiogram (ECG) (see Table 2-6 for differences between organizations).

Often the decisions that determine which monitoring parameters are implemented are based on projected cost of the equipment and personnel. Until there are scientific data to support the exclusion of a specific monitoring parameter, minimal monitoring parameters for the patient receiving moderate sedation and analgesia should include continuous assessment of pulmonary ventilation, oxygenation, blood pressure, cardiac rate and rhythm, level of consciousness, and skin condition (ANA, 1991; AORN, 2002; ASPAN, 2002).

Patient Monitoring

An institution is responsible for defining how monitoring parameters are to be collected through the development of policy and procedures. The policy and procedures should specify the type of equipment and physiologic data to be collected by the monitoring RN to provide continuous assessment of oxygenation, venti-

Table 2-6 | Organizational Differences in Monitoring Parameters for Moderate Sedation

	ANA	AORN	ASA	SGNA	JCAHO	ASPAN	State BON*
Oxygen saturation with use of pulse oximeter	+	+	+	+	+	+	+
Heart rate	+	+	+	+	+	+	+
ECG monitor	+	+	−†	−†	−†	+	+
Monitoring nurse with no other duties	+	+	−‡	−‡	−§	+	+
Level of consciousness	+	+	+	+	+	+	+
Blood pressure	+	+	+	+	+	+	+

Data from ANA, 1991; AORN, 2002; ASA, 2002, ASPAN, 2002; JCAHO, (2004b); SGNA, 2004, Odom-Forren, 2004.

+, Yes; −, no.

*See Appendix A to refer to specific state.

†State that ECG should be used in patients with significant cardiovascular disease or when dysrhythmias are anticipated or detected.

‡State that the individual monitoring the patient may assist the practitioner with interruptible ancillary tasks of short duration (ASA) once the patient's vital signs have stabilized (SGNA); however during deep sedation, individual should have no other responsibilities (ASA & SGNA).

§States that sufficient qualified individuals are present to perform procedure and monitor the patient throughout administration and recovery.

lation, circulation, and level of consciousness for a patient receiving moderate sedation and analgesia medications. The JCAHO (2004b) requires that when a level of sedation may result in the loss of protective reflexes, the same standards used for anesthesia care should be provided. Therefore consideration should be given to the types of medications to be administered by the RN, the desired depth of sedation, appropriate patient acuity level for nurse-monitored sedation, and the types of procedures that allow for a predictable outcome.

The JCAHO recommends that institutional protocols be consistent with professional standards and recommendations. The sources providing professional standards on the role of nonanesthesia RNs administering moderate sedation and analgesia are obtained from the state board of nursing, professional associations, current literature, and the institution's continuous quality improvement data. The JCAHO (2004b) requires protocols for the administration of sedation to address the following (see Chapter 6):

- Sufficient qualified personnel present to perform the procedure and to monitor the patient

- Performing the sedation, including rescuing the patient who slips into deeper level of sedation.
- Appropriate equipment for care and resuscitation
- Appropriate monitoring of vital signs
- Documentation of care
- Monitoring of outcomes

It is important to remember that the same standard of care should be applied to all patients regardless of the location. In no event should reliance on a monitor supersede the continuous observation of a dedicated monitoring RN whose sole responsibility is to monitor the patient. It is not advisable to assign the monitoring RN additional responsibilities that require him or her to leave the patient unattended (i.e., out the room) even for a brief period. This places the patient at potential risk. It is imperative that the patient be appropriately monitored during the procedure to ensure rapid identification and correction of any problem to prevent serious complications and a possible fatal outcome.

The team should conduct a "time out" immediately before the procedure begins to ascertain correct patient, correct procedure, and correct site. The physician should have marked the site if laterality or levels were involved before the start of the procedure (JCAHO, 2003). Initial vital signs, including oxygen saturation, should be obtained immediately before the procedure and administration of any medication.

Ventilatory Function

The principal causes of morbidity associated with sedation and analgesia are drug-induced respiratory depression and airway obstruction. Monitoring ventilatory function during sedation and analgesia decreases the risk of an adverse outcome (ASA, 2002; Odom, 2000). Ventilatory function can be assessed by observing depth and rate of respirations or auscultation of breath sounds. See Box 2-1 for assessment of ventilatory function by inspection, palpation, auscultation, and percussion.

Pulse Oximetry One of the most common and most valuable monitoring devices used to assess oxygenation in a patient receiving moderate sedation and analgesia is the pulse oximeter. Pulse oximetry is used as an adjunct to clinical assessment for detecting hypoxemia (Odom, 2000). This instrument provides a noninvasive measure of the arterial hemoglobin oxygen saturation and pulse rate. Pulse oximeters are portable, easy to use, and may be run by battery, which allows for ease in transporting the patient while providing continuous uninterrupted monitoring. Knowledge of the principles of oxygen transport assists the nurse in interpreting data from the pulse oximeter.

Oxygen saturation (SaO_2) occurs in direct relation to the partial pressure of oxygen (PaO_2), as shown in the oxyhemoglobin dissociation curve (Figure 2-2). PaO_2 is the amount of oxygen that is dissolved in the blood. The normal range of PaO_2 is 80 to 100 mm Hg provided that the pH and the body temperature are

Box 2-1 ASSESSMENT OF VENTILATORY FUNCTION

Inspection

The color of the patient's lips, oral mucosa, nail beds, and extremities should be assessed to determine the presence of cyanosis or pallor. The patient should be observed for signs of labored breathing, such a nasal flaring. Children and males generally are diaphragmatic breathers; observation of abdominal movement is helpful in assessment of rate, depth, and quality. Females tend to move the entire thoracic cage with each breath.

The normal respiratory rate for the adult is between 12 and 20 breaths per minute, with pediatric rates varying by age (see Chapter 8). Fewer than 12 breaths per minute are considered bradypneic, and such a patient should be closely assessed. If moderate sedation and analgesia medications have been administered, oversedation should be ruled out as the cause. More than 20 breaths per minute are considered tachypneic and are most often related to preprocedure anxiety. Respirations should always be counted for one full minute.

Palpation

Following inspection, the patient's chest should be palpated to determine any obvious abnormalities. Respiratory expansion should be assessed by palpating bony structures of the chest. The practitioner's hands are placed over the lower posterior chest wall, and the patient is directed to take a few deep breaths. The assessment of equal lung expansion should be determined. The temperature, moisture, and turgor of the skin should be assessed.

Percussion

The monitoring nurse may percuss the patient's chest by placing the middle finger of one hand (i.e., pleximeter) flat against the chest wall and gently striking the distal portion of the middle finger with the middle finger of the other hand. This causes vibrations that the RN may hear and feel. Resonance is a low-pitched, hollow sound that is heard over the normal lung.

Auscultation

The monitoring RN should listen to the respirations. The patient with normal respirations breathes quietly and without difficulty. Abnormal breath sounds, such as rales, rhonchi, or wheezing, indicate a respiratory problem and should be thoroughly assessed to determine etiology and possible contraindications to nurse-monitored sedation because the sedatives-anxiolytics and opioid analgesics administered for moderate sedation and analgesia have the potential to depress respirations and result in loss of protective reflexes.

Bilateral lung fields are auscultated with a stethoscope. The patient is directed to breathe deeply. A systematic approach should be used to auscultate the anterior, lateral, and posterior chest walls while comparing both sides.

Assessment of the respiratory system allows the monitoring RN to rule out any possible problems related to the administration of medications that may depress the respiratory system. It is essential to provide continuous uninterrupted moni-

---

Box 2-1 ASSESSMENT OF VENTILATORY FUNCTION—cont'd

toring of the respiratory status throughout the entire period of the patient's sedated state. Because of varying degrees of respiratory depression that occur as a result of medications administered, oxygen and oxygen delivery devices should be immediately available. Dyspnea or difficulty in breathing may be exhibited by sudden shallow respirations, nasal flaring, mouth breathing, combativeness, increasing anxiety level, and inability to cooperate during the procedure. Any of these symptoms should be reported to the physician immediately. The etiology (e.g., oversedation, undersedation, pain, idiosyncratic reaction) needs to be determined as soon as possible.

Describes relationship between Pao_2 (arterial oxygen tension) and Sao_2 (arterial hemoglobin oxygen saturation).

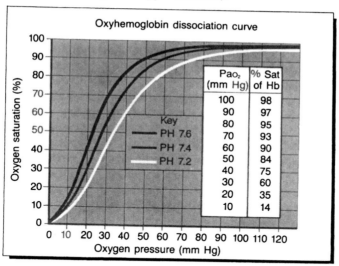

Changes in the affinity of hemoglobin for oxygen shift the position of the oxyhemoglobin dissociation curve.

Standard curve (middle curve above): Assumes normal pH (7.4), temperature, Pco_2, and 2,3-DPG levels

Shift to left (upper curve above): Increases O_2 affinity of Hb: increased pH; decreased temperature, Pco_2, and 2,3-DPG

Shift to right (lower curve above): Decreases O_2 affinity of Hb: decreased pH; increased temperature, Pco_2, and 2,3-DPG

Figure 2-2 Oxyhemoglobin dissociation curve. *(From Wong, D.L. [1995]. Pediatric quick reference. [2nd Ed.]. St. Louis: Mosby, p. 5.)*

normal. This is equivalent to an SaO_2 of 95% to 100%. The curve shifts when changes occur in body temperature, partial pressure of carbon dioxide (PCO_2), and hydrogen ion concentration (H^+). A decrease in body temperature, H^+, and PCO_2 results in the curve shifting to the right. This means that the oxygen attached to the hemoglobin is more easily released into the tissue. An increase in body temperature, H^+, and PCO_2 results in a shift to the left. This means that the oxygen is binding more tightly to the hemoglobin, resulting in less oxygen available to oxygenate tissue.

The use of pulse oximetry has become a standard of care for the patient receiving moderate sedation and analgesia for the single reason that it provides a reliable indication of SaO_2. The monitoring RN should be proficient in interpreting readings from the pulse oximeter. If a saturation level falls below 95% and remains at that level, the nurse should immediately assess the patient's ventilation status, apply supplemental oxygen if not already in place, and notify the physician.

Pulse oximetry provides an early indication of developing hypoxemia. It is an excellent device to assist the RN in monitoring the patient receiving moderate sedation and analgesia. There should always be a clear view of the patient's face, but often the draping, positioning for a procedure, or room lighting makes it nearly impossible to observe the patient's ventilatory status. The use of pulse oximetry offers an added measure of providing continuous uninterrupted monitoring of the patient's arterial oxygenation status. However, the RN should note that monitoring oxygenation by pulse oximetry is not a replacement for monitoring ventilatory function (ASA, 2002).

Capnography Capnography measures ventilation (end tidal carbon dioxide [ETCO2]) by determining the carbon dioxide in every breath as opposed to pulse oximetry that measures oxygen saturation. Capnography provides a graphic representation of exhaled CO_2 levels with a tracing called a capnogram. Capnography provides feedback with each breath and reflects apnea immediately (Carroll, 2002). Each breath results in an individual waveform. See Figure 2-3.

Originally, capnography required the presence of an endotracheal or tracheotomy tube. Today newer devices shaped like a nasal cannula can deliver oxygen and allow capnography on nonintubated patients (Sandlin, 2002).

ASA (2002) were equivocal that capnography was needed during moderate sedation, but agreed that capnography may decrease risks during deep sedation. It is imperative that the RN monitor ventilatory function whether using capnography or assessing with observation and auscultation.

Circulation

Pulse

Assessing the pulse provides a reflection of the overall condition of the heart and the vascular system. The RN may assess the pulse rate by palpating an artery. The radial artery, which is the most commonly used site for older children and

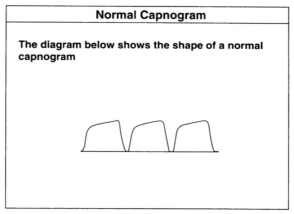

Figure 2-3 Normal capnogram. *(In Sandlin, D. [2002]. Capnography for nonintubated patients: The wave of the future for routine monitoring of procedural sedation patients. Journal of PeriAnesthesia Nursing, 17, 277-281.)*

adults, may be palpated by placing the first two fingers gently on the lateral palmar area of the wrist. Gentle pressure is applied until pulsation is felt, with the artery never fully occluded (i.e., to the point where no pulsation is felt). The apical pulse provides the most accurate assessment for children and adults with known dysrhythmias. To assess the apical pulse, place a stethoscope on the left side of the chest over the apex of the heart, between the fifth and sixth ribs at the midclavicular line.

Pulse Rate

The pulse should be evaluated for a period of at least 30 seconds. If the pulse is irregular, it should be assessed for a full 60 seconds. The pulse rate is initiated by the sinoatrial node, which is located in the right atrium. Normal resting pulse for the adult is 60 to 100 beats per minute. If the pulse is less than 60 beats per minute, it is bradycardic. If the pulse is greater than 100 beats per minute, it is tachycardic. A variety of factors influence the pulse rate. Any heart rate falling below 60 beats per minute should be evaluated. For well-conditioned athletes, many of whom tolerate a rate less than 50 beats per minute without symptoms, no treatment is necessary. However, treatment is indicated if the patient is bradycardic and experiencing symptoms such as chest pain, dizziness, or dyspnea.

Most patients experience fear and anxiety about the impending procedure. This may result in sympathetic stimulation, which increases the pulse rate. Other factors that may cause tachycardia include hyperthyroidism, anemia, hypovolemia, and hypoxia. Also, tachycardia may be related to an increase in oxygen demand (e.g., hypoxemia). When it is suspected that the heart is trying to compensate for the increased demand by increasing the pulse, the cause should be determined.

Medications such as sympathomimetic drugs and beta blockers cause the pulse rate to speed up or slow down, respectively. It is important to know what current medications the patient is taking. Pulse rates also follow a person's circadian rhythm, with rates being slightly higher in the late afternoon.

Pulse Rhythm

Pulse rhythm should be assessed to determine if it is regular or irregular. A regular rhythm has pulsations occurring at regular intervals. A rhythm in which the pulse intervals are unevenly spaced is irregular and indicates a disturbance. An irregular rhythm is commonly referred to as a dysrhythmia or arrhythmia. The two terms are used interchangeably, with both indicating a disturbance in the normal rhythm. Through palpation the only determination that can be made is whether the pulse is regular or irregular. If an irregular rhythm is present, a 12-lead ECG may be ordered by the physician to confirm the dysrhythmia. The most frequent dysrhythmias are premature ventricular contractions and premature atrial contractions.

Pulse Quality

Palpation of the pulse allows assessment of the quality or strength of the pulse. The strength of the pulse can be rated on a scale from 0 to 4 (Table 2-7). The pulse feels stronger in the upper extremities than in the lower extremities. If during the procedure the pulse becomes weak, the patient should be assessed for hypovolemia or hypotension. If the pulse suddenly becomes very strong and bounding, the patient may be hypervolemic or hypertensive or may be experiencing sudden anxiety or pain related to the procedure.

A strong pulse followed by a weak one may indicate pulsus alternans and indicates further patient assessment. A characteristic of pulsus alternans is the palpation of alternate strong and weak beats usually caused by left-sided heart failure, severe hypertension, and coronary artery disease. The patient should be assessed to determine the potential risks for a procedure with the administration of moderate sedation and analgesia agents by a nonanesthesia provider.

Table 2-7 | **Grading of Pulses**

Grade	Description
0	Not palpable
+1	Difficult to palpate, thready, weak; easily obliterated with pressure
+2	Difficult to palpate; may be obliterated with pressure
+3	Easy to palpate; not easily obliterated with pressure
+4	Strong, bounding; not obliterated with pressure

From Wong, D.L. (1995). *Pediatric quick reference. [2nd Ed.].* St. Louis: Mosby.

Blood Pressure

The monitoring RN should employ noninvasive methods for measuring the arterial blood pressure by using an aneroid or mercury type of sphygmomanometer or an automated electronic monitor.

Manual Method This method involves using a stethoscope and a sphygmomanometer with an inflatable blood pressure cuff. The cuff bladder width should be approximately 40% of the upper arm circumference. The length of the cuff bladder should be approximately 80% of the arm circumference. A cuff that is too narrow or too loose provides a falsely elevated or decreased blood pressure reading.

Common Errors

Incorrect application. The most common problem of applying a blood pressure cuff is incorrect position and improper size of the blood pressure cuff. Cuffs that are too short, too long, or too loose may result in an erroneous reading.

Obese arm. If an appropriate-size cuff is not available for the upper arm, an appropriate-size cuff for the forearm may be applied. The stethoscope is placed over the radial artery at the wrist to auscultate systolic and diastolic pressures.

Anxious patient. The most common cause of a high blood pressure reading is anxiety related to the impending procedure. The patient should be allowed time to become relaxed and comfortable before another reading is taken.

Auscultatory gap. A gap that results in the loss of sound between the systolic and diastolic pressures is commonly noted in patients with high blood pressure. Although no sound can be heard, the pulse will be present. It is important for the nurse to palpate the radial pulse and inflate the pressure approximately 30 mm Hg above the point where no pulsations are felt. Otherwise, a false low reading may be obtained.

Automatic Method Arterial blood pressure monitoring of the patient receiving moderate sedation and analgesia is commonly monitored by an oscillometric device. This monitoring device allows for blood pressure readings to be taken at specified intervals. In addition to blood pressure, readings of mean arterial pressure and heart rate are displayed on most models. The cuff contains an actuator and transducer for detection of arterial wall oscillations. The cuff is applied with the same guidelines as used for the conventional method.

Electrocardiogram

The RN responsible for the management of care for the patient receiving moderate sedation and analgesia should have a basic knowledge and understanding of cardiac monitoring and dysrhythmia interpretation. An ECG continuously monitors the heart rate and rhythm and detects cardiac dysrhythmias. The use of an ECG is not considered a universal standard for monitoring the patient receiving moderate sedation and analgesia. In fact, some units monitor heart rate and rhythm by the simple method of palpation, or they use a pulse oximeter monitor to detect dysrhythmias. However, any patient with a history of significant cardiovascular disease or those who are undergoing procedures in

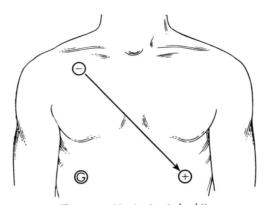

Figure 2-4 Monitoring in lead II.

which dysrhythmias are anticipated must have ECG monitoring (Table 2-6). Many nursing organizations have endorsed position statements that call for ECG monitoring on all patients undergoing moderate sedation (ANA, 1991; AORN, 2002; ASPAN, 2002), and most nurses would rather use EKG monitoring on all patients than determine which patients may or not need it. Continuous ECG monitoring allows rapid detection and intervention in the event of a dysrhythmia (Odom, 2000).

Although various types of cardiac monitors are on the market, most contain an easy-to-locate on-off switch, oscilloscope, brightness control, heart rate display, rate alarms, position control, size control, gain control, mm/sec control, run/hold/freeze control, calibration control, mode control, and lead control. Lead II is commonly selected to monitor the heart's electrical activity because monitoring in lead II is useful in assessing P waves, PR intervals, and atrial dysrhythmias (Figure 2-4). When an ECG is used for monitoring, it is important to remember:

1. A prominent P wave represents atrial activity and should be displayed on the ECG. Leads that easily identify the P wave should be selected.
2. The QRS amplitude should be high enough to trigger the rate meter.
3. Monitoring with an ECG identifies only disturbances in rhythms. If more elaborate ECG interpretation is indicated, a complete 12-lead ECG should be ordered by the physician.
4. Attention should be given to artifact. Because artifact may appear as a wavy baseline resembling ventricular fibrillation, the clinical status of the patient should always be assessed first.

Level of Consciousness

The monitoring RN who administers moderate sedation and analgesia medications should titrate the medications in small increments until the desired seda-

Box 2-2   RAMSAY SEDATION SCALE

Level of Sedation: Moderate (Conscious)

1 = Patient is anxious and agitated or restless or both.
2 = Patient is cooperative, oriented, and tranquil.
3 = Patient responds to commands only.

Level of Sedation: Deep

4 = Patient exhibits brisk response to light glabellar tap or loud auditory stimulus.
5 = Patient exhibits a sluggish response to light glabellar tap or loud response.
6 = Patient exhibits no response.

From Ramsey, M.A.E., et al. (1974). Controlled sedation with alphaxalone-alphadolone. British Medical Journal, 2, 656-659.

tive level is achieved. The optimal sedative level is one in which all the patient's protective reflexes are intact. The patient should be relaxed, easily aroused from sleep, and able to respond to verbal communication and commands.

The Ramsay Sedation Scale (Ramsay, Savage, Simpson, & Goodwin, 1974) is frequently used in intensive care units, but it is limited in clinical application to assessment of a patient's level of consciousness. Its use may be appropriate in areas where moderate sedation and analgesia medications are administered during short-term therapeutic, diagnostic, or surgical procedures. With the scale used as a guide, the medications administered are titrated to the desired level of sedation requested by the physician (Box 2-2). A patient profile for each level might suggest the following:

- Ramsay Sedation Scale 1—Patient is admitted to the preprocedure area experiencing anxiety and fear regarding the impending procedure.
- Ramsay Sedation Scale 2—Patient is alert, talkative, cooperative, calm, and relaxed during the procedure.
- Ramsay Sedation Scale 3—Patient is cooperative, calm, and relaxed with eyes closed. Patient responds to verbal command.
- Ramsay Sedation Scale 4—Patient is asleep. Patient is quick to respond to a light tap between the eyebrows or to calling of his or her name loudly.
- Ramsay Sedation Scale 5—Patient is asleep and more heavily sedated. Patient is slow to respond to a light tap between the eyebrows or to loud calling of name. Stimuli may need to be repeated before patient responds.
- Ramsay Sedation Scale 6—Patient is unresponsive. This level of sedation is beyond the intent and scope of practice for the RN administering moderate sedation and analgesia during short-term therapeutic or diagnostic procedures.

A simple sedation scale, such as that described by McCaffery & Pasero (1999), might be easily implemented (Box 2-3). Implementation of both of these tools

Box 2-3 SEDATION SCALE

S = Sleep, easy to arouse
1 = Awake and alert
2 = Slightly drowsy, easily aroused
3 = Frequently drowsy, arousable, drifts off to sleep during conversation
4 = Somnolent, minimal or no response to physical stimulation

From McCaffery, M., & Pasero, C. (1999). Pain: Clinical manual. St. Louis: Mosby.

provides a more objective assessment of the patient receiving moderate sedation and analgesia. If these tools are used in an institution, both RNs and physicians should be familiar and understand the application and limitation of each one. Understanding the various levels and patient profiles on the moderate sedation and analgesia continuum is key to achieving a standard of administration that is consistent among the various units and disciplines.

Emergency Equipment

Emergency equipment should be immediately available. Each procedure room should have oxygen and suction, oxygen cannulas and/or masks, a positive pressure breathing device, nasal and oral airways, and reversal agents—naloxone and flumazenil—available in the room. A defibrillator and an emergency cart with size appropriate equipment and ACLS drugs should be easily accessible.

Back-up personnel who are experts in airway management, including ACLS, must be available in the event of an emergency. This is especially important in the outpatient setting where the resources normally available in a hospital setting are not present.

POSTPROCEDURE ASSESSMENT

Because the patient has not received general anesthesia, he or she will most likely be transferred to a phase II level of care. The patient may go directly to an ambulatory care unit, a medical-surgical floor, or a recovery area in the unit where the procedure was performed. A verbal report should be given by the monitoring RN to the receiving nurse or caregiver if the patient is transported to another area. It is important for the monitoring RN to report the patient's name, procedure, medical problems, dosage, time of last medication(s) administered for moderate sedation and analgesia, and any adverse reactions. Recovery time depends on the type of medication(s) administered, dose, time of administration, and patient's level of consciousness.

The same monitoring parameters used during the procedure are applicable during the recovery phase. These include assessment of the respiratory rate, ventilatory function, oxygen saturation, blood pressure, cardiac rate and rhythm, level of consciousness, and skin condition. Monitoring the patient is vital during the postprocedure period. The patient is at risk for respiratory depression imme-diately after the procedure because any noxious stimuli have been removed, and the patient is allowed to rest without interference. In addition, if appropriate, the patient should be monitored for operative site bleeding, nausea and vomiting, and appropriate pain management.

The patient receiving moderate sedation and analgesia is discharged when the criteria that have been determined by the physician are met. Although there is no standard set of criteria that must be met for the patient receiving moderate sedation and analgesia, typically the criteria include stable vital signs; stable res-piratory status; level of consciousness; orientation to person, place, and time; ability to dress with minimal assistance; ability to walk without assistance; con-trolled nausea and/or vomiting; minimal discomfort and pain; an understand-ing of postoperative care; and a responsible adult escort available to care for the patient after discharge from the institution. See Chapter 5.

DOCUMENTATION

Documentation of the patient's care throughout the process of moderate seda-tion is imperative. Recording patient data can disclose trends that are critical in determining the development or cause of adverse events. Documentation is also an important tool of communication for all health care workers who take part in the care of the patient (Box 2-4). At a minimum, documentation should occur before the beginning of the procedure, after administration of sedative-analgesic

---

Box 2-4 PROCEDURAL DOCUMENTATION

Preprocedure assessment
Actual and potential nursing diagnoses, such as:
    Anxiety related to the unfamiliar environment and procedure
    Ineffective breathing patterns or impaired gas exchange related to altered level
       of consciousness or airway obstruction
    Knowledge deficit related to poor recall secondary to medication effects
    Increased or decreased cardiac output related to medication effects on the
       myocardium
    Injury related to altered level of consciousness
Nursing interventions and the patient's responses including:
    Dosage, route, time, and effects of all medications and fluids used
    IV site location, type and amount of fluids administered, including blood or
       blood components, monitoring devices, and equipment used
    Level of consciousness/sedation
    Untoward significant patient reactions and their resolution
    Postoperative evaluation based on preoperative assessment data

Modified from Association of periOperative Registered Nurses. (2002). Recommended practices for managing the patient receiving moderate sedation/analgesia. AORN Journal, 75, 649.

agents, at regular intervals during the procedure, during initial recovery, and just before discharge (ASA, 2002).

CONCLUSION

Every patient undergoing a short-term diagnostic, therapeutic, or surgical procedure under moderate sedation and analgesia deserves safe quality care regardless of the provider. The attitude of "It's only a local" has resulted in some patients receiving care that is far below the standard. Minimal monitoring parameters for the patient receiving moderate sedation and analgesia include continuous assessment of the pulmonary ventilation, oxygen saturation, blood pressure, cardiac rate and rhythm, level of consciousness, and skin condition. This chapter has suggested a monitoring process for the patient that includes the following phases:

- Preprocedure Phase: Obtaining the baseline health information (e.g., vital signs, physical examination, medical and medication history).
- Intraprocedure Phase: Continuous monitoring of vital signs (e.g., heart rate and rhythm, respiratory rate, ventilatory function, blood pressure), oxygenation (e.g., oxygen saturation) skin condition, and level of consciousness.
- Postprocedure Phase: Continuation of procedure monitoring parameters until the effects of moderate sedation and analgesia medications have decreased and the patient's level of consciousness is at the preprocedure state.

The intent of monitoring by a nonanesthesia provider is not to sacrifice quality by providing a lesser standard of care than the anesthesia provider but to provide the patient with a quality and standard of care that enhances patient safety and safeguards against an untoward outcome.

REFERENCES

American Nurses Association. (1991). Position statement on the role of the registered nurse (RN) in the management of patients receiving intravenous conscious sedation for short-term therapeutic, diagnostic, or surgical procedures. Retrieved June 2, 2004 from http://nursingworld.org/readroom/position/joint/jtsedate.htm.

American Society of Anesthesiologists. (2002). Practice guidelines for sedation and analgesia by non-anesthesiologists. Anesthesiology, 96, 1004-1017.

American Society of PeriAnesthesia Nurses (2002). Resource 12: The role of the registered nurse in the management of patients undergoing sedation for short-term therapeutic, diagnostic or surgical procedures. In ASPAN, 2002 standards of perianesthesia nursing practice. Cherry Hill, NJ: ASPAN, pp. 47-48.

Association of periOperative Registered Nurses. (2002). Recommended practices for managing the patient receiving moderate sedation/analgesia. AORN Journal, 75, 642-652.

Carroll, P. (2002). Procedural sedation: Capnography's heightened role. Retrieved June 2, 2004, from RNWEB® Archive, October 1, 2002.

Dierdorf, S. F. (1995). ASA practice guidelines for management of the difficult airway. Current Reviews for Nurse Anesthetists, 17(17), 168-171.

Ferrara-Love, R. History and physical examination. In D.M.D. Quinn, & L. Schick (Eds.). Perianesthesia nursing core curriculum: Preoperative, phase I and phase II PACU nursing. St. Louis: Saunders, pp. 235-251.

Flanagan, K. (2001). Preoperative assessment: Safety considerations for patients taking herbal products. Journal of PeriAnesthesia Nursing, 16, 19-26.

Goodwin, S.A., & Dierenfield, J.C. (2004). Complementary and alternative therapies. In D.M.D. Quinn, & L. Schick (Eds.). Perianesthesia nursing core curriculum: Preoperative, phase I and phase II PACU nursing. St. Louis: Saunders, pp. 265-282.

Joint Commission on Accreditation of Healthcare Organizations. (2003). Universal protocol for preventing wrong site, wrong procedure, wrong person surgery™. Retrieved June 1, 2004 from http://www.jcaho.org/accredited+organizations/patient+safety/universal+protocol/universal+protocol.pdf.

Joint Commission on Accreditation of Healthcare Organizations. (2004a). National patient safety goals. Retrieved June 1, 2004, from http://www.jcaho.org/accredited+organizations/patient+safety/npsg.htm.

Joint Commission on Accreditation of Healthcare Organizations. (2004b). Provisions of care, treatment, and services. In JCAHO. Comprehensive accreditation manual for hospitals. Oakbrook Terrace, IL: JCAHO.

Mallampati, S.R., Gatt, S., Gugino, L.D., Desai, S.P., Waraksa, B., Freiberger, D., et al. (1985). A clinical sign to predict difficult tracheal intubation: A prospective study. Canadian Anaesthetists' Society Journal 32, 429-434.

Marenzi, B. (2004). Body piercing: A patient safety issue. Journal of PeriAnesthesia Nursing, 19, 4-10.

McCaffery, M. & Pasero, C. (1999). Pain: Clincal manual. St. Louis: Mosby, pp. 267, 363-367.

Monette, L.F. (2004). Endocrine surgery. In D.M.D. Quinn, & L. Schick (Eds.). Perianesthesia nursing core curriculum: Preoperative, phase I and phase II PACU nursing. St. Louis: Saunders, pp. 814-838.

O'Brien, D. (2003). Care of the perianesthesia patient. In C.B. Drain (Ed.). Perianesthesia nursing: A critical care approach (4th Ed.). St. Louis, Saunders, pp.393-408.

Odom, J. (2000). Conscious sedation/analgesia. In N. Burden, D.M.D. Quinn, L .Schick, & B.S.G. Dawes (Eds.). Ambulatory surgical nursing. Philadelphia: Saunders, pp. 309-330.

Ramsay, M., Savege, T., Simpson, B., & Goodwin, R. (1974). Controlled sedation with alphaxalone-alphadolone. British Medical Journal, 2, 656-659.

Skidmore-Roth, L. (2004). Mosby's handbook of herbs & natural supplements. (2nd Ed.). St. Louis: Mosby.

Society of Gastrointestinal Nurses and Associates. Statement on the use of sedation and analgesia in the gastrointestinal endoscopy setting. Retrieved June 2, 2004 from http://www.sgna.org/resources/Sedationpos.html.

Williams, G.D. (2000). Preoperative preparation of the ambulatory surgery patient. In N. Burden, D.M.D. Quinn, L. Schick, & B.S.G. Dawes (Eds.). Ambulatory surgical nursing. Philadelphia: Saunders, pp. 346-362.

Wren, K.R., Kimbrall, S., & Norred, C.L. (2002). Use of complementary and alternative medications by surgical patients. Journal of PeriAnesthesia Nursing, 17, 170-177.

Ziolkowski, L., & Strzyzewski, N. (2001). Perianesthesia assessment: Foundation of care. Journal of PeriAnesthesia Nursing, 16, 359-370.

3

Pharmacology

One of the main purposes of this book is to provide a resource for the nonanesthesia provider who is responsible for the management of moderate sedation and analgesia in the patient undergoing a short-term therapeutic, diagnostic, or surgical procedure. Providing sedation and analgesia requires vigilance and a knowledge of physiology and pharmacology. The clinician administering sedative and analgesic agents should have no responsibilities other than monitoring the response of the patient to these drugs and rapidly intervening when necessary.

It is important to determine whether a patient needs sedation for anxiolysis, analgesia for painful procedures, or both. The spectrum of pain and anxiety control (Figure 3-1) illustrates various techniques, which include pharmacologic and nonpharmacologic interventions. This chapter focuses on the administration of intravenous (IV) medications to achieve adequate moderate sedation and analgesia.

INTRAVENOUS ADMINISTRATION

Parenteral administration may be required to ensure absorption of the active form of the drug. Systemic absorption after subcutaneous or intramuscular injection is usually more rapid or predictable than after oral administration. The rate of systemic absorption is limited by the surface area of the absorbing capillary membranes and by solubility of the drug in interstitial fluid. The desired concentration of drug in the blood can be achieved more rapidly and precisely by the IV route of administration (Stoelting, 1999 [Table 3-1]).

Administration of medications through IV injection involves rapid onset of action, approximately 20 to 30 seconds from the time the medication is administered until the desired patient effects are observed. The involved times can vary depending on the factors in Table 3-1 and co-existing disease processes in the patient. Because IV injection provides a direct route of entry into the bloodstream, potential adverse effects (e.g., airway obstruction, cardiopulmonary arrest, and allergic reactions) occur rapidly.

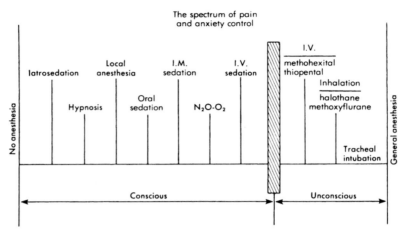

Figure 3-1 Spectrum of pain and anxiety control. Illustration of various techniques available for patient management. Vertical bar represents loss of consciousness. *(From Malamed, S.F. [1995]. Sedation: A guide to patient management. [3rd Ed.]. St. Louis: Mosby.)*

Before any IV medication is administered, the RN should be knowledgeable about each medication. Pertinent information includes recommended dilution, recommended dose, potential adverse reactions, and drug compatibility with other medications and solutions. The RN needs to be aware of any patient drug allergies.

Emergency airway management equipment should be readily available when intravenous sedative and/or analgesic agents are administered. Necessary equipment includes a bag-valve-mask device and oxygen for positive pressure ventilation, functioning suction, oral and nasal airways, age-specific endotracheal tubes, and emergency airway management devices, such as laryngeal mask airways.

IV Push

The technique of IV push is the administration of a medication directly into a vein through a secure IV catheter or other venous access device. The dose and rate of administration should follow the manufacturer's recommendations and those parameters should not be exceeded. Some medications, such as fentanyl, are quite potent (e.g., fentanyl is 100 times more potent than morphine, so morphine 10 mg = fentanyl 100 mcg) and are administered in micrograms (mcg), not milligrams. Therefore the RN should always check the recommended dosage units, appropriate dose, route, and rate of administration for each moderate sedation drug.

Table 3-1 | **Rate and Capacity of Tissue Drug Uptake**

The rate and capacity of tissue uptake for drugs depend on variables that include:

1. Blood flow, which is a function of cardiac output and perfusion of the vital organs, such as the brain, heart, and liver. Perfusion may be impaired in disease states, such as congestive heart failure.
2. Concentration gradient: physical-chemical properties of cell membranes and drugs influence the rate at which drugs achieve their effects at specific receptors.
3. Blood-brain barrier: refers to the limited permeability of brain capillaries. This limited permeability restricts distribution of ionized water-soluble drugs to the central nervous system. The blood-brain barrier is subject to change and can be overcome by the administration of certain drugs.
4. Physicochemical properties of the drug:

   Ionization—a nonionized molecule is usually lipid soluble and can diffuse across cell membranes, including the blood-brain barrier, renal tubules, GI epithelium, and hepatocytes. The ionized portion of a drug is poorly lipid soluble and cannot penetrate lipid cell membranes easily.
   Lipid solubility—may be best understood in the context of drug distribution after systemic absorption. Tissue uptake of drugs is determined by tissue blood flow if the drug can penetrate membranes rapidly. The concentration gradient for the diffusible fraction of drug (nonionized, lipid soluble, and unbound to protein) determines both the rate and direction of net transfer between plasma and tissue.
   Protein binding—a variable amount of most drugs is bound to plasma proteins that include albumin, alpha$_1$-acid glycoprotein, and lipoproteins. Protein binding has an important effect on drug distribution because only the free or unbound portion is readily available to cross cell membranes.
   Drug solubility—the degree to which a drug is soluble in blood or tissue.
   Tissue mass—the mass of tissue to which a drug is bound.
   pH—the acidity or alkalinity of a solution.

From Stoelting, R.K. (1999). *Pharmacology and physiology in anesthetic practice.* Philadelphia: Lippincott-Raven, p. 10.

IV Titration

This technique involves direct intravenous drug administration; small increments of the medication are given until the desired clinical endpoints are achieved (e.g., sedation and analgesia). At the same time, physiologic homeostasis (e.g., oxygenation, ventilation, and circulation) must be maintained. Following the manufacturer's guidelines, the RN slowly administers the drug by pushing the syringe plunger, while observing for the desired patient effects and any adverse reactions.

IV Continuous Infusion

This technique is frequently used in an intensive care unit (ICU) for patients needing sedation and analgesia. Opioids are frequently supplemented by the administration of a benzodiazepine or hypnotic (e.g., propofol, or the centrally acting alpha$_2$-agonist dexmedetomidine (Precedex), which has sedative and analgesic properties [Barash, Cullen, & Stoelting, 2001; Drummond, 2002]). Medications are mixed according to manufacturer guidelines and administered through a controlled-infusion device and titrated to achieve the desired patient effect.

BENZODIAZEPINES

General Pharmacology

The benzodiazepines were developed in the 1950s (Sternbach, 1978). These drugs have amnestic, sedative, muscle relaxant, and anticonvulsant properties. Benzodiazepines, such as midazolam and diazepam, are widely administered to produce sedation and amnesia while maintaining consciousness for therapeutic, diagnostic, or surgical procedures.

Commonly administered benzodiazepines include diazepam (Valium), lorazepam (Ativan), and midazolam (Versed). Desirable pharmacologic characteristics include amnesia, increased seizure threshold to local anesthetic agents, minimal respiratory depression when titrated to individual response, and minimal hemodynamic effects. These drugs are popular because of their antianxiety and sedative properties. In general, benzodiazepines are not recommended during pregnancy. These drugs are pregnancy category D.

Mechanism of Action

The mechanism of action for benzodiazepines is related to specific benzodiazepine receptors found throughout the central nervous system (CNS). These receptor sites are part of the gamma aminobutyric acid (GABA) complex. Benzodiazepine administration facilitates the CNS inhibitory action, allowing increased amounts of GABA at the postsynaptic nerve endings. Increased GABA causes selective inhibition of CNS pathways resulting in anticonvulsant, sedative, muscle relaxant, and anxiolytic properties.

Pharmacokinetics

Compared with diazepam and lorazepam, midazolam has a far shorter elimination half life. Diazepam has pharmacologically active metabolites (oxazepam and desmethyldiazepam) that prolong its effects.

Midazolam and diazepam use hepatic microsomal oxidation for their metabolization. This oxidation process may be slower in the older adult, resulting in a longer duration of action. Both hepatic dysfunction and the administration of drugs known to induce the hepatic microsomal (cytochrome P-450) enzyme system impair the oxidation process. Drugs that induce the cytochrome P-450 system include cimetidine, warfarin, and anticonvulsants. Lorazepam is metabolized by hepatic glucuronide conjugation. Glucuronide conjugation is less affected by age and concurrent medications.

Clinical Uses

The benzodiazepines are frequently used as premedicants and for their sedative, anxiolytic, and amnesic properties during moderate sedation procedures. When titrated appropriately, these drugs produce minimal effects on the cardiovascular and respiratory systems in healthy patients. It is important to note that significant synergy is produced by the addition of opioids to a sedation regimen with benzodiazepines, greatly increasing the potential for respiratory depression. Therefore, oxygen saturation level, adequacy of ventilation, and respiratory rate should all be closely monitored. Airway management skills (e.g., the ability to recognize and correct respiratory obstruction) are essential when these drugs are administered.

Because of its potency and duration of action, midazolam is popular in the perioperative setting. Midazolam has a rapid onset, produces amnesia, and has a shorter duration of action than diazepam or lorazepam. Diazepam and lorazepam have durations of action that exceed many typical diagnostic and therapeutic procedures.

The sedative and respiratory depressant effects of benzodiazepines can be antagonized by flumazenil (Romazicon). The actions of flumazenil are specific to benzodiazepines. Flumazenil administration is not associated with tachycardia and hypertension as seen with naloxone. Analgesia is not affected by flumazenil, and rebound anxiety is not seen (Table 3-2).

DIAZEPAM

Trade Names: Diazemuls, Diazepam, Valium, Valrelease, Vivol, Zetran

Classification: Anticonvulsant, anxiolytic, benzodiazepine, CNS agent

Diazepam was first synthesized in 1959. It was found to have excellent antianxiety, skeletal muscle relaxant, and anticonvulsant properties. During the 1960s, it became one of the most widely prescribed medications in the United

Table 3-2 | Intravenous Benzodiazepines

Drug	Recommended IV Dosage	Peak Effect (Minutes)	Half-Life (Hours)	Duration of Action (Hours)
Diazepam	2.5-5 mg (5-10 mg q2-4 hr)	10-15	20-80	2-4
Lorazepam	0.5-2 mg (2-4 mg q2-4 hr)	15-20	10-20	6-8
Midazolam	0.5-1 mg (2.5-5 mg q1 hr)	3-5	1-12	1.5-2

States. Today, diazepam is a useful premedication for surgical and diagnostic procedures. Following IV administration, anterograde amnesia occurs, which can persist into the postoperative/postprocedure period. Patients should be cautioned not to make major decisions for 24 hours following the administration of this drug.

Parenteral diazepam is nonwater-soluble and contains the preservative propylene glycol. The drug can cause pain on injection and may form precipitate when mixed with incompatible drugs or solutions (Roche, 2004).

Pharmacokinetics: *Onset:* 30 to 60 minutes PO; 15 to 30 minutes IM; 1 to 5 minutes IV. *Peak:* 1 to 2 hours PO; 10 to 30 minutes IV. *Duration:* 2 to 6 hours. *Metabolism:* Occurs in the liver by microsomal oxidation. The oxidation process may be impaired in patients with liver disease, advanced age, or co-administration of medications that inhibit microsomal oxidizing enzymes (cimetidine, warfarin, and anticonvulsants). Active metabolites include desmethyldiazepam and oxazepam, which account for the prolonged effects of this medication. *Elimination:* Half-life is 20 to 40 hours (up to 80 hours in the older adult); excreted in urine.

Contraindications: Do not administer this drug if known hypersensitivity or acute narrow-angle glaucoma exists. Diazepam can be given to patients with open-angle glaucoma if that condition is medically managed. Because diazepam is metabolized in the liver and excreted via the kidneys, it should be administered cautiously in patients with compromised hepatic or renal function. Other CNS-depressant drugs (e.g., opioids, phenothiazines, barbiturates, monoamine oxidase [MAO] inhibitors, and other psychotropic drugs) may potentiate the CNS effects of diazepam.

Adverse Reactions: *CNS:* Drowsiness, confusion, depression, dysarthria, headache, hypoactivity, slurred speech, syncope, tremor, vertigo. Paradoxic reactions (e.g., agitation rather than sedation) may be seen. *GI:* Constipation, nausea. *GU:* Incontinence, libido changes, urinary retention. *CV:* Bradycardia, cardiovascular collapse, hypotension. *EENT:* Blurred vision, diplopia, nystagmus. *Skin:* Urticaria, rash. *Others:* Hiccups, changes in salivation, neutropenia, jaundice.

Dosage and Administration
Premedication
Adult: PO: 2 to 10 mg. *IM:* Inject 5 to 10 mg deeply into muscle using z-track technique approximately 30 minutes before procedure.
Intravenous moderate sedation
Adult: Slowly titrate diazepam until slurred speech noted. The initial dose generally does not exceed 10 mg. Administer slowly over 1 minute for each 5 mg injected. If the patient has not received any premedication, it may be necessary to titrate up to 20 mg to achieve the desired level of sedation. If diazepam is

administered with an opioid, decrease the dose of the opioid by one third and titrate in small increments to achieve the desired effect.

Nursing Considerations
Assessment
- Assess for medications known to inhibit the activity of microsomal oxidizing enzymes (e.g., cimetidine, anticonvulsants).
- Assess for medications known to intensify CNS effects when administered with diazepam (e.g., opioids, barbiturates, phenothiazines, psychotropics).
- Assess for abnormalities in kidney and liver function.
- Assess for respiratory rate, adequacy of ventilation, oxygen saturation, blood pressure, heart rate and rhythm, level of consciousness, and skin condition.

Intervention
- Administer into large veins (e.g., antecubital, with ample [40 cc] flush). Do not administer into small veins (e.g., dorsum of hand or wrist) as phlebitis may result.
- Inject slowly through an infusing, nondextrose-containing IV for more than 1 minute for each 5 mg.
- Administer IM injection into deep muscle mass using z-track technique.
- Avoid intraarterial administration.
- Have suction equipment, a positive pressure breathing device like an Ambu bag, oxygen, and airways in the room when diazepam will be administered.
- Have an emergency cart with defibrillator, ACLS drugs, and airway equipment, such as endotracheal tubes, a functioning laryngoscope, and laryngeal mask airways (LMAs) available.
- Administer cautiously to older adults, debilitated patients, or those with cardiopulmonary disease.
- The nonanesthesia provider who administers diazepam should be skilled at monitoring and supporting ventilation and oxygenation.

Desired outcome
- Patient has decreased anxiety and apprehension during procedure.

LORAZEPAM

Trade Name: Ativan

Classification: Anxiolytic, benzodiazepine, CNS agent, sedative-hypnotic

Lorazepam (Ativan) is a benzodiazepine that is occasionally administered for its sedative effects during a procedure anticipated to last more than 2 hours. The effects produced by lorazepam include sedation, anxiolysis, and amnesia.

Pharmacokinetics: Biotransformation (metabolism) of lorazepam occurs in the liver via a process called conjugation. Conjugation is a principal pathway and is less susceptible to factors such as age, liver impairment, and drugs that inhibit microsomal oxidizing enzymes. *Onset:* 60 to 120 seconds IV; 15 to 30 minutes IM. *Peak:* 60 to 90 minutes IM. *Metabolism:* Occurs in the liver by the principal pathway of glucuronide conjugation. The metabolites in lorazepam are inactive. *Duration:* 6 to 8 hours. *Elimination:* Half-life is 16 hours IM and IV, excreted in urine.

Contraindications and Precautions: Clinical trials reported that patients over 50 experienced more profound, prolonged effects from IV administration. Because of the risk of underventilation and apnea, this drug should be administered with caution to older adults, very ill patients, or patients with limited pulmonary reserve. Lorazepam is contraindicated in patients with known benzodiazepine hypersensitivity or narrow-angle glaucoma.

Adverse Reactions: *CNS:* Excessive sleepiness and drowsiness, hallucinations, dizziness. *CV:* Hypertension or hypotension. *Ear:* Tinnitus. *Eye:* Diplopia, blurred vision. *GI:* Nausea and vomiting. *Respiratory:* Partial airway obstruction. *Skin:* Rash.

Dosage and Administration
Premedication
Adult: PO, IM: 2 to 4 mg (0.05 mg/kg) 2 hours before procedure.
Intravenous moderate sedation
Adult: IV: 0.05 mg/kg or up to 2 mg 15 to 20 minutes before procedure.

Nursing Considerations
Assessment
- Assess for medications known to intensify the CNS effect when administered with lorazepam (e.g., opioids, phenothiazines, barbiturates, psychotropics).
- Assess for any abnormalities in liver and kidney function.
- Assess respiratory rate, adequacy of ventilation, oxygen saturation, blood pressure, heart rate and rhythm, level of consciousness, and skin condition.

Intervention
- For IV administration, dilute medication with equal amounts of compatible solution (e.g., sterile water for injection, saline for injection, or 5% dextrose for injection). Dilution is not recommended for IM injection.
- Inject slowly through an infusing IV line directly into vein. The rate should not exceed 2 mg per minute.
- Administer IM undiluted injection into deep muscle mass.
- Avoid intraarterial administration.

- Have suction and positive pressure breathing device (e.g., Ambu bag), oxygen, and appropriate airways in the room where lorazepam is to be administered.
- Have an emergency cart with defibrillator, ACLS drugs, endotracheal tubes, a functioning laryngoscope, and LMAs immediately accessible.
- The nonanesthesia provider administering lorazepam should be skilled at supporting a patient's oxygenation and ventilation status.

Desired outcome
- Patient has decrease in anxiety and apprehension during the procedure.
- Patient has diminished recall of events during procedure.

MIDAZOLAM

Trade Name: Versed

Classification: Anxiolytic, benzodiazepine, CNS agent, sedative-hypnotic
   Midazolam was first introduced to the U.S. market in 1986. Since that time, it has rapidly replaced diazepam for the sedative component of moderate sedation and analgesia. Midazolam has a rapid onset of action, short elimination half-life, and excellent amnesic effects. Midazolam is metabolized in the liver to inactive metabolites that are excreted in the urine. It is water soluble with a low incidence of venous irritation and injection site discomfort (Roche, 2004).

Pharmacokinetics: *Onset:* 15 minutes IM; 30 to 60 seconds IV. *Peak:* 30 to 60 minutes IM; 10 to 15 minutes IV. *Duration:* One to 2.5 hours IV. *Elimination:* Half-life is 1.2 to 12.3 hours IV; excreted in urine.

Contraindications and Precautions: Contraindicated for patients with known hypersensitivity to midazolam or acute narrow-angle glaucoma. This drug may be administered to patients with open-angle glaucoma if they are receiving appropriate medical therapy. It is not recommended for use during pregnancy or in obstetrics. From clinical studies, guidelines for pediatric administration have been developed. This drug should be administered cautiously in elderly patients, in patients with congestive heart failure, renal impairment, pulmonary disease, or hepatic dysfunction; and in patients receiving concomitant opioids.

Adverse Reactions: Clinical trials on midazolam demonstrated the following findings: fluctuations in vital signs following parenteral administration, including decreased tidal volume and/or decreased respiratory rate in 23.3% of patients following IV administration and in 10.8% of patients following IM administration. Apnea was reported in 15.4% of patients after IV administration along with fluctuations in blood pressure and pulse rate.

The following additional adverse reaction was reported after IM administration: headache (1.3%). At the IM injection site, the following reactions were reported: pain (3.7%), induration (0.5%), redness (0.5%), and muscle stiffness (0.3%).

The following additional reactions were reported subsequent to IV administration: hiccups (3.9%), nausea (2.8%), vomiting (2.6%), coughing (1.3%), oversedation (1.6%), headache (1.5%), and drowsiness (1.2%). At the IV site, the following reactions were reported: tenderness (5.6%), pain during injection (5%), redness (2.6%), induration (1.7%), or phlebitis (0.4%).

Dosage and Administration
Premedication
Adult: IM: 0.07 to 0.08 mg/kg (average dose is 5 mg). Administer 1 hour before procedure.
Intravenous moderate sedation
Healthy adults younger than 60 years: Slowly titrate 1 to 2.5 mg until sedation or slurred speech seen. Initial titrated dose should not exceed 2.5 mg. Administer dose over a 2-minute period. Never administer by rapid or single bolus. If additional medication is needed, titrate small increments (e.g., 0.5 mg) and wait an additional 2 minutes to evaluate the sedative effect. If opioids or other CNS depressants have been administered as a premedication, the patient will require about 30% less midazolam than would a nonpremedicated patient.

Patients older than 60 years, debilitated, or chronically ill: Older adults and those with chronic disease or decreased pulmonary reserve are at increased risk for hypoventilation or apnea. Therefore, titrate in smaller increments and at a slower rate (e.g., 0.5 to 1 mg every minute). If additional medication is necessary, administer no more than 1 mg over 2 minutes. Wait an additional 2 minutes after each increment to evaluate patient effect. Usually no more than 3.5 mg is necessary.
Maintenance dose
If during a procedure additional midazolam doses are needed to maintain the desired sedation level, slowly titrate midazolam in small increments (0.5 mg) to achieve the desired effects. The maintenance dose is usually 25% of the initial dose.

Nursing Considerations
Assessment
- Assess for medications known to inhibit the activity of the cytochrome P-450 microsomal enzyme system (e.g., cimetidine, warfarin, anticonvulsants).
- Assess for medications known to intensify the CNS effect when administered with midazolam: opioids, phenothiazines, barbiturates, psychotropics.
- Assess for any abnormalities in liver or kidney function.
- Assess respiratory rate, adequacy of ventilation, oxygen saturation, blood pressure, cardiac rate and rhythm, level of consciousness, and skin condition.

Intervention
- Slowly titrate to desired effect (e.g., sedation, slurred speech).
- Patients receiving premedication or concurrent treatment with an opioid or other CNS depressant require less midazolam.
- Initial dose should not exceed 2.5 mg administered over at least 2 minutes.
- Do not administer by rapid or single bolus.
- Wait an additional 2 minutes or more to evaluate the effect of midazolam.
- Because the peak effect may take longer to achieve in older adult patients or those with chronic diseases or decreased pulmonary reserve, an additional wait of more than 2 minutes may be necessary.
- Administer IM injection into deep muscle mass.
- Avoid intraarterial administration.
- Have suction and a positive pressure breathing device, oxygen, and appropriate airways in the room where midazolam is to be administered.
- Have an emergency cart with defibrillator, ACLS drugs, endotracheal tubes, a functioning laryngoscope, and LMAs immediately accessible.
- The nonanesthesia provider administering midazolam should be skilled at supporting a patient's oxygenation and ventilation.

Desired outcome
- Patient has decreased anxiety and apprehension during the procedure.
- Diminished intraoperative recall results.

BENZODIAZEPINE ANTAGONIST

FLUMAZENIL

Trade Name: Romazicon

Classification: Benzodiazepine antagonist

Flumazenil was the first benzodiazepine antagonist available in the United States. It is indicated for complete or partial reversal of sedative benzodiazepine effects. Flumazenil antagonizes the sedative, respiratory depressant, and psychomotor effects of benzodiazepines. Flumazenil blocks the benzodiazepine effects by competitive inhibition at the benzodiazepine receptor site. It does not antagonize the effects of opioids and other CNS agents. Flumazenil administered for a high dose of agonist, such as a benzodiazepine overdose, results in rapid reversal of deep CNS depression. Its duration of action is shorter than that of most benzodiazepines.

Pharmacokinetics: *Onset:* 30 to 60 seconds. *Peak:* 6 to 10 minutes. *Duration:* Influenced by the dose administered and the dose of the agonist. *Elimination half-life:* 41 to 79 minutes. For flumazenil doses equal to or less than 1 mg, the duration of action is about 50 minutes. Flumazenil is metabolized in the liver and excreted in the urine.

Contraindications and Precautions: Contraindicated in patients with known hypersensitivity to flumazenil or benzodiazepines, patients undergoing long-term benzodiazepine use for a life-threatening condition (e.g., status epilepticus), and patients showing signs of antidepressant overdose. Use cautiously in patients with impaired hepatic or renal function.

Adverse Reactions: *CNS:* Agitation, dizziness, emotional lability. *CV:* Cutaneous vasodilation. *GI:* Nausea and vomiting. *Other:* Shivering, pain at injection site, fatigue, blurred vision.

Dosage and Administration
Reversal of benzodiazepine sedative effects
Adult: 0.2 mg IV over 15 seconds. If the desired level of consciousness is not achieved after 45 seconds, administer another 0.2 mg. May repeat at 60 second intervals four times up to a maximum total dose of 1 mg.

Treatment of resedation
Adult: May repeat doses administering 0.2 mg IV over 15 seconds at 20 minute intervals as needed. Administer no more than 1 mg at one time and no more than 3 mg in 1 hour.

Benzodiazepine overdose
Adult: Administer 0.2 mg IV over 30 seconds. If desired level of consciousness is not achieved after 30 seconds, administer 0.3 mg over 30 seconds, waiting an additional 30 seconds to evaluate effects. Additional doses of 0.5 mg may be administered over 30 seconds at 1 minute intervals to a maximum cumulative dose of 3 mg if necessary.

Nursing Considerations
Assessment
- Assess patient status for long-term benzodiazepine usage.
- Assess for any abnormalities in liver and kidney function.
- Assess for respiratory rate, adequacy of ventilation, oxygen saturation, blood pressure, heart rate and rhythm, level of consciousness, and skin condition.

Intervention
- Administer intravenously only; may be diluted in 5% dextrose in water, lactated Ringer's solution, and normal saline solution.
- Administer in the recommended increments and rates of administration to the desired endpoint, minimizing the likelihood of adverse effects.
- To minimize patient discomfort, administer into a freely running IV line secured in a large vein.
- Monitor for signs of resedation as appropriate.

Desired outcome
- Patient has rapid return to presedation state.

OPIOID AGONISTS

General Pharmacology

The terms opioid, opiate, and narcotic are used interchangeably to describe potent analgesics, which are controlled substances. Opioid is the more general term and includes the opiates and synthetic narcotic analgesics. Analgesia is a key component of moderate sedation. Opioids that are available for clinical use will vary, depending on institutional formularies. Some of the commonly administered opioids in moderate sedation are morphine, meperidine, and fentanyl.

Mechanism of Action

Opioid actions are determined by target cell receptors, also known as opioid receptor sites. These sites are primarily located in the CNS and include the mu, kappa, delta, and sigma receptors. Mu receptor agonism results in analgesia, respiratory depression, physical dependence, euphoria, and sedation. Kappa receptor agonism causes weak analgesia, respiratory depression, and sedation. Sigma receptor agonism results in dysphoria, delirium, mydriasis, hallucinations, tachycardia, and hypertension. Delta receptor agonism produces weak analgesia and respiratory depression (Stoelting, 1999 [Tables 3-3 and 3-4]).

Opioids are classified as agonists, partial agonists, or mixed agonist-antagonists. There are also specific opioid antagonists available (e.g., naloxone, naltrexone). Opioid effects are dose dependent and occur because of opioid binding at receptor sites. Morphine, Demerol, and fentanyl are pure agonists (e.g., primarily analgesic in action).

Table 3-3 | **Receptor Site Effects**

Effect	μ *Receptor*	κ *Receptor*	Δ *Receptor*
Analgesia	+++	+++	o
Mental status	Euphoria	Sedation Dysphoria	Dysphoria
Respiratory depression	+++	+	+
Gastrointestinal motility	—	–	-
Urinary retention	++		++

From Bennett, J., et al. (2002). Opioid use during the perianesthesia period: Nursing implications. Journal of PeriAnesthesia Nursing, 16, 256.
+++, Large positive effect; ++, moderate positive effect; + small positive effect; —, large negative effect; –, moderate negative effect; -, small negative effect.

Table 3-4 | Sites of Opioid Activity

Medication	μ Receptor	κ Receptor
Morphine	+++	+
Fentanyl	+++	+
Butorphanol	–	+++
Nalbuphine	–	++

From Bennett, J., et al. (2002). Opioid use during the perianesthesia period: Nursing implications. Journal of PeriAnesthesia Nursing, 16, 258.
+, Agonist; –, antagonist.

Agonist-antagonists like butorphanol (Stadol) or nalbuphine (Nubain) do not produce the same effects as agonists. Butorphanol and nalbuphine are mixed agonist-antagonists. These drugs bind as agonists to the kappa receptor and bind as weak agonists at the mu receptor. As a result, analgesia is produced, but patients may experience more dysphoria and psychomimetic effects than when a pure opioid agonist is administered. There is a ceiling or limit on the amount of analgesia and respiratory depression that mixed agonist-antagonist drugs produce.

Antagonists, like naloxone, produce no analgesic affects but displace agonists from opioid receptor sites. The result is dose-dependent reversal of respiratory depression, analgesia, drowsiness, pruritus, and other effects of the agonists and agonist-antagonists (Drain, 2004).

Pharmacokinetics: The pure agonist opioids produce dose-related analgesia and other side effects, such as respiratory depression. Opioids act as agonists at the specific receptors described above, which are located in the brainstem, in the spinal cord, and outside the CNS in peripheral tissue. Most opioids are metabolized in the liver and excreted via the urine. Note that meperidine has an active metabolite, normeperidine, and is not recommended for use in the elderly (Stoelting, 1999).

Pharmacodynamics: Respiratory depression generally occurs within 5 to 10 minutes following IV injection, with duration dependent on the elimination half-life of the involved drug. The patient with ventilatory depression from opioid administration may respond to commands (e.g., "take a deep breath") or stimulation. Patients at greater risk for respiratory depression related to opioids include opioid-naïve individuals who receive large IV doses of these drugs and individuals with histories of sleep apnea.

If respiratory effort is not adequate to maintain adequate oxygenation (SpO_2 > 93%) and ventilation (respiratory rate greater than 10 per minute), a chin lift may be necessary. Supplemental oxygen should be provided, and the involved clinicians may need to provide positive pressure ventilation by mask. An opioid agonist-antagonist, such as nalbuphine—2.5 to 5 mg IV, may be administered to increase respiratory rate and tidal volume. The advantage of this drug is minimal antagonism of mu receptor effects with kappa receptor antagonism and increased tidal volume and respiratory rate.

Clinical Use: Opioids may be administered as premedication or along with other medications, such as benzodiazepines or hypnotics during moderate sedation. To provide optimal analgesia during the procedure, a pain history should be obtained. Elements of a pain history include how the patient reacts to pain; previous effective analgesic methods; attitudes regarding opioids and sedatives; identification of substance abuse; and patient expectations. Numerous scales for pain measurement exist (Figure 3-2). In the perioperative setting, a numeric rating of pain with 0 representing no pain and 10 the worst possible pain can be used.

Opioids alter perceptions of pain. In addition to systemic medications, such as opioids and benzodiazepines, local anesthesia is essential for safe moderate sedation. Overuse of systemic drugs to compensate for inadequate local anesthesia leads to respiratory depression with potentially lethal consequences. Local anesthesia blocks nerve conduction by altering propagation of the action potential in axons. These drugs act on sodium channel receptors, inhibiting sodium ion influx (Sweitzer & Pilla, 1998). Patients receiving local anesthesia and moderate sedation should be aware that they may feel sensations such as tugging, pressure, or pulling during the procedure.

MORPHINE SULFATE

Trade Names: MS Contin, Roxanol

Classification: Narcotic analgesic, opioid agonist

Morphine is a commonly administered opioid. Histamine release, manifested as pruritus and vasodilation, occurs in a dose-dependent fashion. Morphine may be titrated to the desired patient effect (e.g., analgesia). This drug has a high affinity for mu and kappa receptors, and produces altered perceptions of pain and euphoria. Respiratory depression can be antagonized with an agonist-antagonist, such as nalbuphine or naloxone.

Pharmacokinetics: *Onset:* 1 to 3 minutes IV. *Peak:* 10 to 20 minutes IV. *Metabolism:* Occurs in liver. *Duration:* 3 to 4 hours. *Elimination half-life:* 3 to 7 hours. Excreted in urine and bile.

Contraindications and Precautions: Contraindicated in patients with known hypersensitivity to morphine or phenanthrene opioids (e.g., codeine, hydrocodone, hydromorphone, oxycodone, oxymorphone). Administer with

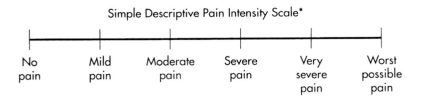

Simple Descriptive Pain Intensity Scale*

No pain | Mild pain | Moderate pain | Severe pain | Very severe pain | Worst possible pain

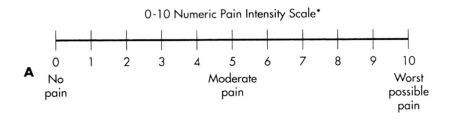

0-10 Numeric Pain Intensity Scale*

A

0 1 2 3 4 5 6 7 8 9 10
No pain / Moderate pain / Worst possible pain

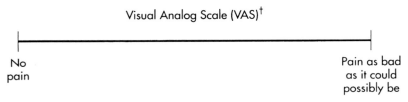

Visual Analog Scale (VAS)†

No pain / Pain as bad as it could possibly be

*If used as a graphic rating scale, a 10-cm baseline is recommended.
†A 10-cm baseline is recommended for VAS scales.

Figure 3-2 A, Pain intensity scales.

caution to any patient with supraventricular dysrhythmias, head injury, or increased intracranial pressure, or to pregnant patients. Also administer with caution to patients with renal or hepatic dysfunction, pulmonary disease (e.g., asthma, COPD), convulsive disorders, or physical addiction to this medication. Concomitant use of other medications that depress the CNS potentiates drug effects, such as respiratory depression. Decrease the normal dose by 25% to 30% if other drugs with CNS-depressant properties are used and when opioids are administered to elderly patients.

Adverse Reactions: *CNS:* Sedation, dizziness, delirium, seizures, euphoria. *GI:* Nausea, vomiting, constipation, biliary tract spasm. *GU:* Urinary retention. *EENT:* Blurred vision, miosis. *CV:* Bradycardia, tachycardia, palpitations, asys-

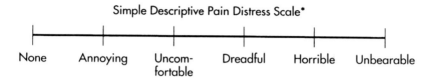

Simple Descriptive Pain Distress Scale*

None   Annoying   Uncom-   Dreadful   Horrible   Unbearable
                    fortable

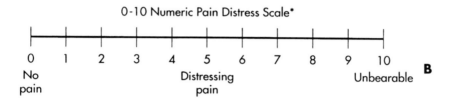

0-10 Numeric Pain Distress Scale*

0   1   2   3   4   5   6   7   8   9   10
No   Distressing   Unbearable   B
pain   pain

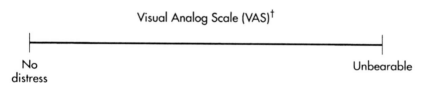

Visual Analog Scale (VAS)†

No   Unbearable
distress

*If used as a graphic rating scale, a 10-cm baseline is recommended.
†A 10-cm baseline is recommended for VAS scales.

Figure 3-2, cont'd. B, Pain distress scales. *(From AHCPR-Acute Pain Management Guideline Panel [February 1992]. Acute pain management: Operative or medical procedures and trauma. Clinical practice guideline. [AHCPR Pub. No. 92-0032]. Rockville, MD: Agency for Health Care Policy and Research, Public Health Service, U.S. Department of Health and Human Services.)*

tole, hypertension, hypotension. *Resp:* Respiratory depression. *Other:* Rash, urticaria, flushing, diaphoresis.

Dosage and Administration
Intravenous moderate sedation
Adult: 1 to 2 mg IV, up to 0.1 mg/kg. *Pediatric:* 0.5 to 1 mg, up to 0.1 mg/kg.

Nursing Considerations
Assessment
- Assess patient medication history for possible interactions with other CNS-depressant medications the patient may be taking.

- Assess for history of drug dependence.
- Assess and choose with patient an appropriate pain intensity scale.
- Assess for kidney and liver dysfunction.
- Assess baseline monitoring data: respiratory rate, adequacy of ventilation, oxygen saturation, blood pressure, heart rate and rhythm, level of consciousness, and skin condition.

Intervention
- Administer slowly over 2 to 3 minutes. May be diluted with sterile water for injection.
- If administering with another CNS-depressant drug, decrease dose by 25% to 30%.

Desired outcome
- Patient demonstrates adequate pain management.
- Side effects, such as respiratory depression, are minimized.

MEPERIDINE

Trade Name: Demerol

Classification: Narcotic analgesic; opioid agonist
  Meperidine has atropine-like effects, and the patient may experience tachycardia following IV administration. Histamine release occurs.

Pharmacokinetics: *Onset:* 1 to 5 minutes IV; 10 minutes IM. *Peak:* 10 to 20 minutes IV; 1 hour IM. *Duration:* 1 to 2 hours. *Elimination half-life:* 2 to 6 hours. Metabolized in liver and excreted via the urine.

Contraindications and Precautions: Contraindicated in patients with known hypersensitivity to meperidine or other phenylpiperidine derivatives. Administer with caution in any patient with supraventricular dysrhythmias, head injury, renal or hepatic dysfunction, pulmonary disease, convulsive disorder, or glaucoma, or in older or debilitated patients. May interact with monoamine oxidase (MAO) inhibitors and result in hypertension, excitation, tachycardia, seizure, and hyperpyrexia.

Adverse Reactions: *CNS:* Drowsiness, dizziness, confusion, headache, sedation, euphoria, convulsions at high doses. *CV:* Tachycardia, asystole, bradycardia, palpitations, hypotension, syncope. *GI:* Nausea, vomiting, anorexia, constipation, cramps. *Skin:* Rash, urticaria, bruising, flushing, diaphoresis, pruritus. *EENT:* Tinnitus, blurred vision, myopia, diplopia. *Respiratory:* Respiratory depression.

Dosage and Administration

Premedication

Adult: 50 to 100 mg IM or SC 30 to 90 minutes before procedure. *Pediatric:* 1 mg/kg IM or SC 30 to 90 minutes before procedure.

Intravenous moderate sedation

Adult: 10 to 20 mg IV, up to 1 mg/kg. *Pediatric:* 5 to 10 mg IV, up to 1 mg/kg.

Nursing Considerations

Assessment

- Assess patient medication history for current use of MAO inhibitors (e.g., isocarboxazid, pargyline, phenelzine, tranylcypromine).
- Assess for history of drug dependence.
- Assess and choose with patient an appropriate pain intensity scale.
- Assess for kidney and liver dysfunction.
- Assess baseline monitoring data: respiratory rate, adequacy of ventilation, oxygen saturation, blood pressure, heart rate and rhythm, level of consciousness, and skin condition.

Intervention

- Administer slowly over 30 seconds or longer into an infusing IV line. Injectable meperidine is compatible with normal saline, 5% dextrose, lactated Ringer's solution, and sodium lactate solution.
- May be administered to some patients with known sensitivity to morphine.
- For drug overdose, administer agonist-antagonist, such as nalbupine or antagonist naloxone.
- Administer 25% to 30% less if other CNS depressant drugs present and when administered to elderly patients.
- For nausea and vomiting, administer an antiemetic (e.g., metoclopramide, ondansetron).

Desired outcome

- Patient demonstrates adequate pain management.
- Side effects, such as excessive sedation and respiratory depression, are minimized.

FENTANYL

Trade Name: Sublimaze

Classification: Opioid agonist, narcotic analgesic

Fentanyl is a popular opioid used as a supplement to inhalational, regional, and monitored anesthesia care (local anesthesia with IV sedation). Fentanyl is often used as the analgesic component of moderate sedation because of its rapid onset and minimal histamine release. This drug is usually given with a benzodiazepine and/or a hypnotic for moderate sedation. Fentanyl is highly lipophilic; when released from fat and muscle tissue back into circulation, delayed-onset respiratory depression may occur. A dose of 100 mcg is equivalent in analgesic activity to morphine 10 mg or meperidine 75 mg.

Pharmacokinetics: *Onset:* 1 to 3 minutes IV; 7 to 8 minutes IM. *Peak:* 5 to 15 minutes IV. *Metabolism:* Occurs in liver. *Duration:* 30 to 60 minutes following single IV dose of less than 100 mcg. *Elimination half-life:* 4 hours; excreted in urine.

Contraindications and Precautions: Contraindicated in patients with known hypersensitivity to fentanyl. Administer with caution to any patient with bradycardia, head injury, renal or hepatic dysfunction, pulmonary disease (e.g., asthma, COPD), convulsive disorders, or physical addiction to this medication. It is not recommended for patients taking MAO inhibitors 14 days before administration. Use cautiously with other CNS depressant medications, and in the elderly, decreasing the dose by 25% to 30%.

Adverse Reactions: *CNS:* Sedation, dizziness, delirium, seizures, euphoria. *GI:* Nausea, vomiting, biliary spasm. *EENT:* Blurred vision, miosis. *CV:* Bradycardia, tachycardia, palpitations, arrest, hypertension, hypotension. *Respiratory:* Respiratory depression, arrest, laryngospasm. *GU:* Urinary retention. *Other:* Apnea, skeletal muscle rigidity.

Dosage and Administration
Premedication
Adult: 50 to 100 mcg (1 to 2 cc) IM 30 to 60 minutes before procedure.
Intravenous conscious sedation
Adult: 25 mcg IV, up to 2 mcg/kg.

Nursing Considerations
Assessment
- Assess patient medication history for current use of MAO inhibitors (e.g., isocarboxazid, pargyline, phenelzine, and tranylcypromine).
- Assess for history of drug dependence.
- Assess and choose with patient an appropriate pain intensity scale.
- Determine if patient is taking beta blockers, calcium channel blockers, benzodiazepines, or tranquilizers, which could cause hypotension.
- Assess for kidney or liver dysfunction.
- Assess baseline monitoring data: respiratory rate, adequacy of ventilation, oxygen saturation, blood pressure, heart rate and rhythm, level of consciousness, and skin condition.

Intervention

- Patient may receive an anticholinergic (e.g., glycopyrrolate, atropine preprocedure to minimize the effect of bradycardia).
- In adults, administer in incremental doses of 25 mcg IV every 2 minutes, carefully titrating to patient response.
- Apnea or muscle rigidity may occur. Be prepared to treat with oxygen, positive pressure ventilation, nalbuphine, or naloxone.
- If administering with another CNS depressant, or when treating elderly patients, decrease dose by 25% to 30%.

Desired outcome

- Patient demonstrates adequate pain management.
- Side effects, such as respiratory depression and muscle rigidity, are minimized.

OPIOID AGONIST-ANTAGONISTS

NALBUPHINE

Trade Name: Nubain

Classification: Narcotic agonist-antagonist
    This drug is a potent analgesic with sedative properties due to its agonist-antagonist receptor agonism. Its analgesic potency is approximately equivalent to that of morphine. Nalbuphine is not a controlled substance. Because of its opioid antagonist properties, nalbuphine is not recommended for patients who are concurrently medicated with opioids. The risk of respiratory depression with this drug is much less than that associated with opioid agonists such as morphine, meperidine, and fentanyl.

Pharmacokinetics: *Onset:* 2 to 3 minutes IV. *Peak:* 30 to 60 minutes IV. *Metabolism:* Occurs in liver. *Duration:* 3 to 6 hours. *Elimination half-life:* 3 to 7 hours; excreted in urine and bile.

Contraindications and Precautions: Nalbuphine is contraindicated in patients with known hypersensitivity to nalbuphine hydrochloride or other phenanthrene opioids (e.g., codeine, hydrocodone, hydromorphone, oxycodone, oxymorphone). Administer with caution to any patient with supraventricular dysrhythmias, head injury, or increased intracranial pressure. Administer cautiously in patients with renal or hepatic dysfunction, pulmonary disease (e.g., COPD or asthma) or physical addiction to opioids (which may precipitate withdrawal). Other CNS depressants may potentiate the effects of the medication.

Adverse Effects: Drowsiness, CNS depression, narcotic withdrawal, histamine release, hypotension, bradycardia, miosis, and respiratory depression.

Dosage and Administration
Intravenous moderate sedation
Adult: 1 to 2 mg IV, up to 0.2 mg/kg.

Nursing Considerations
Assessment
- Assess patient medication history for possible interactions with other CNS-depressant medications that the patient may be taking. Decrease the normal dose by 25% to 30% if other drugs with CNS depressant properties are used and when opioids are administered to elderly patients.
- Assess for allergies to sulfites. Drug contains sodium metabisulfite as a preservative and should not be administered to patients with such an allergy.
- Assess for history of drug dependence.
- Assess and choose with patient an appropriate pain intensity scale.
- Assess for kidney and liver dysfunction.
- Assess baseline monitoring data: respiratory rate, adequacy of ventilation, oxygen saturation, blood pressure, heart rate and rhythm, level of consciousness, and skin condition.

Intervention
- Administer slowly, titrating to effect.
- If administering with another CNS depressant drug, decrease dose by 25% to 30%.

Desired outcome
- Patient demonstrates adequate pain management.
- Side effects, such as respiratory depression, are minimized.

BUTORPHANOL

Trade Name: Stadol

Classification: Narcotic agonist-antagonist; opioid partial agonist
Butorphanol has been available in the United States since 1979. It has both agonist and antagonist properties. Butorphanol is not a controlled substance and is less likely to be abused and cause dependency than an opioid agonist. Butorphanol 2 mg is approximately equivalent to morphine 10 mg in analgesic potency. Butorphanol produces analgesia by working as a kappa and sigma receptor agonist. Due to antagonism at the mu receptor, there is less risk for res-

piratory depression. Because of its opioid antagonist properties, butorphanol is not recommended for patients who are concurrently medicated with opioids. Butorphanol can precipitate withdrawal symptoms in patients who received opioids for a prolonged (>10 days) period. The risk of respiratory depression with this drug is much less than that associated with opioid agonists such as morphine, meperidine, and fentanyl.

Pharmacokinetics: *Onset:* 2 to 3 minutes IV; 10 to 30 minutes IM. *Peak:* 30 minutes IV; 30 to 60 minutes IM. *Duration:* 2 to 4 hours. *Metabolism:* occurs in the liver. *Elimination half-life:* 2.15 to 3.5 hours. Excreted in the urine and bile.

Contraindications and Precautions: Contraindicated in patients with known hypersensitivity to butorphanol tartrate. Administer with caution to any patient with supraventricular dysrhythmias, renal or hepatic dysfunction, pulmonary disease (e.g., asthma, COPD), convulsive disorder, or physical addiction to opioids. The drug may cause biliary spasm and seizures in patients with convulsive disorders. Administer cautiously in hypertensive patients because hypertension may result.

Adverse Reactions: *CNS:* Sedation, headache, vertigo, lethargy, dizziness, confusion, lightheadedness. *CV:* Palpitations, hypotension, hypertension. *Respiratory:* Respiratory depression. *GI:* Nausea, vomiting, dry mouth. *Skin:* Rash, flushing, clamminess, and excessive sweating.

Dosage and Administration
Premedication
Adult: 2 mg IM 60 to 90 minutes before procedure.
Intravenous moderate sedation
Adult: 0.5 to 2 mg IV every 3 to 4 hours.

Nursing Considerations
Assessment
- Assess patient medication history for possible interactions with other CNS-depressant medications that the patient may be taking.
- Assess for history of drug dependence, which can precipitate withdrawal symptoms. Because of its opioid antagonist properties, butorphanol is not recommended for patients who are concurrently receiving opioids for chronic pain because this drug can precipitate withdrawal.
- Assess and choose with patient an appropriate pain intensity scale.
- Assess for kidney and liver dysfunction.
- Assess baseline monitoring data: respiratory rate, adequacy of ventilation, oxygen saturation, blood pressure, heart rate and rhythm, level of consciousness, and skin condition.

Intervention

- If administering with another CNS depressant, or to elderly patients, decrease dose by 25% to 30%.

Desired outcome

- Patient demonstrates adequate pain management.
- Side effects such as excessive sedation, respiratory depression, and nausea are minimized.

OPIOID ANTAGONIST

NALOXONE

Trade Name: Narcan

Classification: Narcotic antagonist

Naloxone (Narcan) was introduced in the 1960s for the rapid reversal of opioid-induced respiratory depression. It is active at the mu, delta, kappa, and sigma receptors. For most patients, naloxone antagonizes the opioid effects of respiratory depression, apnea, and sedation. Its duration of action is shorter than that of most opioids. Rapid naloxone injections IV have been associated with pulmonary edema in otherwise healthy patients (Carlson, 2004). This drug should be used with extreme caution. The drug is supplied as 0.4 mg (400 mcg) in either a 1 milliliter ampule or a multidose vial. The reader is strongly advised to either dilute naloxone 0.4 mg with 9 cc of IV fluid, resulting in a 40 mcg/ml dilution or to administer naloxone with a tuberculin syringe in 0.1 ml (40 mcg) increments.

Pharmacokinetics: *Onset:* 1 to 2 minutes IV; 2 to 5 minutes IM or SC. *Peak:* 5 to 15 minutes IV. *Metabolism:* Occurs in liver by conjugation. *Duration:* 45 minutes. *Elimination half-life:* 90 minutes; excreted in the urine.

Contraindications and Precautions: Contraindicated in patients with known hypersensitivity to naloxone. If this drug is administered to a patient with opioid dependence, severe withdrawal syndrome may result. Administer with caution to patients with cardiovascular disease, head injuries, or convulsive disorders.

Dosage and Administration: *Adult:* Reversal of postoperative opioid depression: 40 mcg IV every 2 minutes, up to 400 mcg. The desired clinical endpoint is spontaneous respiration at a rate that maintains an acceptable SpO_2 (e.g., > 93%).
   Pediatric: 0.005 to 0.01 mg/kg

Nursing Considerations

Assessment
- Obtain a true history from patient to determine opioid addiction.
- Continued assessment is necessary following administration because of the shorter duration of action than that of the opioid and the potential for hypertension and pulmonary edema.

Intervention
- Monitor respiratory and cardiovascular function.
- Document reason for administration.

Desired outcome
- Patient has reversal of respiratory depression related to opioids.

OTHER DRUGS

PROPOFOL

Trade Name: Diprivan

Classification: Sedative-hypnotic

Propofol is a hypnotic drug with antiemetic properties that has been available since 1989. It is used for induction and maintenance of anesthesia, for sedation of the mechanically ventilated ICU patient, and as a supplement to local anesthesia and systemic analgesic drugs (PDR, 2004). Propofol has a rapid onset and short duration of action. It is an emulsion-based product mixed with soybean oil, glycerol, and egg phosphatide. This emulsion can support bacterial growth. Strict aseptic precautions should be followed when handling propofol. Vials or syringes containing propofol should be discarded 6 hours following opening of the original propofol vial or ampule. It is compatible with commonly used IV fluids.

Propofol is available as Diprivan (Zeneca Pharmaceuticals, Wilmington, Del) or in generic form. Generic propofol contains 0.25 mg/ml sodium metabisulfite (see package insert for generic propofol [Gensia, Irvine, Calif]). The incidence of sulfite allergy is estimated at greater than 1 in 1000 patients. The manifestations of sulfite allergy range from mild dermatitis to bronchospasm or anaphylaxis (Langevin, 1999). Clinicians should be aware of these risk factors and be prepared to treat bronchospasm or anaphylaxis when administering generic propofol.

Pharmacokinetics: *Onset:* 30 to 45 seconds. *Peak:* 92 seconds. *Duration:* 1.8 to 8.3 minutes for distribution phase; 34 to 64 minutes for second distribution; and 3 to 8 hours for terminal elimination. *Elimination:* Extrahepatic metabolism and/or extrarenal elimination. Metabolized in the liver and excreted by the kidneys. Metabolites are pharmacologically inactive.

Contraindications and Precautions: Known hypersensitivity to propofol. Allergy to eggs. Should be administered only by anesthesia providers except in critical care areas when the patient is intubated and mechanically ventilated. See Chapter 1 for discussion of nurse-administered propofol sedation. Propofol causes dose-related depression of the protective airway reflexes.

Adverse Reactions

CNS: Movement, headache, dizziness, twitching, clonic/myoclonic movement. *CV:* Hypotension, hypertension, bradycardia. *GI:* Nausea, vomiting, cramping. *Respiratory:* Apnea, cough, hiccup. *Skin:* Flushing. *Other:* Injection site pain.

Dosage and Administration

Continuous infusion for ICU sedation

Adult: IV via a controlled infusion device at a rate of 5 to 50 mcg/kg/min.

Nursing Considerations

Assessment

- Assess for appropriate pain management. Propofol has no analgesic properties.
- Determine that appropriate emergency resuscitative equipment, including airway management supplies, is immediately available.

Intervention

- The drug does not require dilution. May be administered into an infusing IV line with dextrose 5% in water; lactated Ringer's injection; dextrose 5% and lactated Ringer's injection; 5% dextrose and 0.45% saline injection; 5% dextrose and 0.2% saline injection.
- Discard any unused portion after 6 hours.
- Administer into large veins, such as those in the antecubital fossa.
- Use strict aseptic technique. Propofol contains no preservatives or antimicrobial agents.

Desired outcome

- Adequate level of sedation.
- Safe administration of medication.

Phencyclidine Derivative

KETAMINE

Trade Name: Ketalar

Classification: Induction/maintenance agent for general anesthesia; profound analgesic at low doses.

Ketamine produces a state described as dissociation between the thalamus and cortex. The patient is "dissociated" from their environment and may appear to be in a dreamlike cataleptic state (e.g., eyes open with nystagmus). This drug should be administered by anesthesia providers. Emergence reactions, such as hallucinations, may occur without concomitant administration of a benzodiazepine. Profuse oral secretions result if an antisialagogue (e.g., atropine or glycopyrrolate) is not included.

Pharmacokinetics: *Onset:* 30 seconds IV; 3 to 4 minutes IM. *Peak:* 1 minute IV; 5 minutes IM. *Duration:* 5 to 10 minutes IV; 12 to 25 minutes IM. *Metabolism:* Hepatic. *Elimination half-life:* 2 to 3 hours; excreted in urine.

Contraindications and Precautions: Do not administer if known hypersensitivity to ketamine is present. Contraindicated in schizophrenia or other acute psychiatric disorders, hypertension, increased intracranial pressure, aneurysms, congestive heart failure, and thyrotoxicosis.

Adverse Reactions: *CNS:* Confusion, excitement, irrational behavior, hallucinations, excitement, dreamlike state. *CV:* Hypertension, hypotension, tachycardia. *EENT:* Excessive salivation, diplopia, laryngospasm. *GI:* Nausea, vomiting. *Skin:* Rash.

Dosage and Administration: *Adult:* 10 mg IV for analgesia during moderate sedation procedures, or 0.2 to 0.75 mg/kg.

Pediatric: 3 to 5 mg/kg IM (or 0.2 to 1 mg/kg IV) with an antisialagogue and benzodiazepine.

Nursing Considerations
Assessment
- Assess for kidney and liver dysfunction.
- Assess baseline monitoring data: respiratory rate, adequacy of ventilation, oxygen saturation, blood pressure, cardiac rate and rhythm, level of consciousness, and skin condition.
- Assess for patent infusing IV line.

Intervention
- The drug comes in concentrations of 100 mg/ml, 50 mg/ml, and 10 mg/ml. It can be diluted if necessary with commonly used IV fluids.
- Have emergency cart with equipment and medications immediately available.
- Monitor vital signs every 5 minutes.
- During recovery, keep verbal communication and tactile stimulation to a minimum. This can help attenuate emergence reactions, such as hallucinations.
- A benzodiazepine should be available to treat emergence reactions as well as physostigmine (Antilirium).

Desired outcome
- Profound analgesia without observable side effects.

Conclusion

The RN should be knowledgeable about the medications, recommended dosages, and potential adverse effects of the medications that she or he may administer to patients receiving moderate sedation. Each institution should have clearly defined policies and procedures delineating how nonanesthesia providers administer sedative and analgesic medications under the direction of a physician. Safe administration of sedatives and analgesics for moderate sedation requires relevant knowledge of applicable standards of care, anatomy, physiology, and pharmacology.

References

AANA Board of Directors (2003). Considerations for policy guidelines for the registered nurse engaged in the administration of sedation and analgesia. Park Ridge, IL: American Association of Nurse Anesthetists.

American Society of Anesthesiologists (2002). Practice guidelines for sedation and analgesia by non-anesthesiologists. Anesthesiology, 96, 1004-1017.

Barash, P., Bullen, B., & Stoelting, R. (2001). Handbook of clinical anesthesia. (4th Ed.). Philadelphia: Lippincott Williams & Wilkins.

Bennett, J., Wren, K.R., & Hass, R. (2001). Opioid use during the perianesthesia period: Nursing implications. Journal of PeriAnesthesiaNursing, 16, 255-258.

Carlson, K. (2004). Perianesthesia complications. In D.M.D. Quinn, & L. Schick (Eds.). Perianesthesia nursing core curriculum: Preoperative, phase I and phase II PACU nursing. St. Louis: Mosby, p. 659.

Doucet, M.A., Rabbett, P. & Barsanti, F. (1995). Nursing 95, 25(4):32RR-32SS.

Drain, C. (2004). Nonopioid intravenous anesthetics. In C. Drain (Ed.). Perianesthesia nursing: A critical care approach. (4th Ed.). St. Louis: Saunders, pp. 292-303.

Drain, C. (2004). Opioid intravenous anesthetics. In C. Drain (Ed.). Perianesthesia nursing: A critical care approach. (4th Ed.). St. Louis: Saunders, pp. 304-316.

Drummond, G. (2002). Dexmedetomidine may be effective, but is it safe? British Journal of Anesthesia, 88(3), 454.

Langevin, P. (1999). Propofol containing sulfite—potential for injury. Chest, 116, 1140-1141.

Physician's Desk Reference (2004). Diprivan. Retrieved May 26, 2004 from http://www.drugs.com/xq/cfm/pageid_0/htm_04020420.htm/tgid_/bn_ Diprivan%20Injectable%20Emulsion/type_pdr/qx/index.htm.

Roche. (2004). Versed: Complete product information. Retrieved May 26, 2004 from http://www.rocheusa.com/products/versed/pi_iv.pdf.

Roche. (2004). Valium: Complete product information. Retrieved May 26, 2004 from http://www.rocheusa.com/products/valium/pi_iv.pdf.

Sternbach, L.H. (1978). The benzodiazepine story. Progress in Drug Research, 22, 229-266.

Stoelting, R.K. (1999). Pharmacology and physiology in anesthetic practice. Philadelphia: Lippincott-Raven.

Sweitzer, B.J., & Pilla, M. (1998). Local anesthetics. In W.E. Hurford, M.T. Bailin, J.K. Davison, K.L. Haspel, & C. Rosow. (Eds.). Clinical anesthesia procedures of the Massachusetts General Hospital. Philadelphia: Lippincott Williams & Wilkins, pp. 233-241.

4

Management of Complications

Moderate sedation, administered widely in both inpatient and outpatient settings, is in and of itself an anesthesia technique. Administration of moderate sedation by nonanesthesia personnel raises many implications for licensed personnel in all areas of patient care. The role of the practitioner caring for the patient undergoing and recovering from moderate sedation is multifaceted. Crucial elements of this care are the prevention, recognition, and management of patient complications. This chapter will provide an overview of the prevention, recognition, and management of common complications associated with moderate sedation.

COMPLICATION TRENDS

Sedation is generally defined as a continuum of drug-induced states that allow a patient to tolerate an unpleasant procedure while maintaining adequate respiratory and cardiovascular function (American Society of PeriAnesthesia Nurses [ASPAN], 2002). The continuum of sedation can range from minimal sedation (which includes minimal risks) to general anesthesia (Figure 4-1) depending on the level of sedation desired, the type and dose of medications administered, and the reaction of the patient to these medications (American Society of Anesthesiologists [ASA], 2001; ASPAN, 2002; Hooper, 2001a). Complications can arise from a failure to reach an adequate level of sedation; however, they are more commonly associated with incidents in which the patient reaches a deeper level of sedation than intended (ASA, 2001).

Complication rates related to the administration of sedation are relatively low and most are cardiopulmonary in nature. The ASA Task Force on Sedation and Analgesia by Non-Anesthesiologists recognizes drug-induced respiratory depression and airway obstruction as the primary causes of morbidity in patients receiving sedation/analgesia (ASA, 2001). A study by D'Eramo, Bookless, and Howard (2003) examined adverse event rates in oral and/or maxillary surgery patients in Massachusetts. The most common complication in the 57,575 sedation cases analyzed was syncope. Laryngospasm was three times more common than bronchospasm. All of the complication rates, however, were less than 1%. It was

SEDATION CONTINUUM

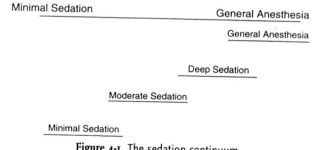

Minimal Sedation   General Anesthesia

General Anesthesia

Deep Sedation

Moderate Sedation

Minimal Sedation

Figure 4-1 The sedation continuum.

interesting to note that phlebitis was rated as a slightly more frequent complication than laryngospasm in this population.

Newman, Azer, Pitetti, and Singh (2003) examined the timing of adverse events in 1367 pediatric procedural sedations. Ninety-two percent of adverse events occurred during the procedure, within $2\frac{1}{2}$ minutes after final medication administration. No primary serious adverse events were noted after 25 minutes of final medication administration; however, three serious adverse events did occur after the 25-minute mark in three children who had already experienced an adverse event in the earlier 25-minute time frame. The most common adverse event was hypoxia (84%). None of the hypoxic events led to intubation or admission. Less serious reactions, such as emesis, agitation, and rash, were the next most common reactions.

A study looking at complications and adverse event rates for colonoscopy patients with selective sedation found that cardiopulmonary events occurred in 2% of the population. All of these events were minor, however, and did not require treatment or early termination of the procedure. Complications requiring medical intervention or prolonged observation were found in only 0.04% of the sample studied. An impaired physical status (elevated ASA class) was the single most common risk factor for all cardiopulmonary complications noted (Eckardt et al, 1999).

Although complication rates for sedation patients are low, failure to recognize and adequately treat any of these complications can lead to greater morbidity or even death. Complications are also related to the general health status of the patient and the timing of drug administration. The greater the co-morbidities for the patient (the higher the ASA status), the greater the risk for complications. Complications also occur more frequently immediately following administration of the sedative agent. All practitioners involved in patient preparation, sedation administration and monitoring, and patient recovery and discharge need to be cognizant of these issues.

PATIENT RISK FACTORS

The key to the successful management of sedation-related complications is to prevent the complications from ever occurring. The prevention of complications is dependent on thorough preprocedure assessment and identification of high-risk patients. Details regarding preprocedure assessment are explored in Chapter 2. Specific issues that are directly related to the prevention of complications include nothing by mouth (NPO) status, neck and airway assessment, and determination of ASA status. High-risk patients should also be identified preprocedure and appropriately evaluated by the sedation team.

NPO Status

The appropriate NPO status should be clearly explained to the patient and their family and/or caregivers as a part of their preprocedure instruction (Hooper, 2001b). Preprocedure fasting decreases aspiration risks that can occur in moderate sedation patients who may progress to deep sedation and lose their protective reflexes. Although rare, aspiration can result in mechanical obstruction and lead to chemical pneumonitis with severe ventilatory perfusion mismatch, a potentially fatal complication (ASA, 2001; Kost, 2003; Martin & Lennox, 2003). ASA Practice Guidelines for Preoperative Fasting are explored in detail in Chapter 2 and recommend a minimum fasting time of 6 hours for solids and nonclear liquids and 2 hours for clear liquids for adults (ASA, 1999). Pediatric fasting times are recommended by age (ASA, 1999); however, a general recommendation is 2 hours for clear liquids, 4 hours for breast milk, and 6 hours for solid food (Malviya, Voepel-Lewis, Tait, & Merkel, 2000). NPO status for all age groups should be verified before the administration of any sedative agents (ASA, 2004). In emergent situations in which recommended preprocedure fasting recommendations cannot be followed, NPO status and patient management should be evaluated by the attending physician in consultation with an anesthesia provider (ASA, 2001; Hooper, 2001b). The risk for pulmonary aspiration should be evaluated in terms of the level of sedation necessary for the procedure, the necessity of the immediate performance of the procedure, and the need for tracheal protection via intubation (ASA, 2001; Martin & Lennox, 2003). Nonanesthesia-administered sedation is generally not recommended in these cases.

Neck and Airway Assessment

Hypoxic and other respiratory complications are most commonly associated with the administration of sedation. Management of this common complication may require the use of airway adjuncts, positive pressure ventilation, and possible intubation. The presence of other airway abnormalities may also compromise spontaneous ventilation, particularly in the sedated patient. Therefore a specific evaluation of the airway in addition to routine preprocedure patient assessment should be conducted before the initiation of sedation. The purpose of this airway-

Table 4-1 | Factors Associated With Sleep Apnea

ETOH consumption	HTN
Use of sedatives	Massively enlarged tonsils or adenoids
Obesity	Anatomically narrowed airways

From Scales, B.A. (2003). *Screening high-risk patients for the ambulatory setting. Journal of PeriAnesthesia Nursing, 18, 307-316.*
ETOH, Ethyl alcohol; HTN, hypertension.

specific assessment is to determine any medical, surgical, or anesthetic risk factors that may indicate the presence of a difficult airway. (ASA, 2001; 2002).
Risk factors associated with difficult airway management include:

- History of problems with anesthesia or sedation
- Advanced rheumatoid arthritis
- Chromosomal abnormalities (i.e., trisomy 21)
- Stridor, snoring, or sleep apnea (ASA, 2001)

Factors contributing to sleep apnea are noted in Table 4-1. Symptoms and other factors that may be associated with sleep apnea and require further investigation include:

- Impairment of daytime functioning
- History of snoring
- Male gender
- Pulmonary hypertension
- Systemic hypertension
- Polycythemia (Scales, 2003).

Physical examination components that may be associated with difficult airway management are noted in Table 4-2. The presence of any of these risk factors or physical examination components indicates the need for further consultation with the attending physician and/or anesthesia provider to determine the appropriateness of nonanesthesia-administered sedation.

ASA Patient Classification Status

One of the primary purposes of the preoperative assessment is to obtain an accurate medical history on the patient. This medical history enables the nurse to establish the ASA Patient Classification Status and thus determine the appropriateness of nonanesthesia-provided sedation. ASA Class I and II patients are usually considered stable and appropriate for nonanesthesia-administered sedation. Class III patients, when well controlled and stable, may also be appropriate; however, any patient with a systemic disease process (e.g., P3 or higher) should be evaluated on an individual basis with the attending physician and/or an anesthesia provider. Class IV and V patients are generally considered inappropriate for registered nurse (RN) administration and monitoring (American

Table 4-2 | Physical Examination Findings Associated With Difficult Airway
         | Management

Examination Component	Finding
Habitus	Significant obesity, particularly involving the neck and facial structures
Head and neck	Short, thick neck
	Limited neck extension
	Inability to touch the tip of the chin to the chest
	Neck mass
	Cervical spine disease or trauma
	Tracheal deviation
	Abnormal or dysmorphic facial features
	Thyromental distance of <3 ordinary finger breadths
Mouth	Small opening (<3 cm in an adult)
	Protruding or relatively long incisors
	Loose or capped teeth
	Dental appliances
	High, arched, or very narrow palate
	Macroglossia
	Tonsillar hypertrophy
	Nonvisible uvula (Mallampati class > II)
	Interincisor distance < 3 cm
Jaw	Prominent "overbite"
	Inability to bring mandibular (lower) incisors anterior (in front of) maxillary (upper) incisors
	Significant malocclusion
	Stiff, nonresilient mandible

From American Society of Anesthesiologists (ASA). (2001). Practice guidelines for sedation and
analgesia by non-anesthesiologists http://www.asahq.org/publicationsAndServices/sedation1017.pdf;
American Society of Anesthesiologists (ASA). (2002). Practice guidelines for management of the
difficult airway http://www.asahq.org/publicationsAndServices/Difficult%20Airway.pdf.

College of Radiology [ACR], 2000; American Dental Association [ADA], 2003;
ASA, 2001; Association of periOperative Registered Nurses [AORN], 2002;
Hooper, 2001b; Malviya et al, 2000; Wyman, 2004).

High-Risk Patients

Patients with significant underlying medical conditions or sedation-related risk
factors should be identified during the preprocedure interview and closely evaluated for the appropriateness for nonanesthesia-administered sedation (ASA,
2001). The following conditions are commonly associated with a higher incidence of complications.

Obesity

Obese patients are at increased risk for gastroesophageal reflux, upper airway obstruction, and oversedation during moderate sedation procedures. The risk for gastroesophageal reflux can be reduced through strict adherence to recommended fasting guidelines. Preprocedure treatment with an oral H_2 antagonist and metoclopramide may also be considered. Because of body mass and composition, obese individuals are also more susceptible to the respiratory depressant effects of sedative agents, leading to possible oversedation and upper airway obstruction. Much care should be taken to administer small incremental doses of sedatives. Adequate time should also be allowed for onset of sedative action before further dosing (Martin & Lennox, 2003).

Chronic Obstructive Pulmonary Disease (COPD)

Patients with COPD are at increased risk for complications because of their preexisting blunted ventilatory response to CO_2. This response can be further compromised by the excessive administration of sedative agents, leading to severe respiratory depression with any type of oversedation. The supine position required for most procedures also compromises this patient by impairing chest wall muscle function, reducing functional residual capacity, and impeding oxygenation. All prescribed bronchodilators should be administered to the COPD patient before initiation of sedation. Supplemental oxygen should also be administered. Sedative agents should be titrated in small incremental doses and used sparingly to effect while monitoring the patient very closely. Supplemental pain control, such as local anesthesia, should also be considered when appropriate (Martin & Lennox, 2003).

Coronary Artery Disease (CAD)

Coronary artery disease can present through multifaceted symptoms or conditions including chest pain, hypertension, exercise intolerance, congestive heart failure, and valvular heart disease. It should also be suspected in any patient undergoing procedures for peripheral vascular or renovascular disease. (Kost, 2003; Martin & Lennox, 2003; National Institutes of Health [NIH], 2000). CAD presents risks to moderate sedation patients in both undersedation and oversedation episodes. Undersedation, as often evidenced by increased pain and anxiety, stimulates the release of catecholamines, which increase the workload and cardiac demand of the heart. Oversedation can trigger cardiac complications related to hypotension and/or hypoxemia. Much care must be taken to adequately balance sedation administration to provide adequate patient comfort and maximal cardiac functioning. All routine cardiac medications, particularly betablockers, should be taken on the day of the procedure. Supplemental oxygen should be a standard for this population, regardless of the preprocedure saturation reading. Adverse events, such as airway obstruction, hypoxia, and hypotension, should they occur, must be rapidly recognized and resolved (Martin & Lennox, 2003).

Chronic Renal Failure (CRF)

Most of the sedative medications and/or their metabolites are dependent on adequate renal function for metabolism and/or excretion; therefore any patient with a history of renal failure will be predisposed to an increased risk for overdose or prolonged medication effect (Kost, 2003; Martin & Lennox, 2003). Care should be taken to avoid the use of longer-acting opioids, such as meperidine and morphine. Fentanyl, however, is thought to be safe for use in this population. CRF patients can also have exaggerated responses to benzodiazepines (BZD). Smaller doses of this class of agents along with incremental dosing is recommended (Martin & Lennox, 2003).

Drug Addiction

Dose requirements in the drug-addicted patient may be difficult to predict because drug intolerance is often encountered. It is also often difficult to distinguish drug-seeking behaviors from a true need for increased analgesia. When at all possible, local anesthesia should be used as a supplement to decrease parenteral analgesic requirements. Short-acting BZDs should be used with incremental dosing. All prescribed replacement medications (e.g., methadone) should be taken the day of surgery. Use of reversal agents should be avoided because severe withdrawal symptoms could occur (Martin & Lennox, 2003).

Elderly Patients

Increased age is an independent risk factor for adverse events associated with sedation. This risk can be exacerbated by coexisting disease states. Because of changes in bioavailability and drug metabolism, sedative and analgesic agents tend to elicit a prolonged and more pronounced effect in the older patient. Conservative incremental dosing and the minimized use of medications is recommended whenever possible (Martin & Lennox, 2003).

Pediatric Patients

Respiratory depression and airway obstruction are the most common complications in pediatric patients, with children age 1 to 5 at the most risk (Martin, Lennox, 2003). Any underlying neurologic disease should be closely evaluated before drug selection. Respiratory depression and hypercapnia should be prevented in patients with increased intracranial pressure (ICP) because both complications will further exacerbate the ICP. Bronchodilators should be continued up until the time of the procedure in children with a history of asthma, and histamine-triggering medications should also be avoided (Malviya et al, 2000). Infants with a history of apnea, premature infants (less than 37 weeks gestation) who are less than 60 weeks postconceptual, or full-term newborns less than 44 weeks postconceptual should be monitored for at least 12 hours postsedation (ASA, 2004).

Other Risks

Patients with a history of smoking, particularly if combined with a respiratory disease history, such as COPD or asthma, are at a greater risk of developing procedural hypoxia, hypercapnia, or hypoventilation. Hepatic dysfunction can affect the metabolism, elimination, and excretion of many sedative agents. Primary neurologic disease that is associated with an overproduction or underproduction of hormones, such as hyperthyroidism or hypothyroidism, can result in an altered stress response. Patients with a history of diabetes should have their blood glucose levels monitored frequently. Morning doses of insulin or oral agents are usually held until the patient fully recovers from the procedure. Procedures in this population should be scheduled early in the morning to allow time for monitoring of blood glucose levels, completion of the procedure, and the administration of the patient's usual morning dose of insulin or oral agent with nutrition (Kost, 2003).

COMPLICATIONS AND THEIR MANAGEMENT

Early recognition and treatment of complications associated with sedation are the keys to decreased morbidity and mortality. The presence of appropriate and functioning emergency equipment along with back-up emergency plans is also crucial to success. Respiratory events make up the majority of complications associated with moderate sedation; however, cardiovascular events and allergic and/or anaphylactic reactions may also arise.

Emergency Equipment

In addition to the appropriate sedative and analgesic agents necessary for successful sedation, appropriate emergency equipment and medications must be immediately available in case of emergency. Recommended equipment and medications include, but are not limited to:

- Oxygen and appropriate delivery devices
- Suction apparatus
- Airway adjuncts to include oral and/or nasopharyngeal airways, endotracheal tubes and laryngoscopes, and bag-valve-mask device
- Noninvasive blood pressure device with appropriate sized cuffs
- Pulse oximetry monitor
- Cardiac monitor
- Opioid and sedative reversal agents
- Fully stocked emergency cart with defibrillator

(American Association of Nurse Anesthetists [AANA], 2003; AORN, 2002; ASA, 2001; ASPAN, 2002; Hooper, 2001b; Kost, 2003; Martin & Lennox, 2003; Wyman, 2004).

In addition to the above emergency equipment and medications, nonhospital facilities should have an emergency assist system established with the nearest hospital emergency facility and ready access to ambulance service for emergency transport (American Academy of Pediatric Dentistry [AAPD], 1998).

Respiratory Complications

Respiratory complications often display a myriad of symptoms that include respiratory depression, hypoxia, hypercapnia, and soft tissue (airway) obstruction. These common respiratory complications are most often caused by oversedation or an untoward patient response to a commonly used medication. This group of complications can be most effectively prevented by titrating small amounts of medication over a period of time until the sedative endpoint is achieved. Laryngospasm and bronchospasm are less common complications that often occur if the patient is having difficulty managing secretions, or if the patient is undergoing a procedure involving the oral cavity and/or respiratory tract. Airway monitoring and management are crucial in preventing these emergencies (Hooper, 2001b)

Respiratory Depression and/or Soft Tissue Obstruction

Benzodiazepines and opioids, when used in combination, are synergistic in their respiratory depressant effect. This respiratory depression is dose dependent and can result in compromised respiratory function as evidenced by a direct depression of the respiratory drive in response to hypoxia, and a diminished ventilatory response to hypercapnia. Muscle tone can also be weakened, leading to a weaker ventilatory effort, resulting in a ventilation and perfusion mismatch. In the unconscious or obtunded patient, the tongue is the most common cause of airway obstruction because airway patency is compromised by a loss of submandibular muscle tone, which normally provides direct support of the tongue and indirect support of the epiglottis. Weakened muscle tone may cause the tongue to be displaced posteriorly and occlude the airway at the level of the pharynx, and the epiglottis may occlude the airway at the level of the larynx. The tongue, epiglottis, or both can occlude the entrance of the trachea (Cummins, 2001; Hotchkiss & Drain, 2003).

Decreased, shallow, or labored respirations and/or snoring are classic symptoms of respiratory depression and/or soft tissue obstruction. This may or may not be accompanied by decreased oxygen saturation. The chest and abdomen should also be observed for coordinated ventilatory efforts; a rocking chest motion is indicative of distress. Movement of air at the nose or mouth area and the presence of breath sounds should be verified. With partial airway obstruction the patient may exhibit a weak, ineffective cough; a high-pitched noise while inhaling; uncoordinated attempts at ventilation; and cyanosis. With complete airway obstruction, the movement of air is absent. Decreasing saturation values, cyanosis, and hypoxia will result if the airway is not rapidly secured (Cummins, 2001; Hotchkiss & Drain, 2003; Martin & Lennox, 2003; Wyman, 2004).

The patient presenting with a deepening level of sedation and snoring respirations requires rapid intervention. Intervention options range from simple and

Table 4-3 | **Recommended Management for Respiratory Depression/Soft Tissue Obstruction**

Steps generally move from least to most aggressive; however more aggressive treatment and/or a combination of intervention strategies may be required depending on patient presentation and response.

Supplemental oxygen
Supine position
Stimulation
Head tilt–chin lift or jaw-thrust maneuver
Airway adjunct
Positive pressure ventilation
Administration of appropriate reversal agents
Intubation

From Hooper, V.D. (2001b). Sedation standards part II. Carrolton, TX: Health & Sciences Television Network

noninvasive to more advanced, (Table 4-3) with the provider typically beginning with the simplest intervention and progressing dependent on patient response (Hooper, 2001b). The patient should initially be placed in the supine position and may be effectively managed through simple patient stimulation (calling the patient by name or gently shaking the patient) and the addition of supplemental oxygen. Should this be ineffective, the airway will have to be repositioned using the head tilt–chin lift maneuver. The goal is to anteriorly displace the mandible. One hand is placed on the patient's forehead, and pressure is applied to tilt the head back (hyperextending the neck). The fingers of the other hand are placed under the bony part of the jaw and lifted to bring the chin forward, assisting the head in tilting back (Figure 4-2). The airway can also be opened using the jaw-thrust maneuver, which involves lifting the jaw by placing the fingers behind the mandible and lifting forward (Figure 4-3). In many cases these actions alone will enable the patient to maintain spontaneous respiration and improved air exchange (Cummins, 2001; Hotchkiss & Drain, 2003).

When airway obstruction persists despite maximal mandibular displacement, insertion of a nasopharyngeal artificial airway may be necessary (Figure 4-4). Nasopharyngeal airways are less stimulating to the irritant receptors in the upper airway, particularly in the awake or lightly sedated patient; however, they must still be used with caution since they might precipitate laryngospasm and vomiting on occasion. After lubricating with a water-soluble lubricant (a local anesthetic water-soluble lubricant is also appropriate), the nasopharyngeal airway can be inserted by gently passing the airway through the naris along the curvature of the nasopharynx to the oropharynx. Insertion should never be forced; if resistance is met, insertion through the other naris should be attempted. Once properly positioned, the airway should rest between the base of the tongue and the posterior pharyngeal wall. Nasopharyngeal airways should never be used in

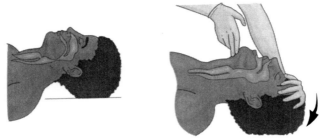

Figure 4-2 Relief of airway obstruction via head tilt–chin lift procedure. *(From Cummins, R. (1994). Textbook of advanced cardiac life support. Copyright American Heart Association.)*

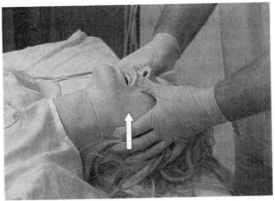

Figure 4-3 Jaw-thrust maneuver. *(From Drain, C.B. [2003] Perianesthesia nursing [4th Ed.]. St. Louis: Saunders.)*

patients with nasal-septal deformities, cerebrospinal fluid leakage from the nose, or coagulation disorders. After inserting the airway, the patient should be monitored for spontaneous respirations. If spontaneous respirations are absent, artificial positive pressure ventilation should be initiated (Cummins, 2001; Hotchkiss & Drain, 2003).

Insertion of an oropharyngeal airway (see Figure 4-4) can relieve an airway obstruction by creating a mechanical conduit for air to pass between the base of the tongue and the posterior oropharynx; however, an oropharyngeal airway is

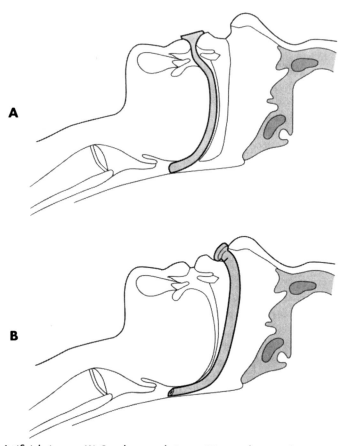

Figure 4-4 Artificial airways: **(A)** Oropharyngeal airway; **(B)** nasopharyngeal airway. *(From Longnecker, D.E., et al. [1997]. Introduction to anesthesia [9th Ed.]. Philadelphia: Saunders.)*

indicated only in the unresponsive, completely obtunded patient because of the risk of injury and laryngospasm (Cummins, 2001; Hotchkiss & Drain, 2003). After clearing the mouth of secretions, the airway can be inserted by one of two methods. In the first method, the airway is placed so that it is turned backward as it enters the mouth. As it passes through the oral cavity and approaches the posterior wall of the pharynx, the airway should be rotated 180° into the proper position (Cummins, 2001). In the second technique, a tongue blade is used to displace the tongue forward, and the airway is slipped in over the tongue blade into the oropharynx. Airway quality and respiratory quality and exchange should be closely assessed after the insertion of the oropharyngeal airway to ensure proper placement and functioning (Cummins, 2001; Hotchkiss & Drain, 2003).

Table 4-4 | Recommended Intubation Equipment
_____

Depending on populations served, pediatric and adult sizes of all equipment may be indicated.

Laryngoscope handle
Macintosh (curved) and Miller (straight) laryngoscope blades
Stylet
Endotracheal tubes of assorted sizes
Water-soluble lubricant
10 ml syringe
Magill forceps
Tongue blades
Oropharyngeal airways of assorted sizes
Commercial endotracheal tube anchoring device
Tape
_____

Modified from Hotchkiss, M.A., & Drain, C.B. (2003). Assessment and management of the airway. In C.B. Drain (Ed.) Perianesthesia nursing: A critical care approach. St. Louis: Saunders, pp. 409-421.

If spontaneous respiration is absent or of poor quality, positive pressure ventilation may be indicated using a bag-valve-mask device. For adequate ventilation and oxygenation, the device should be connected to a high-flow, high-concentration oxygen delivery system, and the caregiver must attain a seal around the patient's face that forces all oxygen into the lungs. An open airway must be maintained under the mask through the head tilt–chin lift maneuver. The mask is applied to the face while the left hand keeps a tight seal around the face. This is best accomplished if the caregiver is positioned near the patient's head. The bag is compressed at a rate of 14 to 16 breaths per minute with a large tidal volume of 10 to 12 ml/kg. To ensure proper technique, the chest should observed for rising and falling during ventilation, and bilateral breath sounds should be confirmed (Cummins, 2001; Hotchkiss & Drain, 2003).

If the patient cannot be adequately ventilated despite the use of airway adjuncts and/or positive pressure ventilation, or if long-term mechanical ventilation is indicated, then endotracheal intubation may be necessary. Other indications for intubation include an inability of the patient to protect his or her airway and respiratory or cardiac arrest. Recommended intubation equipment is noted in Table 4-4. Endotracheal intubation should only be attempted by competent health care providers credentialed in intubation. An anesthesia provider is preferred. All recommended equipment should be at the bedside and tested for proper functioning before intubation. Laryngoscope lights should be tested for brightness (white, bright light is preferred; a yellowish light does not illuminate the landmarks as well and may be about to burn out) and the bulb should be securely attached to the blade. Endotracheal tube cuffs should be tested and then deflated and the stylet should be properly placed so that the end of the stylet does not protrude from the distal end of the endotracheal tube. A working suction device should be at the bedside along with a pulse oximeter, and the patient should be hyperventilated before any intubation attempt. Tube placement should be confirmed via auscultation for breath sounds in all four pulmonary quadrants; the stomach should also be auscultated for the absence of breath sounds or gurgling (Cummins, 2001; Hotchkiss & Drain, 2003).

The administration of reversal agents may be indicated at any point in the treatment of respiratory depression and/or soft tissue obstruction; however, they are typically used judiciously because rapid or overzealous administration of reversal agents may result in both an analgesic and anxiety response (Martin & Lennox, 2003). Naloxone is used to reverse the depressive effects of opioids (Hooper, 2001a; Martin & Lennox, 2003; Messinger, Hoffman, O'Donnell & Dunworth, 1999; Wyman, 2004) and is generally administered by diluting 0.4 mg in 10 cc of saline and then administering 0.02 to 0.04 mg (0.5 to 1 cc of diluted mixture) doses over a period of 30 seconds (Messinger et al, 1999). The agent peaks in 1 to 2 minutes and can be repeated to the desired effect. The duration is 1 to 4 hours and the patient is at greatest risk for resedation at 30 to 60 minutes postadministration (Hooper, 2001a; Martin & Lennox, 2003; Wyman, 2004). Flumazenil is used for BZD reversal and like naloxone should be titrated slowly to effect. Recommended dose is 0.1 to 0.2 mg titrated every 1 to 2 minutes to effect or up to a total of 1 mg. A single dose is effective for 30 to 60 minutes, so the patient should be monitored closely for resedation (Hooper, 2001a; Martin & Lennox, 2003; Messinger et al, 1999; Wyman, 2004). Once a reversal agent is administered, it is unlikely that a procedure can continue without intervention and monitoring by an anesthesia provider (Messinger et al, 1999). Inpatients should be monitored for at least 30 minutes after administration of a reversal agent and before transfer to a hospital room. Outpatients should be monitored at least 2 hours before discharge (Kost, 2003; Martin, Lennox, 2003). More detail on reversal agents and their actions can be found in Chapter 3.

Laryngospasm

A laryngospasm is defined as an airway obstruction secondary to tonic contraction of the laryngeal and pharyngeal muscles (Heffline, 1999). The spasm may be partial, in which the vocal cords are partially closed and the patient displays a loud crowing sound, or complete, in which the vocal cords are completely closed off and there is a complete lack of air exchange; the chest will move up and down, but no air moves in or out. (Drain, 2003b; Hooper, 2001b). The most common risk factors associated with sedation patients include excessive secretions, vomitus, nasal or oral airway placement, mechanical irritation caused by frequent suctioning, laryngoscopy or intubation, smoking history, and the presence of a preexisting respiratory infection (Hannah, 2002; Heffline, 1999; Hooper, 2001b). Rapid recognition and treatment are key in this crisis. On the first sign of laryngospasm, it is recommended that an anesthesia provider be summoned if not already at the bedside (Drain, 2003b). Treatment is dependent on patient presentation and response. A partial laryngospasm often responds well to supplemental oxygen, calming measures, and having the patient attempt to breathe slowly and deeply and try to cough (a patient-generated positive pressure ventilation). If these steps are ineffective, low doses of IV midazolam or lidocaine are sometimes effective in breaking the spasm. If the patient continues to deteriorate (saturations dropping) or progresses to a complete laryngospasm, more aggressive measures are indicated. In addition to positive pressure ventilation with 100% oxygen and suction, small doses of succinyl choline (0.5 mg/kg IV) may be indicated along with possible intubation (Drain, 2003b; Hannah, 2002; Heffline, 1999; Hooper, 2001b).

Bronchospasm

A bronchospasm is a constriction of the bronchial airways caused by an increase in smooth muscle tone, ultimately resulting in airway obstruction (Drain, 2003b). Although a less common complication than laryngospasm (D'Eramo et al, 2003), a bronchospasm can be equally as dangerous if undiagnosed and untreated. Risk factors for bronchospasm include preexisting bronchospastic disease; airway irritation caused by excessive secretions, aspiration, intubation, suctioning, etc.; histamine release; allergic reaction; environmental factors, such as odors or perfumes; and a history of smoking. Patient presentation is dependent on the extent of the bronchospasm. A bronchospasm affecting only a few smaller bronchioles may present with symptoms of mild wheezing that is audible only by stethoscope. The greater the area of lung and number of bronchi affected, however, the more obvious the symptoms and the greater the risk to the patient. Assessment findings can include audible wheezing, tachypnea, dyspnea, decreased lung compliance, decreased oxygen saturation, accessory muscle use, restlessness, and tightness in the chest (Hannah, 2002; Heffline, 1999). The ideal treatment is to pick up on risk factors during the preprocedure assessment and intervene to prevent complications (Heffline, 1999). Patients with a history of bronchospastic disease should be pretreated with bronchodilators. Histamine-triggering medications, such as morphine, should be avoided in patients with a history of multiple allergies. Smokers should be encouraged to avoid smoking for at least 24 hours before the procedure (Heffline, 1999). Patients having multiple risk factors should be closely evaluated by the attending physician and/or an anesthesia provider before nonanesthesia-administered sedation. Treatment of a bronchospasm includes decreasing airway irritability and administration of bronchodilators and humidified oxygen (Hannah, 2002; Heffline, 1999; Hooper, 2001b).

Aspiration

Aspiration is defined as the entry of a foreign body, blood, or gastric contents into the tracheobronchial tree (Heffline, 1999). Because sedation may compromise a patient's ability to maintain their protective reflexes, patients are at particular risk for aspiration, particularly as a result of postoperative (postprocedure) nausea and vomiting (PONV). The incidence of nausea and vomiting as a side

Table 4-5 | Risk Factors for Aspiration
_____
Obesity
Hiatal hernia
Pregnancy
Peptic ulcer disease
Loose teeth
Diminished pharyngeal reflexes
Full stomach
Laparoscopic insufflation
Trendelenburg position
Surgical manipulation of the airway
Trauma
_____

From Hannah, B. (2002). Airway management. In B. Gooden (Ed.). Compentency based orientation credentialing program: 2002 edition. Cherry Hill, NJ: ASPAN, pp. 47-48. Heffline, M. (1999). Cardiopulmonary care and emergency support. In D.M.D. Quinn (Ed.), Ambulatory surgical nursing core curriculum. Philadelphia: Saunders, pp. 167-195.

effect of anesthesia is 20% to 30% (Islat, 2003; Ku, Ong, 2003); however, the incidence of aspiration is relatively low at less than 1% (Islat, 2003; Tham & Koh, 2002). Risk factors associated with aspiration are noted in Table 4-5. As with most complications, the best treatment is prevention.

Prevention of aspiration is first accomplished by ensuring that preoperative fasting guidelines have been appropriately followed. The unconscious and/or sedated patient should be closely monitored for airway patency and PONV; they should also be placed in the side-lying, head-down position whenever possible. Suction should be immediately available at the bedside. If airway adjuncts are necessary for airway support or to conduct the procedure, they should be removed as soon as possible to prevent gagging and regurgitation. Protective reflexes should be well established before any intake of oral fluids after a procedure, particularly if a topical anesthetic was used. Medications may also be indicated to decrease secretions (anticholinergics), neutralize gastric secretions (nonparticulate antacids), decrease acidity and volume of gastric contents (histamine H_2-receptor antagonists), foster gastric emptying (metoclopramide), and/or reduce the incidence of nausea and vomiting (Heffline, 1999).

Treatment for aspiration will depend on the amount and type of aspirate. Foreign body aspiration requires the immediate removal of the foreign body, proper head position, and implementation of the stir-up regimen with ventilation (Hannah, 2002). Aspiration of blood or gastric contents requires immediate establishment of a patent airway with suctioning to remove the blood or gastric contents. Hypoxemia should be corrected with the use of supplemental oxygen, continuous positive airway pressure (CPAP), or intubation with mechanical ventilation. Antibiotics, bronchodilators, and/or steroids may

Table 4-6 | Risk Factors for NPPE in the Moderate Sedation Patient

Laryngospasm
Vocal cord paralysis
Choking
Foreign body aspiration
Young, healthy male with increased muscle mass
Narcotic use
Short neck
Obesity
Obstructive apnea

From Tarrac, S.E. (2003). Negative pressure pulmonary edema: A postanesthesia emergency. Journal of PeriAnesthesia Nursing, 18, 317-323.

be administered depending on severity and patient presentation (Hannah, 2002; Heffline, 1999). The outpatient will most likely require at least an overnight admission for extended monitoring.

Negative Pressure Pulmonary Edema (NPPE)

Negative pressure pulmonary edema, also known as postobstructive or noncardiogenic pulmonary edema, is a life-threatening complication that can occur after any acute obstruction of the airway, as occurs in all of the above emergencies. The incidence of NPPE has been reported to be as high as 11% of posttriggering episodes. Common risk factors seen with the moderate sedation population are noted in Table 4-6. The cause of this complication is thought to revolve around the patient's attempt to breathe against an obstructed airway, creating highly negative intrathoracic pressure, eventually resulting in the formation of pulmonary edema (see Figure 4-5). Diagnosis is usually made based on the precipitating event and symptomatology. Presenting signs and symptoms may include agitation, tachypnea, tachycardia, frothy pink sputum, rales, and progressive oxygen desaturation. Symptoms usually occur within 1 hour of the event but may be delayed, requiring extended observation of the patient. Outpatients, in fact, may warrant an overnight stay after an obstructive event. Standard treatment includes CPAP and diuretics with the goal of maintaining an open airway and supporting the patient until the condition resolves, usually within 24 hours (Tarrac, 2003).

Cardiovascular Complications

D'Eramo et al (2003) noted that the most common complication associated with sedation was syncope. The physiology contributing to the development of syncope is generally cardiovascular in nature and commonly associated with hypotension or a rhythm disturbance. As with respiratory complications, rapid

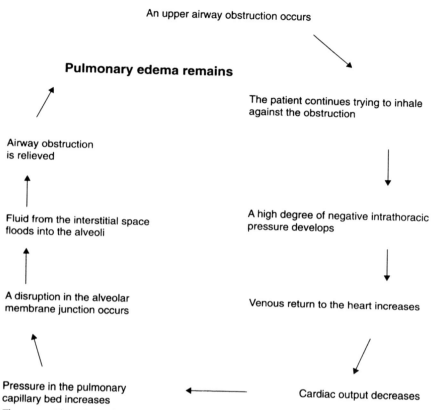

An upper airway obstruction occurs

Pulmonary edema remains

The patient continues trying to inhale against the obstruction

Airway obstruction is relieved

Fluid from the interstitial space floods into the alveoli

A high degree of negative intrathoracic pressure develops

A disruption in the alveolar membrane junction occurs

Venous return to the heart increases

Pressure in the pulmonary capillary bed increases

Cardiac output decreases

Figure 4-5 Physiology of NPPE. *(From Tarrac, S.E. [2003]. Negative pressure pulmonary edema: A postanesthesia emergency. Journal of PeriAnesthesia Nursing, 18, 317-323.)*

recognition and response to cardiovascular events are crucial to decreased morbidity and mortality.

Hypotension

Hypotension in the sedated patient can be procedural or pharmacologic in origin. Procedure-related causes of hypotension include hemorrhage, sepsis, dehydration, vasovagal reactions, and anaphylaxis. Pharmacologic causes are related to the vasodilatory effects associated with many opioid and sedative agents and are more commonly associated with deeper sedation levels (Martin & Lennox, 2003). Any drop in blood pressure of greater than 20% for longer than 2 minutes should be investigated (Messinger et al, 1999). Hypotension may be easily corrected by placing the patient in the Trendelenburg position (Wyman, 2004). Concurrent in-depth evaluation is warranted; however, Figure 4-6 illustrates a hypotension algorithm that, although designed for use in the

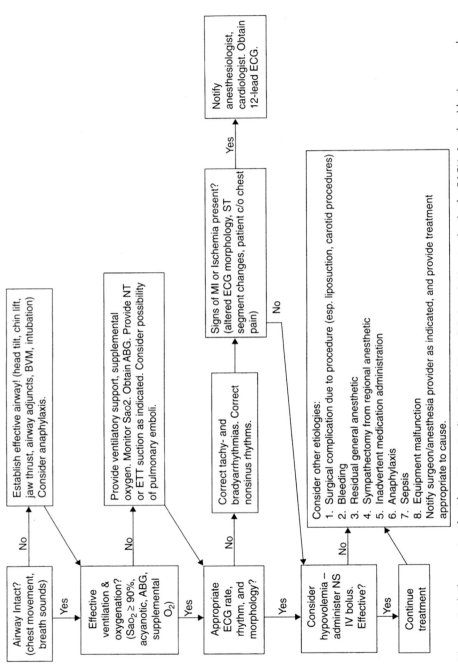

Figure 4-6 The hypotension algorithm. *(From Cowling, G.E., & Haas, R.E. [2002]. Hypotension in the PACU: An algorithmic approach. Journal of PeriAnesthesia Nursing, 17, 159-163.)*

postanesthesia care unit (PACU), is equally effective for the analysis of hypotension in the sedated patient.

Assessment of hypotension, as with any other emergency, should begin with assessment of the ABCs and should include confirmation of an intact airway and adequate ventilatory effort and oxygenation. This should be followed by confirmation of an appropriate electrocardiogram (ECG) rate, rhythm, and morphology (Cowling & Haas, 2002). The presence of hypovolemia should then be considered and can be ruled out by the administration of a 200 cc rapid IV bolus of 0.9% normal saline in the absence of specific contraindications, such as congestive heart failure (CHF). If the patient responds with a rise in blood pressure, the presence of hypovolemia can be assumed and further fluid replacement may be indicated (Cowling & Haas, 2002; Messinger et al, 1999; Wyman, 2004). If the pressure remains unresponsive to a fluid challenge, other causes should be considered and a call for assistance should be placed. Residual medication effect can be ruled out by the judicious administration of appropriate reversal agents. Decreased vascular resistance can be treated with the administration of vasopressive agents, such as ephedrine or phenylephrine (Cowling & Haas, 2002; Martin & Lenox, 2003; Wyman, 2004). An anaphylactic reaction is generally characterized by respiratory distress and hypotension and usually occurs within minutes of the exposure to the triggering agent, although delayed reactions of 15 minutes or longer have been reported. Early administration of epinephrine (0.3 to 0.5 mg IV over 3 to 5 minutes) is indicated for anaphylaxis to counteract both vasodilation and bronchoconstriction. Sepsis may be suspected in any patient presenting with symptoms of gangrenous extremities, pressure ulcers, or ischemic or infarcted bowel. Procedure-specific causes should also be examined. (Cowling, Haas, 2002).

Cardiac Dysrhythmias

Cardiac dysrhythmias should be recognized promptly and aggressively treated according to Advanced Cardiac Life Support (ACLS) protocols (Cummins, 2001; Wyman, 2004). Tachycardias are most commonly associated with undersedation in the moderate sedation population. During frightening or uncomfortable procedures, patients are under stress both mentally and physically. Mental and physical stress causes the activation of the fight-or-flight response from the autonomic nervous system. This defensive reaction assists the body in physiologically coping with noxious stressors. During the fight-or-flight response, catecholamines are released that increase heart rate, cardiac output, and blood pressure in an attempt to provide more blood flow to vital organs to allow the body to withstand any deleterious assault (Guyton & Hall, 1997). During the fight-or-flight response the heart works more vigorously, and myocardial oxygen consumption is increased, potentially causing myocardial ischemia and dysrhythmias. Pain also exacerbates anxiety and subsequently exacerbates pain. Sinus tachycardia, a heart rate of greater than 100 beats per minute, results from any stressful situation, including procedural stress, anoxia, hypovolemia, pain, anxiety, apprehension, or any combination of these factors. Supraventricular dys-rhythmias and premature atrial contractions (PACs) can also be related to stress. The patient should be closely evaluated for their ability to tolerate the increased rate. Patients with healthy hearts may tolerate rates up to 160 beats per minute without signs or symptoms; a compromised myocardium, however, is much less tolerant of the increased workload and oxygen demand placed on the heart. All tachycardias should be fully evaluated and the cause ascertained before treatment, which should be focused on the removal of the underlying cause (Drain, 2003a).

Bradycardias are defined as a heart rate of less than 60 beats per minute. Bradycardias associated with moderate sedation procedures are generally sinus in nature and can be triggered by several possible causes, including vasovagal reactions to the procedure, depressant effects of the sedative medications, hypoxia, and excessive parasympathetic stimulation caused by uncontrolled pain. As with tachycardia, the cause and patient response to the dysrhythmia should be closely evaluated before determining treatment. A symptomatic patient who is hypotensive and showing other signs of decreased cardiac output should be immediately treated with atropine. Nonsymptomatic patients often require no treatment and respond well to stimulation (Cummins, 2001; Drain, 2003a) Type II second-degree atrioventricular (AV) block or third-degree AV block should be immediately treated as per ACLS protocol, which includes administration of atropine for symptom control and preparation for the insertion of a transvenous pacemaker (Cummins, 2001).

Premature ventricular contractions (PVCs) involve an earlier than expected ventricular contraction from an irritable area in the ventricle. Occasional PVCs are common—particularly related to procedures—can occur in any patient, and generally do not require treatment. Multiple PVCs, however, are often related to inadequate oxygenation and require close assessment of the patient's ventilatory status. Other causes of PVCs include unrelieved pain, electrolyte disturbances, acid-base imbalance, drug toxicity, and myocardial hypoxemia. Treatment should be aimed at the underlying cause and obliteration of the irritable focus. PVCs that occur at a rate of greater than 6 per minute, occur in runs of two or more, are multifocal, occur in patterns (i.e., every other beat), or occur during the vul-nerable period of the ECG complex require immediate treatment because they are precursors to more lethal ventricular dysrhythmias. Lidocaine is the drug of choice according to ACLS protocol. PVCs that are present with bradycardia, however, should first be treated with atropine or overdrive pacing to eliminate ventricular escape rhythms (Cummins, 2001; Drain, 2003a). Life-threatening ven-tricular dysrhythmias (ventricular tachycardia and fibrillation) and asystole should be immediately treated using current ACLS protocols (Cummins, 2001).

Allergic Reactions and/or Anaphylaxis

Anaphylactic reactions, although rare, can present life-threatening scenarios. Opioids are the most common moderate sedation class of drugs associated with allergic reactions; however, reactions have also been associated with various

Table 4-7 | Clinical Manifestations of Anaphylaxis

Type	Clinical Manifestations
Cutaneous	Urticaria, erythema, wheals, flaring, angioedema, edema
Cardiovascular	Hypotension, tachycardia, dysrhythmia, absence of pulse
Respiratory	Coughing, wheezing, stridor, hoarseness, dysphagia, pulmonary edema, bronchospasm, arterial hypoxemia, hypercapnia
Hematologic	Clotting defects

From Golembiewski, J.A. (2002). *Allergic reactions to drugs: Implications for perioperative care. Journal of PeriAnesthesia Nursing, 17, 393-398.*

classes of antibiotics, aspirin and nonsteroidal antiinflammatory drug (NSAIDs), barbiturates, propofol, local ester anesthetics, radiocontrast dye, and drug preservatives or other additives. Drug allergies can occur in any age group but are more common in patients between 20 and 49 years of age; they are also more common in women. The most common reaction seen in the moderate sedation environment is a Type I (anaphylactic, immediate hypersensitivity) reaction. Symptoms generally occur within 60 minutes of medication administration and can range from urticaria to bronchoconstriction, laryngeal edema, hypotension, and circulatory collapse. A systematic breakdown of anaphylactic symptoms is found in Table 4-7. Other reactions can include drug fever, vasculitis, serum sickness syndrome, and gastrointestinal symptoms, such as nausea, abdominal pain, diarrhea, and vomiting. Mild reactions can be treated by stopping the offending agent and administering diphenhydramine. Life-threatening reactions, however, require immediate treatment that includes supplemental oxygen, IV crystalloids for volume expansion, and epinephrine. Aminophylline may be considered for persistent bronchospasm. Diphenhydramine and ranitidine administration will block any unoccupied histamine receptors; hydrocortisone and methylprednisolone may also be administered, although their exact physiologic role is unclear (Golembiewski, 2002).

CONCLUSION

Moderate sedation is in and of itself an anesthesia technique. Although complication rates are relatively low, those complications that do occur can easily lead to increased morbidity and mortality if not rapidly recognized and properly treated. Comprehensive preprocedure assessment; vigilant assessment and monitoring during and after sedation administration; and competent, aggressive intervention when emergencies do arise are the keys to positive patient outcomes.

References

American Academy of Pediatric Dentistry (AAPD). (1998). Clinical guideline on elective use of conscious sedation, deep sedation, and general anesthesia in pediatric dental patients [On-line]. Available: http://www.aapd.org/members/referencemanual/pdfs/02-03/G_Sedation.pdf.

American Association of Nurse Anesthetists (AANA). (2003). Considerations for policy guidelines for registered nurses engaged in the administration of sedation and analgesia [On-line]. Available: http://www.aana.com/practice/conscious.asp.

American College of Radiology (ACR). (2000). ACR practice guideline for adult sedation/analgesia [On-line]. Available: http://www.acr.org/dyna/?doc=departments/stand_accred/standards/dl_list.html.

American Dental Association (ADA). (2003). Guidelines for the use of conscious sedation, deep sedation and general anesthesia for dentists [On-line]. Available: http://www.ada.org/prof/resources/positions/statements/anesthesia_guidelines.pdf.

American Society of Anesthesiologists (ASA). (1999). Practice guidelines for preoperative fasting and the use of pharmacologic agents to reduce the risk of pulmonary aspiration: Application to healthy patients underging elective procedures [On-line]. Available: http://www.asahq.org/publicationsAndServices/NPO.pdf.

American Society of Anesthesiologists (ASA). (2001). Practice guidelines for sedation and analgesia by non-anesthesiologists [On-line]. Available: http://www.asahq.org/publicationsAndServices/sedation1017.pdf.

American Society of Anesthesiologists (ASA). (2002). Practice guidelines for management of the difficult airway [On-line]. Available: http://www.asahq.org/publicationsAndServices/Difficult%20Airway.pdf.

American Society of Anesthesiologists (ASA). (2004). JCAHO compliance kit: Sedation model policy [On-line]. Available: http://www.asahq.org/clinical/toolkit/sedmodelfinal.htm.

American Society of PeriAnesthesia Nurses (ASPAN). (2002). Resource 12: The role of the Registered Nurse in the management of patients undergoing sedation for short-term therapeutic, diagnostic or surgical procedures. In ASPAN, 2002 standards of perianesthesia nursing practice. Cherry Hill, NJ: ASPAN, pp. 47-48.

Association of periOperative Registered Nurses (AORN). (2002). Recommended practices for managing the patient receiving moderate sedation/analgesia. AORN Journal, 75, 642-652.

Cowling, G.E., & Haas, R.E. (2002). Hypotension in the PACU: An algorithmic approach. Journal of PeriAnesthesia Nursing, 17, 159-163.

Cummins, R.O. (Ed.). (2001). ACLS provider manual. Dallas, TX: American Heart Association.

D'Eramo, E.M., Bookless, S.J., & Howard, J.B. (2003). Adverse events with outpatient anesthesia in Massachusetts. Journal of Oral and Maxillofacial Surgery, 61, 793-800.

Drain, C.B. (2003a). Assessment and monitoring of the perianesthesia patient. In C.B. Drain (Ed.). Perianesthesia nursing: A critical care approach. St. Louis: Saunders, pp. 360-408.

Drain, C.B. (2003b). The respiratory system. In C.B. Drain (Ed.). Perianesthesia nursing: A critical care approach. St. Louis: Saunders, pp. 150-188.

Eckardt, V.F., Kanzler, G., Schmitt, T., Eckardt, A.J., & Bernhard, G. (1999). Complications and adverse effects of colonoscopy with selective sedation. Gastrointestinal Endoscopy, 49, 560-565.

Golembiewski, J.A. (2002). Allergic reactions to drugs: Implications for perioperative care. Journal of PeriAnesthesia Nursing, 17, 393-398.

Guyton, A.C., & Hall, J.E. (Eds.). (1997). Human physiology and mechanisms of disease (6th Ed.). Philadelphia: Saunders.

Hannah, B. (2002). Airway management. In B. Gooden (Ed.). Compentency based orientation credentialing program: 2002 edition. Cherry Hill, NJ: ASPAN, pp. 47-48.

Heffline, M. (1999). Cardiopulmonary care and emergency support. In D. M. D. Quinn (Ed.), Ambulatory surgical nursing core curriculum. Philadelphia: Saunders, pp. 167-195.

Hooper, V.D. (2001a). Sedation standards part I. Carrolton, TX: Health & Sciences Television Network.

Hooper, V.D. (2001b). Sedation standards part II. Carrolton, TX: Health & Sciences Television Network.

Hotchkiss, M.A., & Drain, C.B. (2003). Assessment and management of the airway. In C. B. Drain (Ed.), Perianesthesia nursing: A critical care approach. St. Louis: Saunders, pp. 409-421.

Islat, G. (2003). Anesthesia machine [On-line]. Available: http://www.mpasohio.com/faq.htm.

Kost, M. (2003). Administration of conscious sedation/analgesia. In Nursing Spectrum [On-line]. Available: http://nsweb.nursingspectrum.com/ce/ce159.htm.

Ku, C.M., & Ong, B.C. (2003). Postoperative nausea and vomiting: A review of current literature. Singapore Medical Journal, 44, 366-374.

Malviya, S., Voepel-Lewis, T., Tait, A.R., & Merkel, S. (2000). Sedation/analgesia for diagnostic and therapeutic procedures in children. Journal of PeriAnesthesia Nursing, 15, 415-422.

Martin, M.L., & Lennox, P.H. (2003). Sedation and analgesia in the interventional radiology department. Journal of Vascular and Interventional Radiology, 14, 1119-1128.

Messinger, J.A., Hoffman, L.A., O'Donnell, J.M., & Dunworth, B.A. (1999). Getting conscious sedation right. American Journal of Nursing, 99(12), 44-49.

National Institutes of Health (NIH). (2000). Monitoring of patients undergoing conscious sedation. Critical care medicine department: Critical care therapy and respiratory section [On-line]. Available: http://clinicalcenter.nih.gov/ccmd/pdf_doc/Clinical%20Monitoring/09-conscious%20Sedation.pdf.

Newman, D.H., Azer, M.M., Pitetti, R.D., & Singh, S. (2003). When is a patient safe for discharge after procedural sedation? The timing of adverse effect events in 1,367 pediatric procedural sedations. Annals of Emergency Medicine, 42, 627-635.

Scales, B.A. (2003). Screening high-risk patients for the ambulatory setting. Journal of PeriAnesthesia Nursing, 18, 307-316.

Tarrac, S.E. (2003). Negative pressure pulmonary edema: A postanesthesia emergency. Journal of PeriAnesthesia Nursing, 18, 317-323.

Tham, C., & Koh, K.F. (2002). Unanticipated admission after day surgery. Singapore Medical Journal, 43, 522-526.

Wyman, C. I. (2004). Conscious sedation: A self study guide [On-line]. Available: http://www.gasnet.org/protocols/sedation/.

5

Patient Discharge

Apatient who has received moderate sedation and analgesia during a short-term therapeutic, diagnostic, or surgical procedure should be monitored until discharge criteria have been met. The Association of periOperative Registered Nurses' (AORN) Recommended Practice VIII regarding moderate sedation states: "Patients who receive moderate sedation/analgesia should be monitored postoperatively, receive verbal and written discharge instructions, and meet specified criteria before discharge" (AORN, 2004). Specific criteria for discharge are determined by the physician or are set according to standardized criteria developed by a multidisciplinary team. These criteria assist the physician and the registered nurse (RN) in assessing that the patient is ready to go home or ready for discharge to an appropriate skilled nursing unit. Documentation should clearly reflect that the patient has met each of the specified criteria.

Following a procedure for which moderate sedation and analgesia has been administered, the patient is usually transferred to a recovery area until determined home ready. The physical location and type of unit used for patient recovery vary and are determined by the institution. Some patients recover on the unit where the procedure was performed (e.g., emergency department), whereas others are transferred to a different area, such as short stay or postanesthesia care unit (PACU). The type of monitoring and criteria for discharge are determined by the procedure performed, the type and amount of medications administered, and the patient's health status.

THE REPORT

When care of the patient is transferred from the monitoring RN to a discharge RN or unit RN, the monitoring RN is responsible for providing a concise and detailed report. This information allows the receiving RN to make a more accurate initial, ongoing, and discharge assessment of the patient.

The monitoring RN's report may be phoned in or given in person (verbally) to the receiving RN before unit transfer. The report should include, but is not limited to, the following information (ASPAN, 2002):

Patient name and age. The RN should know the patient's age and should address the patient with his and/or her preferred name.

Preexisting medical conditions and preprocedure vital signs. The RN is responsible for total assessment of the patient. Information should include any history of conditions such as respiratory problems, cardiovascular disease, diabetes, hypertension, substance abuse, and posttraumatic stress syndrome. Baseline vital signs should be communicated, and any significant changes should be reported to the physician.

Type of therapeutic, diagnostic, or surgical procedure and physician. Identification of the type of procedure allows the RN to monitor the patient's response to the diagnostic, therapeutic, or surgical intervention. The RN should be aware of the responsible physician in the event that immediate consultation is necessary.

Type of medications, dosage, route, and times. The RN should be informed of all medications administered, total dosage administered, route, time of last dose, and length of time sedation is administered. Medications reported include sedative and analgesic agents, reversal agents, and local agents administered during the procedure and any other medications taken the day of the procedure. The RN should be aware of any medications used at home and the location of any prescriptions written by the physician following surgery, which should be attached to the chart.

Allergies. The RN should be aware of any allergies to medications, latex, prepping solutions, foods, and environmental allergies.

Intraprocedure monitoring parameters. The RN should be aware of monitoring parameter ranges (e.g., heart rate, respirations, blood pressure, level of consciousness, oxygen saturation, and skin condition) and any significant deviation from preprocedure baseline ranges. This information is critical for continuous assessment of the patient throughout the postprocedure period. The RN should notify the physician of any significant changes from preprocedure and intraprocedure monitoring ranges.

Drains and dressings. The RN should be informed of any type of drain, packing, reservoir, and dressing. This information allows the RN to anticipate the type and the usual amount of drainage.

Fluid intake and output. The RN should be provided information regarding the amount of intravenous (IV) fluids, irrigation type and amount used, blood loss, and urinary output as appropriate.

Complications. The RN should be apprised of any complications that occurred during the procedure, interventions, and patient outcome.

Pain management intervention. The RN should be aware of the patient's preprocedure pain score and pain scores documented during the procedure.

The monitoring RN's report may vary by institution. The preceding listing is minimal information that should be communicated to the RN to allow for an accurate patient assessment for facilitation of quality care.

POSTPROCEDURE ASSESSMENT

The patient is monitored for continued assessment of respiration, circulation, level of consciousness, skin color, and level of voluntary activity. This information should be documented in the patient record. Documentation should reflect continuous evaluation of expected patient outcomes. Patients are most at risk for residual sedation and cardiorespiratory depression immediately after admission to the recovery area (ASA, 2002). One reason for this risk may be that the patient is moved to a quiet environment with no noxious stimuli present. The patient must be assessed thoroughly and often during this period to ensure airway patency and respiratory adequacy. The length of postprocedure recovery to discharge will vary based on type and amount of medication administered, procedure performed, and the policy of the institution (Odom, 1997). In a study to determine recovery time and safe discharge of endoscopy patients after conscious sedation, patients above the age of 70 had significantly longer recovery stays than patients below the age of 70 (Lugay et al, 1996).

Criteria should be established for discharge that is consistent throughout the institution (AORN, 2004). Objective parameters are used instead of time restrictions as in the past (Odom, 2000). Multiple scoring systems are available to standardize documentation (e.g., Aldrete & Kroulik, 1970; Aldrete & Wright, 1992; Chung, 1992). However, most of these scoring systems were developed for use in phase I of recovery for inpatients recovering from general anesthesia. Generally, these scoring systems reflect assessment and documentation of the patient's respirations, circulation, level of consciousness, skin color or oxygenation, and level of voluntary activity.

The PostAnesthesia Discharge Scoring System (PADSS) is specifically designed to measure phase II recovery and to determine discharge readiness for outpatients (Box 5-1). A score of 2, 1, or 0 is assigned to the main criteria of the PADS system, which include (1) vital signs (i.e., blood pressure, heart rate, respiratory rate, and temperature); (2) activity and mental status; (3) pain, nausea, and/or vomiting; (4) surgical bleeding; (5) intake and output. A score of 9 or 10 indicates that the patient is ready for discharge. The PADSS has been clinically validated. Because a score of 9 is indicated for discharge, the patient must either void or take fluids. Institutions that have eliminated intake and output from discharge criteria may use another scoring system, such as the Modified PADSS or modified Postanesthetic Recovery (PAR) Score for Outpatient's Street Fitness. The MPADSS does not require the patient to void or take fluids before discharge (Box 5-2). The Modified PAR scoring system was adapted from the Postanesthetic Recovery (PAR) Score that was developed in 1970. The establishment of outpatient surgery outdated the PAR scoring system, and in 1992 it was modified to reflect additional assessment factors: oxygen saturation, dressing, pain management, coordination, urinary output, fasting, and feeding (Box 5-3). Whatever scoring system an institution uses, documentation should reflect objective data supporting the assessment that the patient is stable and suitable for discharge.

Box 5-1 POSTANESTHESIA DISCHARGE SCORING SYSTEM (PADSS)

Vital Signs

2 = Within 20% of preoperative value
1 = 20%-40% of preoperative value
0 = > 40% of preoperative value

Activity and Mental Status

2 = Oriented × 3 and a steady gait
1 = Oriented × 3 or a steady gait
0 = Neither

Pain, Nausea, and/or Vomiting

2 = Minimal
1 = Moderate, requiring treatment
0 = Severe, requiring treatment

Surgical Bleeding

2 = Minimal
1 = Moderate
0 = Severe

Intake and Output

2 = Postoperative fluids and void
1 = Postoperative fluids or void
0 = Neither

The total score is 10. Patients scoring > 9 are considered fit for discharge.

From Chung, F. (1995). Discharge process. In Twersky, R. (Ed.). The ambulatory anesthesia handbook. St. Louis: Mosby, p. 438.

The patient is encouraged to participate in activities that assist the RN in determining home readiness and appropriateness for discharge. Typical goals of nursing care in phase II are summarized in Box 5-4.

The ASPAN (2002) recommends the following initial, ongoing, and discharge assessment for a patient admitted to a phase II recovery area. These Standards of PeriAnesthesia Nursing Practice (2002) are applicable for any RN managing the recovery of a patient receiving IV moderate sedation and analgesia medications and should be documented (Box 5-5).

PATIENT DISCHARGE

The discharge planning process begins when the decision to perform a procedure is made by the patient and physician. The goal is to provide for an organized plan of care based on the patient's needs and health status. The discharge planning process should be responsive to the patient, physicians, and RNs involved in the

> **Box 5-2** A MODIFIED POSTANESTHETIC DISCHARGE SCORING SYSTEM
>   (MPADSS)
>
> **Vital Signs**
>
> 2 = within 20% of preoperative value
> 1 = 20-40% of preoperative value
> 0 = 40% of preoperative value
>
> **Ambulation**
>
> 2 = steady gait/no dizziness
> 1 = with assistance
> 0 = none/dizziness
>
> **Nausea/Vomiting**
>
> 2 = minimal
> 1 = moderate
> 0 = severe
>
> **Pain**
>
> 2 = minimal
> 1 = moderate
> 0 = severe
>
> **Surgical Bleeding**
>
> 2 = minimal
> 1 = moderate
> 0 = severe
>
> The total score is 10. Patients scoring >9 are considered fit for discharge.

From Chung, F. (1995). Discharge process. In Twersky, R. (Ed.). The ambulatory anesthesia handbook. St. Louis: Mosby, p. 440.

management of the patient's care. Most patients receiving moderate sedation and analgesia are undergoing a procedure that is relatively short in duration. In establishing a discharge plan for the patient, there must be clear discharge criteria to determine that the patient can safely recover at home. Discharge criteria decrease the likelihood of adverse outcomes for the patient (ASA, 2002).

The Joint Commission on Accreditation of Healthcare Organizations (JCAHO, 2004) has developed anesthesia care standards applicable to the patient receiving IV moderate sedation and analgesia. These are excerpted as follows:

Standard PC.13.40 Patients are monitored immediately after the procedure and/or administration of moderate or deep sedation or anesthesia. Elements of Performance include:

1. The patient's status is assessed on arrival in the recovery area.

2. Each patient's physiological status, mental status, and pain level are monitored.

Box 5-3 Modified Postanesthesia Recovery (PAR) Score for Outpatient's Street Fitness

Activity

2 = Able to move four extremities voluntarily on command
1 = Able to move two extremities voluntarily on command
0 = Able to move no extremities voluntarily on command

Respiration

2 = Able to breathe deeply and cough freely
1 = Dyspnea or limited breathing
0 = Apneic

Circulation

2 = BP +20 of preanesthesia level
1 = BP +21-49 of preanesthesia level
0 = BP +50 of preanesthesia level

Consciousness

2 = Fully awake
1 = Arousable on calling
0 = Not responding

O₂ Saturation

2 = Able to maintain O_2 saturation > 92% on room air
1 = Needs O_2 inhalation to maintain O_2 saturation > 90%
0 = O_2 saturation < 90% even with O_2 supplement

Dressing

2 = Dry
1 = Wet but stationary
0 = Wet but growing

Pain

2 = Pain free
1 = Mild pain handled by oral meds
0 = Pain requiring parenteral meds

Ambulation

2 = Able to stand up and walk straight*
1 = Vertigo when erect
0 = Dizziness when supine

Fasting-Feeding

2 = Able to drink fluids
1 = Nauseated
0 = Nausea and vomiting

Urine Output

2 = Has voided
1 = Unable to void but comfortable†
0 = Unable to void and uncomfortable

Data from Aldrete, J., & Wright, A. Anesthesia News, Nov. 1992, pp. 16-17.
*May be substituted by Romberg's test, or picking up 12 clips in one hand.
†Aldrete, J.A. & Kroulik, D. (1970). A post anesthetic recovery score. Anesthesia and Analgesia, 49, 924-928.

Box 5-4   TYPICAL PHASE II UNIT GOALS

- To provide close assessment of and attention to the patient's physical, emotional, and educational needs in the postoperative period.
- To provide an environment and the personnel who are prepared for emergency interventions at all times.
- To provide family oriented care that stresses the concept of wellness and acknowledges the integral relationship of the patient and family or other supporting adult.
- To encourage the patient toward as much self-sufficiency as possible, given the type of surgery and anesthesia performed.
- To respect the patient's right to confidentiality, privacy, and respectful, compassionate nursing care.
- To maintain accurate records of patient-related care and environmental preparedness.
- To interact with physicians and other health care providers in a professional manner that results in high-quality patient care.
- To provide patients and families with a resource for questions, comments, and nursing information during their stay and in the immediate period after discharge.
- To offer an environment that encourages the professional growth of nursing personnel.

From Smith, S. (2002). Progressive postanesthesia care: Phase II recovery. In Burden, N. (Ed.). Ambulatory surgical nursing. Philadelphia: Saunders, p. 482.

3. Monitoring is at a level consistent with the potential effect of the procedures and/or sedation or anesthesia.

4. Patients are discharged from the recovery areas and the hospital by a qualified Licensed Independent Practitioner (LIP) or according to rigorously applied criteria approved by the clinical leaders.

5. Patients who have received anesthesia in the outpatient setting are discharged in the company of a responsible, designated adult.

It is required that all institutions develop specific written criteria for discharge that have been approved by the medical and surgical staff to ensure that the same standard of care is provided to all patients. Although the physician is ultimately responsible for patient discharge, it is usually the RN who is responsible for determining that the patient has met the standardized discharge criteria and that it is reasonable to discharge the patient.

The following parameters for discharge are frequently used to assess readiness for discharge and assist the RN in determining that the patient has returned to a safe physiologic level: stable vital signs, level of consciousness, mobility, airway patency, intact protective reflexes, skin color and condition, condition of dressing and surgical site, absence of protracted vomiting, and ability to urinate

Box 5-5 DATA REQUIRED FOR INITIAL, ONGOING, AND DISCHARGE ASSESSMENT: PHASE II

Initial Assessment: Phase II

Initial and documentation include, but are not limited to:

1. Integration of data received at transfer of care
2. Vital signs
   a. Respiratory rate and status
   b. Blood pressure
   c. Pulse
   d. Temperature/route
   e. Pain assessment
3. Level of consciousness
4. Position of patient
5. Patient safety needs
6. Condition and color of skin
7. Neurovascular assessment as applicable
8. Condition of dressings, drains, and tubes as applicable
9. Muscular response and strength/mobility status if applicable
10. Fluid therapy: location of lines, condition of IV sites, and amount of fluid infusing
11. Level of physical and emotional comfort
12. Numerical score, if used

Ongoing Assessment: Phase II

Ongoing assessment and management include, but are not limited to, the following:

1. Monitor, maintain, and/or improve respiratory function
2. Monitor, maintain, and/or improve circulatory function
3. Promote and maintain effective pain management
4. Promote and maintain physical and emotional comfort
5. Monitor surgical/procedural site and continue procedure-specific care
6. Administer medication as ordered, document results
7. Promote patient safety
8. Encourage fluids by mouth as indicated
9. Progress to preprocedure level of mobility as appropriate
10. Review discharge planning with patient, family/accompanying responsible adult as appropriate; provide written discharge care instructions
11. Provide follow-up for extended care as indicated

Discharge Assessment: Phase II

Data collected and documented to evaluate the patient's status for discharge include, but are not limited to:

1. Adequate respiratory function
2. Stability of vital signs
3. Hypothermia resolved as defined by Resource 14
4. Level of consciousness and muscular strength

Box 5-5 DATA REQUIRED FOR INITIAL, ONGOING, AND DISCHARGE ASSESSMENT:
PHASE II—cont'd

5. Ability to ambulate consistent with developmental age level
6. Ability to swallow
7. Minimal nausea/vomiting
8. Skin color and condition
9. Adequate pain control
10. Adequate neurovascular status of operative extremity
11. Ability to void as indicated
12. Patient and home-care provider understand discharge instructions
13. Written discharge instructions given to patient/accompanying responsible adult
14. Verify arrangements for safe transportation home
15. Provide additional resource to contact if any problems arise
16. The professional perianesthesia nurse will complete a discharge follow-up to assess and evaluate patient status

From Standards of perianesthesia nursing practice, 2002, pp. 29-30. Copyright ASPAN, 10 Melrose Avenue, Suite 110, Cherry Hill, NJ 08003-3696.

(AORN, 2004). Box 5-6 identifies typical criteria for common discharge parameters. If the patient fails to meet the identified discharge criteria, the RN should notify the physician and document appropriate interventions as indicated. Box 5-6 lists guidelines for discharge suggested by the ASA.

DISCHARGE TEACHING AND INSTRUCTIONS

Most patients receiving moderate sedation and analgesia are in the institutional setting for a very short time and are discharged with a responsible escort to continue their recovery. Because the medications administered may result in drowsiness and amnesia, discharge instructions should be explained to both patient and escort. Ideally, discharge instructions were begun preprocedure and reinforced to the patient and responsible escort after the procedure. General discharge instructions include basic information such as medications (including scheduled medications, prescribed medications with names, purpose, route, dosage, frequency, duration, and significant or expected side effects); dietary regimen; activity and limitations as appropriate; instructions related to postprocedure care; signs and/or symptoms related to care that may require medical attention; emergency numbers and physician's number; expected follow-up care with the physician; instructions regarding driving limitations; appropriate referral sources for continuing care needs. Postprocedure instructions may be specific to the type of procedure and possible complications (Figure 5-1).

> **Box 5-6** GUIDELINES FOR DISCHARGE
>
> - Patients should be alert and oriented; infants and patients whose mental status was initially abnormal should have returned to their baseline status. Practitioners and parents must be aware that pediatric patients are at risk for airway obstruction if the head falls forward while the child is secured in a car seat.
> - Vital signs should be stable and within acceptable limits, including adequate respiratory function and temperature.
> - Patient should have minimal nausea and vomiting, adequate pain control, and ability to urinate (if appropriate).
> - Use of scoring systems may assist in documentation of fitness for discharge.
> - Sufficient time (up to 2 hours) should have elapsed after the last administration of reversal agents (naloxone, flumazenil) to ensure that patients do not become resedated after reversal effects have worn off.
> - Outpatients should be discharged in the presence of a responsible adult who will accompany them home and be able to report any postprocedure complications.
> - Outpatients and their escorts should be provided with written instructions regarding postprocedure diet, medications, activity restrictions, care of surgical or procedure site (if applicable), possible complications, and a phone number to use in case of emergency.

Data from ASA (2002). Practice guidelines for sedation and analgesia by non-anesthesiologists: An updated report by the American Society of Anesthesiologists task force on sedation and analgesia by non-anesthesiologists. Anesthesiology, 96:1012; Redmond, M.C. (2004). Postanesthesia assessment phase II. In D.M.D. Quinn & L. Schick (Eds.). Perianesthesia nursing core curriculum: Preoperative, phase I and phase II PACU nursing. Philadelphia: Saunders, pp. 1235-1251; Schick, L. (2004). Discharge planning: Home and phase III. In D.M.D. Quinn & L.Schick (Eds.). Perianesthesia nursing core curriculum: Preoperative, phase I and phase II PACU nursing. Philadelphia: Saunders, pp. 1262-1265.

Information should be documented to reflect patient and escort understanding of discharge instructions (e.g., patient and escort complete successful return demonstration of emptying a drain). A copy should be given to the patient, and a copy should be retained as part of the patient record. Hayes and Buffum (2000) discovered that written instructions can go unread even with a memory reminder used in the study. In their study, age seemed to be a marker for memory problems. Patients older than age 65 had more problems with memory of instructions and may require more educational attention.

POSTPROCEDURE PHONE CALL

In some areas the accepted standard of care is a postprocedure phone call (Burden, 2000). This phone call is usually made within 24 hours after the procedure. This allows the RN to assess the patient's health status and determine any immediate needs the patient may have. It also alerts the RN of any

Lowery A. Woodall, Sr.
OUTPATIENT SURGERY FACILITY
A Division of Forrest General Hospital

POST INSTRUCTIONS FOR LOCAL ANESTHESIA WITH SEDATION

The medication or sedation which was used to calm you will be acting in your body for the next 24 hours, so you might feel a little sleepy. This feeling will slowly wear off. Because the medicine or sedation is still in your system, for the next twenty-four (24) hours, the adult patient:

    SHOULD NOT -- Drive a car, operate machinery or power tools.

    SHOULD NOT -- Drink any alcoholic beverages (not even beer).

    SHOULD NOT -- Make any important decisions (such as sign important papers).

PAIN:

    You may have some pain. A prescription for pain may be given by your doctor. This should be taken as directed on the label. If your doctor does not prescribe any pain meds, you may take non-prescription medication, which can be purchased at your drugstore.

DIET:

    You may resume your normal diet when you arrive home, unless you are instructed otherwise by your doctor.

ACTIVITY LEVEL:

    We strongly suggest you have a responsible adult with you the rest of today and also during the night for your protection and safety. Rest the remainder of today and tonight.

ADDITIONAL INSTRUCTIONS:_____

_____

_____

_____

_____

See Dr. _____ on _____ at _____ in his office.

If you have any questions or concerns, call Dr. _____ at phone _____.

If you are unable to reach him/her or his/her partner, call or come to the Forrest General Hospital Emergency Department at 288-2100.

The information/instructions above have been discussed with and a copy given to me or a significant other who demonstrates an adequate level of understanding and will give these instructions for care to the individual responsible for my care.

_____   _____
    Patient/Significant Other   Physician/Nurse

_____ AM _____ PM
    Date/Time

Revised 2/6/95
FGH 211020

Figure 5-1 Post instructions for local anesthesia and sedation. (*Courtesy Forrest General Hospital, Hattiesburg, Miss.*)

complications related to moderate sedation. The patient should be informed of the postprocedure phone call during discharge teaching. Specifically the patient should be told that once he or she is at home to write down any questions he or she would like to discuss during the call. The RN should document any signs and symptoms on the patient chart. Any follow-up, such as immediate referral of the patient to the attending physician and calling the physician with a direct report, also has to be documented. The postprocedure phone call conveys a positive message to the patient that the health care providers are truly interested in the individual's follow-up care and leads to positive patient satisfaction.

CONCLUSION

The manner in which a patient is discharged is determined by institution policy and procedure. RNs should fully understand their role in the discharge process. Written discharge instructions should be given to the patient, and accurate documentation should be completed to reflect the patient's achievement of discharge criteria. The overall goal of well-established discharge criteria is to ensure that the patient has adequately recovered from the effects of the procedure and the medications administered to achieve a state of moderate sedation and analgesia and may safely continue recovery at home.

REFERENCES

Abeles, G., Warmuth, I.P., Sequeira, M., Swenson, R.D., Bisaccia, E., & Scarborough, D.A. (2000). The use of conscious sedation for outpatient dermatologic surgical procedures. Dermatologic Surgery, 26, 121-126.

Aldrete, J. A., & Kroulik, D. (1970). A post anesthesia recovery score. Anesthesia and Analgesia, 49, 924.

Aldrete, J., & Wright, A. (1992). Post anesthesia scores. Anesthesia News, Nov. 1992, pp. 16-17.

American Society of Anesthesiologists. (2002). Practice guidelines for sedation and analgesia by non-anesthesiologists: An updated report for the American society of anesthesiologists task force on sedation and analgesia by non-anesthesiologists. Anesthesiology, 96, 1004-1017.

American Society of PeriAnesthesia Nurses. (2002). 2002 standards of perianesthesia nursing practice. Cherry Hill, NJ: ASPAN.

Association of periOperative Registered Nurses (2004). Recommended practices for managing the patient receiving moderate sedation/analgesia, In Standards, recommended practices and guidelines. Denver, Col: AORN, pp. 211-218.

Chung, F. (1995). Discharge process. In Twersky, R. (Ed.). The ambulatory anesthesia handbook. St. Louis: Mosby, pp. 438-440.

Hayes, A., & Buffum, M. (2001). Educating patients after conscious sedation for gastrointestinal procedures. Gastroenterology Nursing, 24, 54-57.

Joint Commission for Accreditation of Healthcare Organizations. (2004). Hospital accreditation standards. Oakbrook Terrace, IL: JCAHO.

Lugay, M., Otto, G., Kong, M., Mason, D., & Wilets, I. (1996). Recovery time and safe discharge of endoscopy patients after conscious sedation. Gastroenterology Nursing, 19, 194-200.

Odom, J. (2000). Conscious sedation/analgesia. In Burden, N. (Ed.). Ambulatory surgical nursing (2nd Ed.). Philadelphia: Saunders, p. 318.

Odom, J. (1997). Conscious sedation in the ambulatory setting. Critical Care Nursing Clinics of North America, 9, 361-370.

6

Institution Policy and Guideline Development: Standard of Care

The administration of moderate sedation and analgesia is a common practice among settings throughout an institution, including the various interventional suites, diagnostic laboratories, and departments—such as radiology, emergency, surgical services, endoscopy, special procedures, cardiac catheterization, electrophysiology, labor and delivery suites, and others. The Joint Commission on Accreditation of Healthcare Organizations (JCAHO) clearly defines the standards of care for sedation and anesthesia care and clearly articulates that they apply across the continuum in a facility.

Because sedation is a continuum, it is not always possible to predict how an individual patient receiving sedation will respond (JCAHO, 2004). Therefore each hospital develops specific, appropriate protocols for the care of patients receiving sedation. These protocols are consistent with professional standards and address at least the following:

- Sufficient qualified individuals present to perform the procedure and to monitor the patient throughout administration and recovery
  - Presedation evaluation
  - Monitoring of patient during the procedure
  - Appropriate equipment
- Appropriate equipment for care and resuscitation
- Appropriate monitoring of vital signs
  - Including, but not limited to, heart rate and oxygenation using pulse oximetry
  - Respiratory rate and adequacy of pulmonary ventilation
  - Monitoring of blood pressure (BP) at regular intervals
  - Cardiac monitoring in patients with significant cardiovascular disease or when dysrhythmias are anticipated or detected
- Documentation of care
- Monitoring of outcomes (JCAHO, 2004)

Institutions must work collaboratively to develop policy, documentation tools, and quality monitors that can be applied in all areas in which nonanesthesia-provider sedation is delivered.

The JCAHO standards have been refined in the section of the manual entitled Provision of Care, Treatment, and Services (JCAHO, 2004). The guidelines state the standard, the rationale for the standard, and the elements of performance for each standard.

PC.13.20 states "Operative or other procedures and/or the administration of moderate or deep sedation or anesthesia are planned" (JCAHO, 2004) and addresses the following:

- Sufficient qualified personnel present to perform the procedure, monitor, and recover the patient
- Qualified staff must be credentialed
- A registered nurse supervises the perioperative nursing care
- Appropriate equipment is available
- Resuscitation capabilities are available
- The components of the preprocedure assessment
- The requirement to articulate a plan of care

PC.13.30 addresses monitoring of patients during the procedure stating that appropriate methods are used to continuously monitor oxygenation, ventilation, and circulation, and that the information is documented. PC.13.40 addresses the monitoring of patients in the immediate postprocedure period. This standard also includes discharge planning.

In addition, the 2004 Patient Safety Goals have been incorporated into the standards. Of particular importance in the development of policy are the following patient safety goals (JCAHO, 2004):

Goal #1: Improve the accuracy of patient identification
Goal #2: Improve the effectiveness of communication among caregivers
Goal #4: Eliminate wrong-site, wrong-patient, wrong-procedure surgery

PROCESS FOR DEVELOPING A SINGLE STANDARD OF CARE

Well-written, collaboratively developed policies establish a standard of care and often serve as templates for the development of care delivery models. It is essential that the unique characteristics of the institution, its patient populations, and its articulated mission are communicated through the policies. It is also essential that the critical elements of assessment are consistent throughout a facility.

Step 1: Selection of Team Members

Ongoing monitoring of standards of care is essential to provide safe, seamless patient care. A multidisciplinary team is essential to ensure that the policies and guidelines are consistent with practice across an institution. The person selected to chair the project team should have a proven record as a leader and the ability to move a group forward. It is helpful if the chairperson and other members of the project team are well respected among their peers and are knowledgeable and experienced in the administration of moderate sedation and analgesia.

It is imperative that at least one member of the team is a representative of the anesthesia department. Other members might include staff nurses from areas that monitor patients undergoing moderate sedation, clinical nurse specialists, pharmacists, surgeons, or other interested parties or disciplines. Familiarity with national guidelines and recommendations is desirable.

Some institutions report that revisions to the standard of care for the administration of moderate sedation and analgesia have taken years to make or have not occurred at all because of the turf battles that occur among departments. Therefore the leader must stay focused on the overall goal of the institutionwide standard of care (i.e., to deliver safe, high-quality patient care). This individual may guide the group through the process of evaluating the existing standard of care by asking:

1. Are we keeping our practices current and correct?
2. Do our practices keep us in line with our organizational mission?
3. What practices do the national nursing and medical associations recommend, and what is the community standard?
4. What are the risks of practicing within these guidelines, and how should they be addressed?
5. Are any recommendations currently not being practiced at the local level and can these be incorporated into the current guidelines?
6. Are there any systems issues that have to be addressed in the guidelines to ensure that safe patient care is delivered?
7. Are we measuring quality of care and its improvement?

Any data that have been collected should be analyzed. This should include any sentinel events or "near miss" data. Plans for improvement should be discussed.

Step 2: Evaluation of Nationally Endorsed Position Statements, Recommended Practices, and Guidelines

The project team should review available nationally endorsed position statements, recommended practices, and guidelines on the administration of moderate sedation and analgesia (see Chapter 1). Each should be evaluated to determine recommended practices versus actual practices of the institution. Do actual practices vary from national recommendations? If an institution has a practice that differs from national nursing and medical association recommendations, is there any documentation in the literature or other sources to provide support for the local practice? If the project team decides to follow local practice versus the national recommendation, the reasons should be justified, supported, and documented.

The project team members should review any patient teaching pamphlets (that may be distributed), standardized patient documentation form or flow chart used for documenting the administration of moderate sedation and analgesia, standardized discharge criteria, required patient assessments, patient education instruction, and informed consent as appropriate. Figure 6-1 shows a sample procedure record.

Step 3: Determining Policy Format

Each institution should have a designated format for developing policy and procedures, protocols, and standards of care. The following benchmarks could be included in any existing protocol:

Scope of Practice

This section should identify the intended health care provider of the protocol. For example, "This protocol applies to all registered nurses at the University Medical Center." A sample policy and guideline are presented in Figure 6-2.

Definition of Moderate Sedation and Analgesia

A concise and well-defined definition should be included to assist in determining appropriate patient populations. The most widely accepted definition from the literature is the one illustrated in Table 6-1. The definitions of the levels of sedation that are published in the JCAHO manual are identical to those published in the American Society of Anesthesia (ASA) guidelines.

Purpose

This section should describe the intent of the protocol, for example:

1. To establish one standard of care for administering and monitoring sedation administered by nonanesthesia providers for all patients throughout the medical center.
2. To delineate the practice for safe and effective administration of moderate sedation by a nonanesthesia provider (BIDMC, 2004).

Implementation

This section should include necessary supplies and equipment, assessment and monitoring parameters, medication guidelines, discharge criteria, and documentation requirements.

Education and Competency

This section should identify ongoing education and competency requirements for health care providers responsible for managing the care of patients receiving moderate sedation and analgesia.

Preprocedure Assessment and Documentation

This section should describe the preprocedure assessment and documentation of that assessment. It should include validation of consent and language that

Text continued on p. 140.

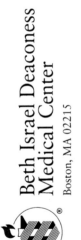

Beth Israel Deaconess Medical Center
Boston, MA 02215

PROCEDURE RECORD

Patient Identification Area

Pre-Procedure Check List

Chart preparation	✓	Patient preparation	✓	Allergies
H&P within 30 days of procedure		Patient identified using two indicators		
H&P update if > 7 days old		ID Band Applied		**Precaution Status**
General admission consent		IV access site		
Consent for procedure/conscious sedation		Procedure explained to patient		Weight
NPO since		Patient has escort home		Height

Patient has Health Care Proxy ☐ Yes ☐ No   If no, Proxy Explained & Patient Advised how to Obtain

Advanced Directives ☐ Yes ☐ No   If no, Directives Explained & Patient Advised how to Obtain

Pre-Procedure Assessment

Past Medical History:
☐ Heart Disease   ☐ Bleeding/Clotting
☐ Hypertension   ☐ Digestive/Reflux
☐ Angina   ☐ Kidney/Liver
☐ CVA   ☐ Diabetes
☐ Dyspnea   ☐ Anemia
☐ Asthma   ☐ Cancer
☐ Previous anesthesia problems?   ☐ Yes ☐ No

Comments: _____

Habits
Smoking ☐ Yes ☐ No _____ ETOH ☐ Yes ☐ No
Recreational drug use ☐ Yes ☐ No

Psycho/Social
Lives: ☐ Alone ☐ w/Family ☐ w/Spouse ☐ Other
Occupation: _____
Cultural/Religious Preference: _____
Do you feel safe in your relationships? ☐ Yes ☐ No
If patient answers no, contact ☐ Safe Transitions (#31389) and/or
                              ☐ Social Work for assistance

Cognitive/Perceptual
Visual/Hearing Deficit ☐ Yes ☐ No
Primary language: _____ Interpreter requested ☐

Past Surgical History: _____

Routine Medications: _____

Pre-Procedure Physician Assessment

☐ Refer to patient record

☐ Patient examined, chart reviewed, history as above.

Mental Status _____

Neck: _____

Chest/lungs: _____

Heart _____

Comments _____

_____ MD   Date: _____   Pager# _____

MC 1155-IP-OP (Rev.6/04)

Pain

Baseline Pain score(0-10): _____ Location: _____

Quality: _____

Daily Narcotic use: ☐ Yes ☐ No

Type and amount/day: _____

Preoperative plan: _____

Activity

H/O slips and falls ☐ Yes ☐ No   Balance ☐ Steady ☐ Unsteady

Elimination _____

Bladder/bowel problems ☐ Yes ☐ No

Nutrition/Metabolic

Reflux ☐ Yes ☐ No   Recent weight loss ☐ Yes ☐ No

Diagnosis _____

ASA _____   **AIRWAY** _____

Vital Signs: T _____ BP _____ HR _____ RR _____

02 Sat _____

Relevant Labs: _____

Continued

Figure 6-1 Nursing procedure record. *(Courtesy Beth Israel Deaconess Medical Center, Boston, 2004.)*

Date: ____ / ____ / ____

Procedure suite: ☐ Cath Lab ☐ Radiology ☐ GI lab ☐ Derm
Other _____

Planned monitoring: ☐ EKG ☐ BP cuff ☐ Pulse oximeter
☐ Other _____

Procedure _____
Physician _____
RN performing conscious sedation _____
Other _____

Time-Out

Initiated by: _____ Initials of staff participating in "Time-Out" _____ Time: _____

☐ Identity of the patient
☐ Verification of procedure
☐ Verification of Site and Side .... ☐ N/A
☐ Correct patient position .... ☐ N/A

☐ Verification of implants or special equipment ...... ☐ N/A
☐ Radiological images .... ☐ N/A
☐ Patient Stable and appropriate for planned anesthetic

Discrepancy noted, Surgeon notified _____ date _____ time
Physician's final side/site directive with Physician's signature _____

INTRAPROCEDURE

| TIME |
| MEDICATION |

| IVF |

| EBL/U.O. |
| SEDATION |
| PAIN |
| O₂ Source |
| O₂ SAT |

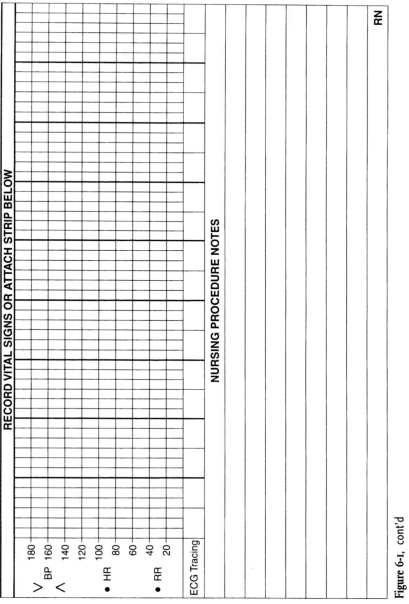
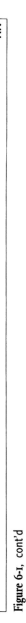

Figure 6-1, cont'd

Continued

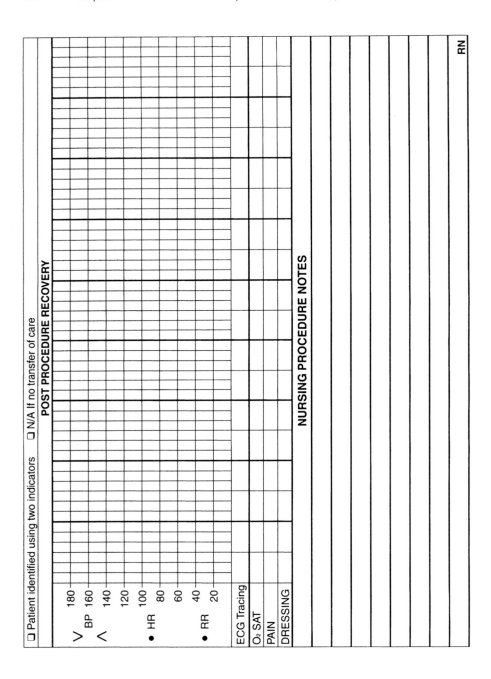

RECOVERY SCORE

	TIME
ACTIVITY	
Able to move 4 extremities voluntarily or on command	2
Able to move 2 extremities voluntarily or on command	1
Unable to move extremities voluntarily or on command	0
RESPIRATION	
Able to breathe deeply and cough freely	2
Dyspnea, limited breathing or tachypnea	1
Apneic or on mechanical ventilator	0
CIRCULATION	
BP plus or minus 20% of pre-anesthetic level	2
BP plus or minus 20% - 40% of pre-anesthetic level	1
BP plus or minus 40% of pre-anesthetic level	0
CONSCIOUSNESS	
Fully awake	2
Arousable on calling	1
Not responding	0
O₂ SATURATION	
Able to maintain O₂ saturation > 92% on room air	2
Needs O₂ inhalation to maintain O₂ saturation > 90%	1
O₂ saturation < 90% even with O₂ supplement	0

TOTAL PAR ____ / **SCORE** ____

SCORE = ≥ 8 RETURN TO INPATIENT UNIT.

PHASE 2 OUTPATIENT

	TIME
VITAL SIGNS	
BP and pulse within 20% of preoperative baseline	2
BP and pulse 20%-40% of preoperative baseline	1
BP and pulse >40% of preoperative baseline	0
ACTIVITY LEVEL	
Steady gait, no dizziness, or meets preoperative level	2
Requires assistance	1
Unable to ambulate	0
NAUSEA & VOMITING	
Minimal to none	2
Moderate	1
Severe	0
PAIN	
Minimal to pain free	2
Moderate pain handled by oral medication	1
Severe pain requiring parenteral medication	0
SURGICAL BLEEDING	
Minimal to none	2
Moderate	1
Severe	0

TOTAL PADS ____ / **SCORE** ____

SCORE = 9 OR 10 DISCHARGE HOME.

OUTPATIENT DISCHARGE CRITERIA

- ❏ PADS score ≥ 9
- ❏ Able to void   ❏ N/A
- ❏ Instructions reviewed
- ❏ Emergency contact given
- ❏ Patient demonstrates understanding
- ❏ Discharged with an adult escort
- ❏ Discharged Home

Time _____

- ❏ Transferred to unit report given

_____ RN

NURSING DIAGNOSES AND PATIENT OUTCOMES

OUTCOME CRITERIA MET	YES	NO	REASON
1. Anxiety Outcome: The patient participates in decisions affecting his/her plan of care; The patient's right to privacy is maintained.			
2. Alteration in Comfort: Pain Outcome: The patient demonstrates knowledge of pain management; The patient demonstrates and/or reports adequate pain control throughout the procedure.			
3. Knowledge Deficit Outcome: The patient demonstrates knowledge of physiological and psychological responses to medications and procedure.			
4. Potential for Injury Outcome: The patient is free from signs and symptoms of physical injury; The patient receives appropriately prescribed medications, safely administered by a qualified practitioner, during the procedure.			
5. Ineffective Breathing Pattern Outcome: The patient's respiratory pattern is consistent with the baseline level established pre-procedure.			

Figure 6-1, cont'd

Continued

American Society of Anesthesiologists
Physical Status Classification

Class I

There is no organic, physiological, biochemical or physical disturbance. The pathologic process for which operation is to be performed is localized and not a systemic disturbance.

Class II

Mild to Moderate systemic disturbance caused either by the condition to be treated surgically or by other pathophysiological processes.

Class III

Severe systemic disturbance or disease from whatever cause, even though it may not be possible to define the degree of disability with finality.

Class IV

Indicative of the patient with severe systemic disorder already life threatening, not always correctable by the operative procedure.

Class V

The moribund patient who has little chance of survival but is submitted to operation in desperation.

E

The letter "E" should be appended in cases where the patient was not scheduled for an elective procedure.

CONSCIOUS SEDATION DRUG DOSAGE INFORMATION

The Recommendations included here are generally acceptable guidelines and may require modification for individual patients at the discretion of the physician operator. Dosages provided are generally acceptable, but may need to be revised downward in a given patient in order to avoid serious cardiorespiratory depression or other undesired side effects. Furthermore, many of these medications have synergistic respiratory depressant effects; when administered in combination, lower dosages may be required.

Drug	Dose	Total	Onset	Duration	Caution
Benzodiadepine Sedatives					
DIAZEPAM (Valium)	1.25-2.5mg over 30 sec into rapidly infusing IV line; may repeat @ 5 min intervals	0.1mg/kg to 0.2mg/kg	1 to 5 minutes	3 to 4 hours may be much increased in pts >60y/o	Hepatic and renal insufficiency increase duration of effect
MIDAZOLAM (Versed)	<60y/o 1.0 to 2.5mg over 5 min (wait 2 min to evaluate) Titrate in small increments at 2 min intervals	Total maximum dose 5.0mg	1 to 5 minutes	60 to 90 minutes	Hepatic insufficiency increases duration of effect; 30% dose reduction with concomitant use of opiate agonists or CNS depressants
	>60y/o, debilitated, or chronically ill 0.5mg (wait 3 min to evaluate) Titrate 0.5mg increments at 2-3 min intervals	Total maximum dose 3.5mg			50% dose reduction with concomitant use of opiate agonists or CNS depressants

Opiate Agonists (Narcotics)					
MORPHINE	1-2mg at 3-5 min intervals	up to 0.1mg/kg - 0.15mg/kg	1 to 5 minutes	4 to 5 hours	Hepatic or renal insufficiency increases duration of effect
FENTANYL (Sublimaze)	25-50mcg at 3-5 min intervals	1.5mcg-2.0mcg/kg	1 to 5 minutes	1/2 to 1 hour	Hepatic insufficiency increases duration of effect
MEPERIDINE (Demerol)	12.5mg at 5-10 min intervals	up to 1mg/kg	1 to 5 minutes	2 to 4 hours	Should not be used in patients with renal failure or pts on MAO inhibitors. Caution with hepatic insufficiency
Opiate Antagonist	*Pts who receive reversal agents should be observed closely for an additional 2 hours*				
NALOXONE (Narcan)	0.1 mg to 0.2mg IV prn at 1 min intervals until respiratory function is restored		1 to 2 minutes	Variable: up to 45 minutes	Narcotic effects my last longer than Versed. Must monitor at least 2 hours after Narcan
Benzodiazepine Antagonist					
FLUMAZENIL (Mazicon)	0.1mg to 0.2mg over 30 sec into rapidly infusing IV line	Maximum dose 1mg	30 to 60 seconds	60 minutes	Pts on chronic benzodiazepines or with acute head injury

SEDATION RATING SCALE

The patient experiences:

0 - No sedation, awake

S - Sleepy (normal to arouse)

1 - Mild sedation (occasionally sleepy, easy to arouse, responds to verbal stimuli)

2 - Moderate sedation (frequently drowsy, responds to gentle shake)

3 - Severe or deep sedation (somnolent, difficult to arouse, responds to sternal rub)

4 - Unresponsive

Volume of oropharyngeal cavity
(Mallampati Class)

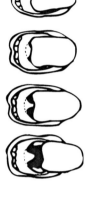

- Tongue size
- Palate narrow/high arch

Can J Anaesth 32:429-34.1985

Figure 6-1, cont'd

Beth Israel Deaconess Medical Center
BIDMC Manual

Title: **Conscious Sedation (Non-Anesthetist Moderate Sedation)**

Policy #: **CP-03**

Purpose:
- To establish one standard of care for administering and monitoring conscious sedation for all patients throughout the medical center.
- To delineate the practice for the safe and effective administration of conscious sedation (IVCS) in the absence of an anesthesia provider.

Procedure(s) for Implementation:

I. **AUTHORITY**
- Authority for the application of the Beth Israel Deaconess Medical Center *policy* resides with the Beth Israel Deaconess Medical Center Medical Executive Committee.
- Privileging of operators and monitors is under the authority of the BIDMC Medical Executive Committee. Individual practitioners and department leaders are responsible for ensuring that those who provide conscious sedation are privileged to do so.
- Appropriate Quality Improvement efforts and complications review will be performed and reported to PCAC annually.

II. **INTENT**
These guidelines are intended to address patients who receive moderate sedation (see below) by non-anesthesiologists (IVCS). The following populations are excluded from this policy:
- Patients sedated by a qualified anesthesia provider.
- Intubated patients receiving intravenous conscious sedation (IVCS) for diagnostic and therapeutic procedures.
- The care of the pediatric patient. (Neonatal sedation is discussed in the policies of the Neonatal Intensive Care Unit).

III. **DEFINITIONS**
Sedation progresses on a continuum. The following definitions illustrate that continuum.
- **Minimal sedation (anxiolysis)**
A drug-induced state during which patients respond normally to verbal commands. Although cognitive function and coordination may be impaired, ventilatory and cardiovascular functions are unaffected;

- **Moderate sedation/analgesia ("conscious sedation")**

Figure 6-2 Policy and procedure. *(Courtesy Beth Israel Deaconess Medical Center, Boston, 2004.)*

A drug-induced depression of consciousness during which patients respond purposefully to verbal commands, either alone or accompanied by light tactile stimulation. No interventions are required to maintain a patent airway, and spontaneous ventilation is adequate. Cardiovascular function is usually maintained.

- **Deep sedation/analgesia**
  A drug-induced depression of consciousness during which patients cannot be easily aroused but respond purposefully following repeated or painful stimulation. The ability to independently maintain ventilatory function may be impaired. Patients may require assistance in maintaining a patent airway and spontaneous ventilation may be inadequate. Cardiovascular function is usually maintained.

- **General Anesthesia**
  Consists of general anesthesia and spinal or major regional anesthesia. It does *not* include local anesthesia. General anesthesia is a drug-induced loss of consciousness during which patients are not arousable, even by painful stimulation. The ability to independently maintain ventilatory function is often impaired. Patients often require assistance in maintaining a patent airway, and positive pressure ventilation may be required because of depressed spontaneous ventilation or drug-induced depression of neuromuscular function. Cardiovascular function may be impaired.

IV. **SEDATION RATING SCALE**
In order to assess a patient's response to sedative or analgesic use, the following rating scale is applied:

The patient experiences:
  0- No sedation, awake
  S- Sleepy (normal to arouse)
  1- Mild sedation (occasionally sleepy, easy to arouse, responds to verbal stimuli)
  2- Moderate sedation (frequently drowsy, responds to gentle shake)
  3- Severe or deep sedation (somnolent, difficult to arouse, responds to sternal rub)
  4- Unresponsive

V. **PERSONNEL**
- At least two clinicians (Operator and Monitor) privileged in IVCS shall be present whenever IVCS is administered. Both of these two personnel will be available to the patient from the time of sedative/analgesic medication administration until recovery is judged adequate, or the care of the patient is transferred to personnel performing recovery care.

Figure 6-2, cont'd

Continued

- Operator

  The physician who administers the conscious sedation must have clinical privileges to perform IVCS. Privileging requires training in the safe use of these drugs and appropriate "rescue training." Documentation of training will be maintained in the physician's credentialing and reappointment file.

- Monitor

  The monitor must also have privileges in IVCS. S/he must have knowledge and experience in the use of oximetry, cardiac monitoring equipment and in the recognition of cardiac arrhythmias. The Nurse Manager shall certify that the nurse monitor is trained in the safe use of these drugs and appropriate rescue training. Documentation of biannual training will be maintained in the nurse's educational record. During the administration of IVCS, the monitor should have no other significant responsibilities.

- When IVCS is administered by non-anesthetists without ACLS or ATLS training, a physician with current training in advanced cardiac life support should be readily available (i.e., in the same or contiguous building) in case of medical complications and emergencies.

- The means for notifying additional support services such as Respiratory Therapy and for calling cardiac arrest pages should be clearly identified in procedure/sedation areas.

- When the patient has been identified as "high risk," or when the procedure to be carried out is particularly complex, a member of the anesthesia care team should be present to assist with the procedure. In elective cases, this must be scheduled with an anesthesiologist at least 24 hours in advance by requesting an Anesthesia Consultation (ext. 7-3112).

VI.   **TRAINING AND PRIVILEGING OF PERSONNEL:**
- The training requirements below pertain to the administration of moderate sedation. No specific training is required to administer minimal sedation (anxiolysis). Only clinicians with privileges in Anesthesia may administer deep sedation or general anesthesia.

- Training requirements for privileging in moderate sedation include education in the safe use of sedation drugs, appropriate rescue training and evidence of clinical experience. As with all Medical Center privileging, the individual practitioner and relevant department leaders are responsible to ensure that those who provide moderate sedation are appropriately trained. The training must be completed at least every 2 years in accordance with the re-credentialing requirements. When these training requirements are met, privileges to administer Moderate Sedation may be requested.

Figure 6-2, cont'd

- Training in airway management will be accomplished every two years through completion of ACLS, ATLS, CCMALS or BCLS certification. Those who provide sedation to ASA III or IV patients must obtain ACLS or ATLS certification as cardiovascular instability during sedation is more common among these patients. As an alternative, airway management skills can be obtained through training provided by the Department of Anesthesia and approved by the MEC.

- Training in the safe use of these drugs shall be achieved through a course offered by the Department of Anesthesia and Critical Care in the use of drugs and monitoring modalities used during conscious sedation. Alternatively, the videotape of this training may be viewed to fulfill the course requirements or an on-line training module can be completed.

VII. **EQUIPMENT**
- The room where the procedure USING IVCS is scheduled to take place should have adequate, uncluttered floor space to accommodate emergencies.

- The following monitoring and emergency resuscitation equipment should be available and in good working order prior to beginning the procedure.
  1. An airway and a self-inflating positive-pressure oxygen delivery system capable of delivering 100% oxygen at a 15 liter/minute flow rate for at least 60 minutes must be available. Various appropriate bag and mask sizes must be available.

  2. Supplemental oxygen source

  3. Nasal prongs and non-rebreathing or rebreathing oxygen masks

  4. A source of suction (portable or wall)

  5. An emergency cart or kit including the necessary drugs (including appropriate reversal agents) and equipment to resuscitate an apneic or unconscious patient and provide continuous support while that patient is being transported to another area

  6. A pulse oximeter with an alarm

  7. A manual or automatic device for measuring blood pressure

  8. Cardiac monitor with alarm. The Board of Registration in Medicine recommends the use of cardiac monitors for patients with an ASA classification of III or greater or with a history of cardio-pulmonary disease.

  9. All equipment shall be inventoried and maintained on a regularly scheduled basis, in conjunction with policies established by the hospital's Biomedical Engineering Department.

Figure 6-2, cont'd

Continued

VIII. **INFORMED CONSENT**
- The informed consent for any short-term therapeutic, diagnostic or surgical procedure in which conscious sedation is to be administered should include the risks of conscious sedation, benefits and alternative options.

IX. **PRE-PROCEDURE ASSESSMENT AND DOCUMENTATION**

Prior to the procedure and the initiation of conscious sedation, it shall be ascertained that the patient is an appropriate candidate for conscious sedation utilizing the following criteria:

1.   The patient's state of consciousness and medical condition are appropriate for the use of conscious sedation.

3.   Preparatory studies appropriate to the procedure and the patient have been done, including a determination of the need for blood or blood products or other additional diagnostic data.

3.   There is a sedation plan and order written by the physician with clinical privileges to perform the procedure (or his designee), unless that physician will be administering the medication him/herself.

4.   The patient has no known allergies or sensitivities to the prescribed medication.

5.   The patient has been NPO for at least six hours prior to the planned procedure except for clear liquids, which may be given up to two hours before the procedure. Patients considered to be at risk for aspiration may require a longer NPO period. Medications may be administered with a sip of water. In cases of emergency, where the patient has not been NPO, IVCS may be dangerous. It should either not be administered or administered judiciously to avoid unconsciousness or suppression of protective airway reflexes.

6.   The patient/guardian has been informed by the physician of the risks and alternatives to sedation as a component of the planned procedure, and documentation of the patient's consent has been placed in the patient's record prior to the procedure.

7.   The patient has been instructed:
     a.   In the concepts of conscious sedation and about the sedation planned for the procedure, and
     b.   To report any problems associated with the procedure or conscious sedation (e.g., pain, tender site, itching, difficulty in breathing) to the individual responsible for monitoring the patient.

Figure 6-2, cont'd

8. A physical examination has been conducted which includes assessing/measuring the patient's:

   a. Actual or estimated height and weight
   b. Vital signs (baseline blood pressure; heart rate; respiratory rate, pattern and quality)
   c. Baseline oxygen saturation
   d. Airway (i.e., an evaluation performed in anticipation of possible intubation, e.g. checking condition of teeth; range of neck motion; ability to open mouth)
   e. Chest and cardiac status
   f. General neurologic status (e.g., assessing mental status; presence of stroke deficits) and
   g. Physical status (ASA physical status category)

9. Health evaluation has been documented including:

   a. Allergies and previous adverse drug reactions
   b. Current medications
   c. Diseases, disorders and abnormalities
   d. Prior hospitalizations
   e. Pertinent family history of diseases or disorders
   f. Review of systems

10. The patient has a functioning IV line or saline lock.

11. The patient's oxygen requirements are evaluated. The need for administration of supplemental oxygen via nasal prongs should be considered.
    Patients who are over the age of 60 or who have a medical history significant for heart, lung or kidney disease should be routinely given supplemental oxygen unless specifically contraindicated.

12. A rationale for sedation, sedative plan, and plan for post procedure care are documented.

13. Physician operator shall sign immediate preprocedure assessment and include phone number or page ID.

Such an assessment may be abbreviated as appropriate in emergencies.

X. **MONITORING**
The Board of Registration in Medicine recommends use of a standard real-time form to be included in the medical record, in which the patient's management and monitoring during IVCS would be documented.

Figure 6-2, cont'd

Continued

1.   During the procedure the designated monitor shall record:

a.   Heart rate, respiratory rate, blood pressure, sedation score, pain level. If the patient has been classified ASA III or greater, or has a history of cardiopulmonary disease, heart rate, and rhythm should be displayed continuously on a cardiac monitor. The oxygen saturation should be continuously displayed and recorded at 5-*minute* intervals.

b.   Medication given (route, site, time, drug, and dose), including oxygen therapy in liters/minute and means of delivery (e.g., nasal prongs).

c.   The patient's head position should be checked frequently to ensure a patent airway.

d.   If the patient becomes unstable during the procedure, appropriate medical consultation should be sought immediately.

2.   Following the procedure:

- The nurse in the post procedure area should continuously monitor the patient, and document vital signs (heart rate, blood pressure, respiratory rate, oxygen saturation, pain level) at 15-*minute* intervals for a minimum of 30 minutes following the end of the procedure.
- Beyond this thirty minute period, and, if stable, the above parameters should be monitored every 15 minutes until the patient has returned to preprocedure condition, or is transferred to other personnel performing recovery care.
- Functioning suction apparatus and capability for delivering more than 90% oxygen with bag and mask must be readily available in the post procedure recovery area.
- The patient must be observed for a minimum of 30 minutes following the procedure, and for two hours if reversal agents including flumazenil or naloxone have been given to reverse sedative/analgesics.

XI.   **POST-PROCEDURE PATIENT CARE AND DISCHARGE PLANNING**

1. Transfer to a nursing unit will only be permitted when the patient's PAR score is 8 or above or at baseline.
- Patient has stable vital signs (blood pressure, pulse, respiratory rate) and oxygen saturation (SaO_2).
- Patient's swallow, cough, and gag reflexes are present as appropriate to baseline.
- Patient is alert or appropriate to baseline.
- Patient's activity level is at pre-sedation baseline.

Figure 6-2, cont'd

2. Discharge to home will be permitted when the patient's PADS score is 9 or above or at baseline.
   - Patient has stable vital signs.
   - Patient can sit unaided if appropriate to baseline and procedure.
   - Patient can walk with assistance if appropriate to baseline and procedure.
   - Nausea and dizziness are minimal.
   - Hydration is adequate. Dressing/procedure site have been checked if applicable.
   - Discharge order has been written by the physician, or readiness for discharge has been determined by the RN using established criteria.

3. For patients being discharged to return home, the following apply:
   a. The ambulatory care patient may not leave the premises unless they are under the care of a competent adult.
   b. Written patient instructions include an explanation of potential or anticipated post sedation effects and limitations on activities and behavior including dietary precautions. Patients should be advised to refrain from operating heavy machinery, driving a car, consuming alcohol, and making important decisions for 12 to 24 hours. A 24-hour emergency contact telephone number should be provided.

4. If the patient is being transferred for further care within the facility, standard criteria for inter-unit transfer should be met.

Vice President Sponsor: Ken Sands, MD, VP, Health Care Quality

Approved By:

☒ **Medical Executive Committee: 5/26/04**   **Mary Anne Badaracco, MD**
                                                                              Chair, MEC

Requestor Name: Steven Pratt, MD

Date Original Approved: 10/01

Next Review Date: 05/01/07

Revised: 5/26/04

Eliminated:

References: See Conscious Sedation in the BIDMC Manual of Clinical Practice. Changes made to this document must also be made in the Manual of Clinical Practice.

Figure 6-2, cont'd

Table 6-1 | **ASA: Continuum of Depth of Sedation Definitions of General Anesthesia and Levels of Sedation/Analgesia**

Minimal sedation (anxiolysis)	A drug-induced state during which patients respond normally to verbal commands. Although cognitive function and coordination may be impaired, ventilatory and cardiovascular functions are unaffected.
Moderate sedation/ analgesia (conscious sedation)	A drug-induced depression of consciousness during which patients respond purposefully to verbal commands, either alone or accompanied by light tactile stimulation. No interventions are required to maintain a patent airway, and spontaneous ventilation is adequate. Cardiovascular function is usually maintained.
Deep sedation/analgesia	A drug-induced depression of consciousness during which patients cannot be easily aroused but respond purposefully following repeated or painful stimulation. The ability to independently maintain ventilatory function may be impaired. Patients may require assistance in maintaining a patent airway, and spontaneous ventilation may be inadequate. Cardiovascular function is usually maintained
General anesthesia	A drug-induced loss of consciousness during which patients are not arousable, even by painful stimulation. The ability to independently maintain ventilatory function is often impaired. Patients often require assistance in maintaining a patient airway, and positive pressure ventilation may be required because of depressed spontaneous ventilation or drug-induced depression of neuromuscular function. Cardiovascular function may be impaired.

From *American Society of Anesthesiologists. (2002). Practice guidelines for sedation and anesthesia by non-anesthesiologists, Anesthesiology, 96, 1004-1017.*

ensures that patient identification and site identification are in line with the JCAHO Universal Protocol (JCAHO, 2004). The process should clearly indicate that the patient has been an active participant in developing the plan of care, and that the plan has been communicated between providers.

Intraprocedural Care and Documentation

This section describes the monitoring process and includes its duration and the communication that is essential when a "hand-off" occurs from one care provider to another. The "time-out" should be documented as well.

Postprocedure Care and Discharge Planning

This section should include the recovery score, (e.g., Modified Aldrete PAR Score) that will be implemented in the care of the patient; duration of care; modifications in care related to the administration of reversal agents, if any are administered; discharge teaching; and plans for communication between the agency and the patient in the event of an emergency.

Signoff and Approvals

This section should include information such as the owner of the policy or guideline, the approval bodies and dates, and the next scheduled review date for the policy.

Bibliography

This section should identify any documents that have been used or referenced in the policy development or revision.

Step 4: Communication

A request for multidisciplinary input of comments and suggestions on the draft version should be sent out to all departments before final administrative approval. The accepted process for administrative approval of the protocol and methods for informing and educating staff should be identified. All health care providers who may be affected by the revised standard of care should be informed and educated as appropriate. One of the most common forms of communication is the development of a required in-service educational program for all staff who are responsible for the management of patients receiving moderate sedation and analgesia. Web pages and other electronic methods of communication have facilitated dissemination within a system and should be encouraged as a preferred way to give easy access to policies and procedures to all care providers throughout a facility.

Step 5: Outcome Evaluation

Part of the continuous quality improvement process should include a plan to monitor any variation from identified indicators and patient outcome. For example, if NPO status or airway assessment was not obtained before the procedure, such an occurrence should be identified, and any effects on patient outcome and treatment should be documented and forwarded to appropriate channels for review (e.g., anesthesia committee).

Management of a patient receiving moderate sedation and analgesia is identified by the JCAHO as high volume, high risk, and problem prone. A plan should be in place to measure and determine that the care delivered is attaining the desired patient effect. An institution should measure the outcome of patient care and identify the impact of the existing standard of care to determine if there are any opportunities for improvement (Figure 6-3).

Performance Manager

Interdisciplinary Conscious Sedation Use Documentation Review

Rate the overall legibility of record (All providers of care)

  ◌ Excellent   ◌ Good   ◌ Fair   ◌ Poor

Date of Service

Care Area/Unit

Medical Record Number

Encounter Number

Attending MD (Last name, first)

Date of Birth

Reviewed by

Review Date

ASA category patient

  ◌ Class I
  ◌ Class II
  ◌ Class III
  ◌ Class IV
  ◌ Class V

Informed consent, including conscious sedation, is documented

  ◌ Yes ◌ No

There is a complete pre-procedure assessment by the MD that is done within 30 days prior to the procedure and includes an update note within 7 days of the procedure.

  ◌ Yes ◌ No

The patient's airway has been assessed prior to the procedure.

  ◌ Yes ◌ No

The patient has been NPO for 6 hours for solid food and 2 hours for liquids.

  ◌ Yes ◌ No

Figure 6-3 Interdisciplinary conscious sedation use documentation review. *(Courtesy Beth Israel Deaconess Medical Center; Boston, Ma, 2004.)*

There is a pre-procedure plan for use of the conscious sedation with the procedure.　　○ Yes　○ No

There is an immediate pre-procedure assessment just prior to the administration of the sedation.　　○ Yes　○ No

Patient identification using 2 indicators is documented.　　○ Yes　○ No

The site/side is marked and/or confirmed prior to the procedure, if applicable.　　○ Yes　○ No　○ N/A

Images, implants and equipment are validated.　　○ Yes　○ No　○ N/A

There is a nursing pre-procedure assessment.　　○ Yes　○ No

There is baseline assessment of patient's vital signs prior to the procedure.　　○ Yes　○ No

Documentation of "time out" is documented immediately prior to start of procedure.　　○ Yes　○ No

Monitoring of the patient during the procedure shows heart rate of more than 120 or less than 40.　　○ Yes　○ No

Monitoring of the patient during the procedure shows systolic blood pressure rate of more than 200 or less than 90.　　○ Yes　○ No

There is monitoring of the patient's respiratory rate during the procedure.　　○ Yes　○ No

Monitoring of the patient during the procedure shows oxygen saturation rate less than 90%.　　○ Yes　○ No

Monitoring of the patient during the procedure shows sedation rate of less than 2 is achieved.　　○ Yes　○ No

Midazolam used is greater than 5 mg　　○ Yes　○ No

Fentanyl used greater than 250 mcg　　○ Yes　○ No

A reversal agent was required to recover the patient.　　○ Yes　○ No

Figure 6-3, cont'd

Continued

There is monitoring of the patient in the recovery area for at least one hour that reassesses vital signs, heart rate, blood pressure, respiratory rate, O2 saturation until the discharge criteria are met.	☐ Yes ☐ No
There is an assessment of pain during the recovery period.	☐ Yes ☐ No
The patient is given verbal and written discharge instructions just prior to discharge.	☐ Yes ☐ No
The patient is discharged with an escort (patient may not drive).	☐ Yes ☐ No
NO prohibited abbreviations are documented.	☐ Yes ☐ No ☐ N/A

Submit Survey   Clear Form

Back

Figure 6-3, cont'd

CONCLUSION

An institution's standard of care during a procedure requiring the administration of moderate sedation and analgesia by a nonanesthesia provider should be written clearly and concisely. The care provided to the patient should be based on both national and local recommendations. Ongoing continuous process improvement initiatives should be in place and included on Quality Improvement Dashboards. Compliance with the JCAHO patient care guidelines, the Universal Protocol and incorporation of the Patient Safety Goals throughout the continuum of care are essential to provide safe, seamless patient care.

REFERENCES

American Society of Anesthesiologists. (2002). Practice guidelines for sedation and anesthesia by non-anesthesiologists, Anesthesiology, 96, 1004-1017.

Association of periOperative Registered Nurses. (2004). "Recommended practices for managing the patient receiving moderate sedation/analgesia" in Standards, recommended practices and guidelines. Denver, CO: AORN, pp. 211-218.

Beth Israel Deaconess Medical Center. (2004). Procedure record. Boston: BIDMC, p. 1.

Joint Commission on Accreditation of Healthcare Organizations. (2004). 2004 national patient safety goals. Retrieved March 15, 2004 from http://www.jcaho.org/accredited+organizations/patient+safety/04+npsg/index.htm

Joint Commission on Accreditation of Healthcare Organizations. (2004) Provisions of care, treatment and services. In Comprehensive accreditation manual for hospitals, 2004 CAMH Refresher Core (PC 41-43). Oakbrook Terrace, IL: JCAHO.

Joint Commission on Accreditation of Healthcare Organizations. (2004). Universal protocol for preventing wrong site, wrong procedure, wrong person surgery. Retrieved March 15, 2004 from http://www.jcaho.org/accredited+organizations/patient+safety/universal+protocol/universal+protocol.pdf

7

Competence in Patient Management

Competence is a contemporary issue that has been addressed in the education, nursing, and health care literature for well more than 15 years. These disciplines have taken different approaches to assessing, developing, and maintaining competence in practitioners, and each has designed activities and mechanisms to establish, facilitate, enhance, monitor, and measure competence in practitioners. Increasing public awareness of health care issues and problems has further reinforced the necessity for an adequate number of professional, competent health care providers. This mandate is supported by all major accrediting (including the Joint Commission on Accreditation of Healthcare Organizations [JCAHO] and the Accreditation Association for Ambulatory Health Care [AAAHC]) and specialty organizations who demand that health care facilities show evidence of initial and ongoing demonstrations of staff competency (Hooper, 2002). Nowhere is competent care more crucial to positive patient outcome than in nonanesthesia-administered moderate sedation. The purpose of this chapter is to discuss the various concepts of competency in the practice setting and to describe techniques to determine appropriate unit and/or procedure-specific competencies. Sedation-specific competencies will then be addressed and a recommended program for implementation described.

AN OVERVIEW OF COMPETENCE

Speers and Ziolkowski (1996) define competence as "the capacity to perform job functions by an individual who has the knowledge, skills, behaviors, and personal characteristics necessary to function well in a given situation." Competence, regardless of environment, is a multifaceted concept that involves the realms of technical (cognitive and psychomotor), interpersonal, and critical thinking activities (Epstein & Hundert, 2002; Flanagan, Baldwin, & Clarke, 2000; LaDuke, 2000; Redman, Lenburg, & Walker, 1999). Competence is holistic in nature and involves both skill and knowledge, action, and critical thinking. As such, competence within a profession is often difficult to define and even more difficult to measure.

Competency-based practice in nursing integrates the knowledge, attitudes, skills, and behaviors necessary to maintain consistent standards of care within a specialty or practice setting. The competent nurse should:

- Maintain personal accountability for professional competency
- Participate in professional continuing educational activities
- Adhere to national, state, and specialty standards of nursing practice
- Comply with institutional policies and procedures regarding competence
- Accept responsibility and accountability for his or her specific area of nursing practice
- Participate in performance improvement activities
- Use competency-based orientation and annual review processes
- Remain current on new products and procedures affecting practice
- Practice with compassion and respect toward each individual patient/ family/significant other (American Society of PeriAnesthesia Nurses [ASPAN], 2002a).

Individualized competency-based practice in any employment setting develops over time as a result of personal education, continuing education, professional literature, and practice. Every nurse competent to care for the patient receiving moderate sedation brings to the bedside individualized practice standards that have been, and continue to be, molded by environmental changes such as new equipment, time constraints, staffing patterns, patient acuity levels, and payer and accreditation agency demands. Individual nurses may safely and effectively achieve the same patient outcomes via different routes or approaches in competent practice (Bargagliotti, Luttrell, & Lenburg, 1999). Competency assessment therefore must encompass more than a "skills checklist" but must be designed to incorporate individual practice differences. Competency in the practice setting must determine if the nurse carries out a procedure properly, but it must also determine if the nurse reacts to the complexities of patient care with responses that are contextually appropriate (Bradley & Huseman, 2003; LaDuke, 2000). Competency assessment must also be specific to the unit and to the patient population for whom the care is given.

DETERMINING APPROPRIATE COMPETENCIES

The first step in developing and measuring competency in the practice setting is to establish those practices or competencies that are unique to the particular practice environment, both from an orientation and an annual credentialing perspective. This should be a collaborative effort that involves the bedside nurse, management, and education. The emphasis for orientation competencies should be those competencies that require the minimal level of skill and knowledge to practice in a particular setting. Annual credentialing competencies should include those issues that are problem prone, high risk, and/or infrequently implemented (Hooper, 2002; Quinn, 2003).

The Competency Outcomes and Performance Assessment (COPA) model (Lenburg, 1999a; 1999b) recommends that the following four questions be answered.

1. What are the essential/core competencies and outcomes for the area of practice?
2. What are the indicators that define those competencies?
3. What are the most effective ways to learn those competencies?
4. What are the most effective ways to document achievement of the desired competencies?

The essential competencies and outcomes determined by answering question 1 tend to fall within one or more of eight core practice areas applicable to all practice settings. Each core practice area incorporates a flexible array of subskills that further specifies required practice abilities (Table 7-1). The core practice areas will help to shape the development of indicators for education and evaluation of the essential competencies (Lenburg, 1999a; 1999b). An example of how core practice areas can be grouped with an identified essential competency is noted in Table 7-2.

Once the essential competencies are grouped with core practice areas, then competency outcome statements can be developed. The outcome statements should be practice based and learner oriented. The language should be clear, concise, and action oriented; the statement should begin with the verb that most precisely describes the actual, preferred outcome that is desired (Lenburg, 1999b). Competency statements can be supported by specific criteria that allow for specific measurement or observation. An example is provided in Table 7-3.

SEDATION-SPECIFIC COMPETENCIES

The JCAHO (2004) standards clearly state that those health care providers administering sedation "must be qualified to manage the patient at whatever level of sedation or anesthesia is achieved, either intentionally or unintentionally." Therefore the practitioner administering moderate sedation should be qualified to rescue the patient from deep sedation. If the goal is to administer deep sedation, then the practitioner should be qualified to rescue the patient from the depth of general anesthesia. Health care providers administering both moderate and deep sedation should be competent to manage whatever level of sedation is achieved (Hooper, 2001). Competencies for all levels of health care providers involved (including physicians) should include comprehensive knowledge of medication administration and interaction, proven skills in airway management, and documented competence in dysrhythmia recognition and management (American Association of Nurse Anesthetists [AANA], 2003; American College of Radiology [ACR], 2000; American Dental Association [ADA], 2003; American Society of Anesthesiologists [ASA], 2002; ASPAN, 2002b;

Table 7-1 | COPA 8 Core Practice Areas With Subskill Examples

Core Practice Area	Subskill Examples
Assessment and intervention	Safety and protection
	Assessment and monitoring
	Therapeutic treatments and procedures
Communication	Oral skills
	Writing skills
	Computing skills
Critical thinking	Evaluation, integrating pertinent data from multiple sources
	Problem solving, diagnostic reasoning, creating alternatives
	Decision making, prioritizing
	Scientific inquiry, research process
Human caring and relationships	Morality, ethics, legality
	Cultural respect, cooperative interpersonal relationships
	Client advocacy
Management	Administration, organization, coordination
	Planning, delegation, supervision of others
	Human and material resource usage
	Accountability and responsibility, performance appraisals
Leadership	Collaboration, assertiveness, risk taking
	Creativity, vision to formulate alternatives
	Planning, anticipating, supporting with evidence
	Professional accountability, role behaviors, appearance
Teaching	Individuals and groups, clients, coworkers, others
	Health promotion, health restoration
Knowledge integration	Nursing, health care, and related disciplines
	Liberal arts, natural and social sciences, and related disciplines

Modified from Lenburg, C.B. (September 30, 1999b). The framework, concepts and methods of the competency outcomes and performance (COPA) model. Online Journal of Issues in Nursing [On-line]. Retrieved May 28, 2004 from http://www.nursingworld.org/ojin/topic10/tpc10_2.htm.

Association of periOperative Nurses [AORN], 2002; Martin & Lennox, 2003; Society of Gastroenterology Nurses and Associates [SGNA], 2001).

Medication Administration and Interaction

Competencies addressing medication administration and interaction must encompass all sedation and analgesic medications administered in the institu-

Table 7-2 | **Essential Competencies Grouped With Core Practice Areas**

Competency	Core Practice Areas
Airway management	Assessment and intervention Critical thinking Knowledge integration
Discharge teaching	Assessment and intervention Communication Critical thinking Human caring and relationships Teaching Knowledge integration

Table 7-3 | **Competency Statement With Supportive Criteria**

Competency Statement	Criteria
Demonstrate basic airway management	Perform a respiratory assessment on admission and discharge as per unit protocol and patient condition Identify signs and symptoms of respiratory distress or airway obstruction Identify existing and/or select airway adjunct and oxygen delivery systems based on adequacy of oxygenation and patient condition Determine level of consciousness Initiate the steps of basic life support if indicated Demonstrate use of bag-valve-mask apparatus Maintain patent airway as indicated Assess oxygen saturation via pulse oximetry Communicate and document all pertinent information per institution/unit specific policy/protocol

From Hannah, B. (2002). Airway management. In B. Gooden (Ed.). Competency based orientation credentialing program: 2002 edition. Cherry Hill, NJ: ASPAN, pp. 47-48.

tion for moderate sedation and all related reversal agents. Documented knowledge of adverse reactions, dosage, and route of administration should also be included. These competencies can be easily accomplished through the completion of a class or self-study module (SSM) that reviews all of the required information. Successful completion of a posttest provides documented evidence of successful knowledge acquisition (Hooper, 2001).

Airway Management

The most common emergencies associated with the administration of both moderate and deep sedation involve airway management. Therefore it is crucial that all parties involved in the administration and monitoring of the patient undergoing sedation demonstrate both didactic and skill-based competency regarding routine and emergency airway management. Competency recommendations addressing airway management are shown in Table 7-4.

Basic Dysrhythmia Recognition and Management

Cardiac dysrhythmias are commonly associated with hypoxia and respiratory depression and may also occur as a result of the actual procedure. For this reason, competence in basic ECG interpretation and dysrhythmia management is also crucial to the safe administration and management of sedation at all levels. Documented competencies should include basic ECG interpretation, dysrhythmia recognition and management, and the management of life-threatening dysrhythmias. These competencies, like medication administration and interaction, can also be accomplished through the successful completion of a dysrhythmia class or SSM reviewing all of these areas (Hooper, 2001).

Table 7-4 | Recommended Airway Management Competencies

Basic airway assessment	Oral cavity inspection
	Mallampati classification
	Presence of a patent airway
	Monitoring of the rate, depth, and general quality of respiratory effort
Pulse oximetry	Basic use and monitoring
	Troubleshooting
Basic airway management	Airway maneuvers
	Lateral head lift
	Chin lift/support
	Jaw thrust
	Airway adjuncts
	Nasal airway insertion
	Oral airway insertion
	Endotracheal tube insertion
	Oxygen delivery devices
Advanced airway management	Use of a positive pressure ventilation device
	Establishment of an airway via intubation

From Hooper, V.D. (2001). *Sedation standards part I*. Carrolton, TX: Health & Sciences Television Network. From Kost, M. (2004). Moderate sedation/analgesia. In D.M.D. Quinn & L. Schick (Eds.). *PeriAnesthesia nursing core curriculum: Preoperative, Phase I, and Phase II PACU nursing*. St. Louis: Saunders, pp. 432-433.

Emergency Management

In addition to individual competencies in all of the above areas, it is also recommended that competency in emergency management be documented. This competency can be easily documented through successful management of a mock code situation involving both respiratory and cardiac arrest (Hooper, 2001).

PROGRAM IMPLEMENTATION

All health care providers involved in the administration and management of patients undergoing procedures involving sedation should complete competency programs in moderate sedation. Although health care institutions have traditionally focused heavily on nursing competencies in the administration and management of moderate sedation, competencies must also be evident in the privileging and credentialing process for all nonanesthesia physicians involved in these procedures. This physician credentialing process is most commonly managed by the department of anesthesia (Hooper, 2001).

All sedation competency programs will contain similar elements; however, the administration of these programs should be geared to fit the requirements of the institution. Most health care facilities will develop and administer competency programs within their institution. However, smaller facilities may find it more cost effective to contract with other facilities or health care providers and/or educators to provide these programs. The airway and dysrhythmia management components of a sedation competency program can be addressed by successful completion of an Advanced Cardiac Life Support (ACLS) class. Supplementation of this class with the successful completion of SSM addressing all pharmacologic agents involved in sedation should arm the health care provider with all of the necessary knowledge and skills to manage emergent situations involved in the administration of and recovery from procedures involving sedation.

CONCLUSION

Competent care is crucial to positive patient outcome in nonanesthesia-administered moderate sedation. Sedation competencies should be established in a collaborative effort with the bedside provider (nurse, physician, etc.), management, and education involved, and should reflect those practices unique to the particular practice environment. These competencies should be holistic in nature and involve skill and knowledge, action, and critical thinking. Moderate sedation competencies should be didactic and skill based in nature and at a minimum should cover medication administration and interaction, airway management, dysrhythmia recognition and treatment, and emergency management. Completion of an orientation sedation competency program and continued annual competence evaluation should enable the health care provider to provide safe, quality care in the sedation environment.

REFERENCES

American Association of Nurse Anesthetists (AANA). (2003). Considerations for policy guidelines for registered nurses engaged in the administration of sedation and analgesia [On-line]. Available: http://www.aana.com/practice/conscious.asp.

American College of Radiology (ACR). (2000). ACR practice guideline for adult sedation/analgesia [On-line]. Available: http://www.acr.org/dyna/?doc=departments/stand_accred/standards/dl_list.html.

American Dental Association (ADA). (2003). Guidelines for the use of conscious sedation, deep sedation and general anesthesia for dentists [On-line]. Available: http://www.ada.org/prof/resources/positions/statements/anesthesia_guidelines.pdf.

American Society of Anesthesiologists (ASA). (2001). Practice guidelines for sedation and analgesia by non-anesthesiologists [On-line]. Available: http://www.asahq.org/publicationsAndServices/sedation1017.pdf.

American Society of PeriAnesthesia Nurses (ASPAN). (2002a). Perianesthesia standards for ethical practice. In ASPAN, 2002 standards of perianesthesia nursing practice. Cherry Hill, NJ: ASPAN, pp. 8-10.

American Society of PeriAnesthesia Nurses (ASPAN). (2002b). Resource 12: The role of the registered nurse in the management of patients undergoing sedation for short-term therapeutic, diagnostic or surgical procedures. In ASPAN, 2002 standards of perianesthesia nursing practice. Cherry Hill, NJ: ASPAN, pp. 47-48.

Association of periOperative Registered Nurses (AORN). (2002). Recommended practices for managing the patient receiving moderate sedation/analgesia. AORN Journal, 75, 642-652.

Bargagliotti, T., Luttrell, M., & Lenburg, C.B. (1999). Reducing threats to the implementation of a competency-based performance assessment system. Online Journal of Issues in Nursing [On-line]. Retrieved May 28, 2004, http://www.nursingworld.org/ojin/topic10/tpc10_5.htm.

Bradley, D., & Huseman, S. (2003). Validating competency at the bedside. Journal for Nurses in Staff Development, 19(4), 165-173.

Epstein, R.M., & Hundert, E.M. (2002). Defining and assessing professional competence. Journal of the American Medical Association, 287, 226-235.

Flanagan, J., Baldwin, S., & Clarke, D. (2000). Work-based learning as a means of developing and assessing nursing competence. Journal of Clinical Nursing, 9, 360-368.

Hannah, B. (2002). Airway management. In B. Gooden (Ed.). Competency based orientation credentialing program: 2002 edition. Cherry Hill, NJ: ASPAN, pp. 47-48.

Hooper, V. (2002). Introduction. In B. Gooden (Ed.). Competency based orientation credentialing program: 2002 edition. Cherry Hill, NJ: ASPAN, pp. 3-5.

Hooper, V.D. (2001). Sedation standards part I. Carrolton, TX: Health & Sciences Television Network.

Joint Commission on Accreditation of Healthcare Organizations (JCAHO). (January 1, 2004). Moderate sedation medication and patient monitoring. JCAHO FAQs [On-line]. Retrieved May 28, 2004 from http://www.jcaho.org/accredited+organiza-

tions/hospitals/standards/hospital+faqs/provision+of+care/anesthesia+care/sed+m
ed_pat+med.htm.

Kost, M. (2004). Moderate sedation/analgesia. In D.M.D. Quinn & L. Schick (Eds.). Peri-Anesthesia nursing core curriculum: Preoperative, Phase I, and Phase II PACU nursing. St. Louis: Saunders, pp. 432-433.

LaDuke, S. (2000). Competency assessments: A case for the nursing interventions classification and the observation of daily work. Journal of Nursing Administration, 30, 339-340.

Lenburg, C.B. (September 30, 1999a). Redesigning expectations for initial and continuing competence for contemporary nursing practice. Online Journal of Issues in Nursing [On-line]. Retrieved May 28, 2004 from http://www.nursingworld.org/ojin/topic10/tpc10_1.htm.

Lenburg, C.B. (September 30, 1999b). The framework, concepts and methods of the competency outcomes and performance (COPA) model. Online Journal of Issues in Nursing [On-line]. Retrieved May 28, 2004 from http://www.nursingworld.org/ojin/topic10/tpc10_2.htm.

Quinn, D.M.D. (2003). Perianestheia nursing as a specialty. In C.B. Drain (Ed.). Perianesthesia nursing: A critical care approach. St. Louis: Saunders, pp. 11-29.

Redman, R.W., Lenburg, C.B., & Walker, P.H. (September 30, 1999). Competency assessment: Methods for development and implementation in nursing education. Online Journal of Issues in Nursing [On-line]. Retrieved May 28, 2004 from http://www.nursingworld.org/ojin/topic10/tpc10_3.htm.

Society of Gastroenterology Nurses and Associates (SGNA). (2001). Standards of clinical nursing practice: Performance and standards of care for the gastroenterology and/or endoscopy setting. Chicago: SGNA.

Speers, A.T., & Ziolkowski, L. (1996). Preparing for the future: Perianesthesia orientation. Journal of PeriAnesthesia Nursing, 11, 133-142.

8

Pediatric Sedation

The patient undergoing sedation and analgesia has a "drug induced depression of consciousness during which the patient responds purposefully to verbal commands, either alone or accompanied by light tactile stimulation. No interventions are required to maintain a patent airway, and spontaneous ventilation is adequate" (American Society of Anesthesiologists [ASA], 2002). In the past, patient selection for nurse-monitored sedation generally included clinical conditions that allowed for a wide safety margin and predictability. Patients were healthy, over the age of 18, and without compromising systemic problems. Today registered nurses (RNs) and other nonanesthesia health care providers are monitoring acutely ill patients and those younger than 18 years. Proper education, experience, competence, and adherence to appropriate guidelines allow the nonanesthesia provider and physician to collaborate in the delivery of a safe sedation level for the pediatric patient undergoing diagnostic, therapeutic, or minor surgical procedures.

The process of sedating a pediatric patient begins with an approach that is appropriate for the child's developmental status, both psychologically and physiologically. Communication that is appropriate to the child's developmental stage enhances patient learning and reduces anxiety. Communication on the child's level and encouragement of parenteral participation can increase the child's level of trust in the health care provider (Box 8-1).

The pediatric population presents many challenges for the nonanesthesia provider responsible for monitoring and administering medications. Scarcity of information regarding pediatric drug dosages is further complicated by the fact that the level of sedation achieved by any given dose of medication is unpredictable and varies from patient to patient (Dial et al, 2001). Therefore providers must be knowledgeable about how the pediatric population differs from adult patients anatomically and physiologically and be prepared for the unpredictability of the effect of medications given.

Health care personnel caring for the pediatric sedation and analgesia patient must have a clear understanding of the desirable effects of moderate sedation and analgesia. These effects include alteration in perception of pain, maintenance of intact protective reflexes, initiation of slurred speech, easy arousal from

Box 8-1 GUIDELINES FOR COMMUNICATING WITH CHILDREN

Allow children time to feel comfortable.
Avoid sudden or rapid advances, broad smiles, extended eye contact or other
gestures that may be seen as threatening.
Talk to the parent if the child is initially shy.
Give older children the opportunity to talk without the parents present.
Assume a position that is at eye level with the child.
Speak in a quiet, unhurried, and confident voice.
Speak clearly, be specific, use simple words, and short sentences.
Offer choices only when they exist.
Be honest with children.
Allow them to express their concerns and fears.
Use a variety of communication techniques.

sleep, and minor variations in vital signs. Certain procedures call for a more
deeply sedated patient. Because the risks of deep sedation are similar to those
of general anesthesia, the patient should be monitored by professionals trained
in pediatric basic life support and pediatric airway management (Agency for
Healthcare Policy and Research [AHCPR], 1992; Lawson, 2000).

Deep sedation is "a drug-induced depression of consciousness during which
patients cannot be easily aroused but responds purposefully following repeated
or painful stimulation. The ability to independently maintain ventilatory function may be impaired. Patients may require assistance in maintaining a patent
airway, and spontaneous ventilation may be inadequate" (ASA, 2002). Administration of medications for the purpose of deep sedation may be specifically
regulated by individual state nurse practice acts. It is the individual nurse's
responsibility to be familiar with laws regarding the practice of nursing in the
state where the nurse is licensed. Lawson (2000) states that if deep sedation is
required, it should be performed by someone who is working to an accepted
guideline; whose sole responsibility is monitoring the sedated patient; who has
been trained to an acceptable level (such as pediatric advanced life support
[PALS]); who is familiar with drugs, dosages, monitoring equipment, and requirements; and who is supported by other skilled staff, such as a pediatric nurse.

Sedation is a continuum. Patients may pass from moderate to deep sedation
at any given time during a procedure. It is for this reason that children undergoing sedation require additional skilled personnel for careful monitoring.
Sedation practice guidelines (American Academy of Pediatrics [AAP], 1992) recommend that one assistant, generally a nurse who is skilled in airway management, devote exclusive attention to patient monitoring and not share in other
responsibilities of the procedure. A minimum of two assistants is therefore
required when sedation is administered for procedures in children. One assistant supports the airway and assesses vital signs, and the other prepares or

administers additional medication and assists with collection of specimens or other procedural interventions. Continuous assessment includes observation, monitoring, administering medications, and documenting the effects of these medications on the patient. Minimal monitoring parameters include respiratory rate, oxygen saturation, blood pressure (BP), cardiac rate and rhythm, level of consciousness, and skin condition. Documentation should occur at 5- to 15- minute intervals, depending on the patient's level of sedation (AAP, 1992) and should include monitoring parameters, medications administered, time, route, and level of consciousness (e.g., crying, awake and peaceful, drowsy, sleeping but arousable).

Children who demonstrate normal oxygen saturation by pulse oximetry may simultaneously have significant carbon dioxide retention. Capnography is a new technology that allows the accurate, real-time graphic display of ventilatory wave-forms in nonintubated patients by measuring their end-tidal carbon dioxide. Microstream capnography has been shown to provide a highly reliable meas-urement of abnormal ventilation in the adult population (Colman, 1999). Capnography may reveal that abnormal ventilation is occurring during proce-dures in children at rates higher than expected. One recent pilot study by Light-dale, Sethna, Heard, Donovan, and Fox (2002) found abnormal capnograms in 20% of children monitored by capnography and standard means. However, no patients in this pilot study had desaturation detected by pulse oximetry.

Although there are suggestions that microstream capnography may become a standard of care in the monitoring of the sedated patient, clinical effectiveness of this new technology for improving ability of staff to monitor children under-going moderate sedation has not yet been determined. Clinical trials are war-ranted to test the effectiveness of capnography at improving the safety of children undergoing sedation.

GUIDELINES

The following guidelines incorporate recommendations from the American Academy of Pediatrics (1992), the American Society of Anesthesiologists (2002), and the guidelines endorsed by 23 specialty nursing organizations (see Appen-dix C). These recommendations provide for an optimal achievable level of care for the RN monitoring the pediatric patient. The types of procedures vary and may be performed with or without local anesthesia in a variety of settings (e.g., emergency department, operating surgical suite, medical-surgical unit, catheter-ization laboratory, pediatric unit, endoscopy laboratory, and critical care unit). Medications should be administered under the direction and in the presence of a licensed independent provider. Serious complications may arise at any time during the administration of medications for sedation and analgesia. Therefore care is directed toward the prevention of these complications, which include (but are not limited to) hypoventilation, apnea, respiratory arrest, hypotension, aller-gic reaction, and cardiac depression.

Box 8-2 AAP ADDENDUM RECOMMENDATIONS

The AAP guidelines apply regardless of the setting where the sedation is performed.

Sedative or anxiolytic medications should not be administered at home preprocedure.

Sedative or anxiolytic medications should not be administered by anyone who is not medically skilled or supervised by skilled medical personnel.

When children are deeply sedated, at least one individual must be present who is trained in pediatric BLS and skilled in airway management, with PALS preferred.

Age- and size-appropriate resuscitation equipment and medications should be immediately available.

Children who receive sedative medication with long half-life may require extended observation.

Some children may best be served by sedation in a hospital setting.

From AAP Committee on Drugs. (2002). Guidelines for monitoring and management of pediatric patients during and after sedation for diagnostic and therapeutic procedures: addendum. Pediatrics, 110, 836-838.

Hoffman, Nowakowski, Troshynski, Berens, and Weisman (2002) tested whether use of an AAP/ASA-structured guideline model would reduce the risk of sedation-related adverse events. They discovered that the adverse event rate was 0 if all process guidelines were followed and concluded that there is direct evidence that AAP/ASA guidelines can reduce the risk of pediatric procedural sedation. The American Academy of Pediatrics revisited their guidelines on sedation for pediatric patients and continued to affirm that sedation of children is different from sedation of adults. In the addendum (AAP, 2002), they emphasized specific recommendations (Box 8-2).

Goals

The RN should be familiar with the goals of sedation for the pediatric patient, which are similar to those for the adult patient. These include (AAP, 1992) the following:

Ensure patient safety and welfare. Safe sedation of the pediatric patient is of primary concern. Consideration must be given to patient selection, skilled nursing staff, appropriate monitoring equipment, selective administration of medications, and preparedness to intervene in the event of an untoward effect.

Minimize physical discomfort or pain. How the RN manages the child's pain will influence the child's reaction to future procedures. During a painful procedure, opioids are frequently administered to alter the pain threshold by providing analgesia during and following the procedure.

Minimize negative psychologic responses. The patient should be provided with proper analgesia and emotional support throughout the sedation process to minimize the potential for negative psychologic responses.

Maximize potential for amnesia. Many medications are selected for their amnesic effects. Benzodiazepines are frequently administered for the excellent anxiolysis and amnesic effects they provide to the patient.

Control behavior. Administration of selective medications can often control pain and thus behavior, lessening the necessity for physical restraint.

Discharge safely. The patient receiving moderate sedation and analgesia should be monitored for an appropriate period of time. Recommended discharge criteria should be determined and met before the child is allowed to return to the unit or home. The American Academy of Pediatrics (1992) recommends the following criteria for discharge:

1. Cardiovascular function and airway patency are satisfactory and stable.
2. The patient is easily arousable, and protective reflexes are intact.
3. The patient can talk (if age appropriate).
4. The patient can sit up unaided (if age appropriate).
5. For a very young or disabled child incapable of the usual expected responses, the presedation level of responsiveness or a level as close as possible to the normal level for that child should be achieved.
6. The state of hydration is adequate.

Children who receive sedative medication with a long half-life may require extended observation (AAP, 2002; Malviya Voepel-Lewis, Prochaska, et al, 2000).

Patient Selection

Appropriate patient selection is critical. Requiring staff to monitor a patient who is beyond their skill and knowledge level places the patient at risk for a negative outcome and represents significant legal risk for the nurse, physician, and institution. Patient selection criteria or categories must be part of an institution's policy and procedure on sedation and analgesia. Patient selection for RN-monitored pediatric sedation and analgesia should include patients who are healthy or have only mild systemic disease. The classification system of patient physical status by the American Society of Anesthesiologists (ASA) is commonly used to determine appropriate patient categories for RN-monitored sedation (see Chapter 2). A normal healthy patient and a patient with mild systemic disease that is medically controlled and presents no contraindications to sedation and analgesia or for the procedure to be performed are appropriate candidates for nurse-monitored sedation. Very young children and children with co-morbid conditions are at a notably higher risk for adverse events (Shobha, Voepel-Lewis, & Tait, 1997) and should be individually assessed to determine if RN-monitored sedation is appropriate.

Personnel and Facility

Both the physician and the RN managing the care of the patient must be trained and adequately prepared to deal with life-threatening emergency situations. A minimum of three persons should attend to the pediatric patient, including a monitoring RN or anesthesia provider, who provides continuous uninterrupted monitoring of physiologic parameters throughout the procedure, an additional provider to assist during the procedure as necessary, and the physician performing the therapeutic, surgical, or diagnostic procedure. The physician performing the procedure is unable to provide uninterrupted monitoring of the patient because of the necessity to focus on the procedure itself. Therefore the physician cannot be responsible for monitoring the sedated patient. Depending on the type of procedure, the assistance of a fourth person—such as an RN, first assistant, or physician assistant—may be required.

The physician should be skilled in the appropriate selection of medications and trained in the management of complications related to sedation and analgesia. Training should include at minimum pediatric basic life support and, ideally, PALS, which includes skills for the management of a pediatric airway, use of positive-pressure ventilation, insertion of oropharyngeal and nasopharyngeal airways, and endotracheal intubation (AAP, 2002).

To minimize risks to the patient, the monitoring RN should be knowledgeable about all medications that might be administered to the pediatric patient. These medications include single doses or combinations of sedatives, hypnotics, anxiolytics, and opioids. The RN should be familiar with each medication; understand the indications, contraindications, potential adverse reactions and their management; drug interactions; acceptable pediatric dose ranges; and the use of antagonists. The RN providing care for the pediatric patient should be competent in the following areas:

Pediatric basic life support (cardiopulmonary resuscitation)
Pediatric airway management with documented competency
Patient assessment
Recognition of potential complications
Cardiac dysrhythmia interpretation
Pediatric advanced cardiac life support (recommended)

Emergency medications and emergency equipment to treat life-threatening complications should be immediately available. Essential equipment that should be present in the room includes a positive-pressure oxygen delivery system capable of delivering 90% oxygen or greater for a period of at least 60 minutes and an appropriate source of suction. Emergency equipment must be available in a range of sizes appropriate for the population of patients being treated. The emergency medication supply should include drugs in concentrations appropriate for use in children and a reference for calculation of dosages by weight. Antagonists for the medications used should also be immediately available in the room. If the facility is free standing, written protocols should include patient transportation to an acute care facility (e.g., ambulance) in the event of an adverse reaction.

The environment in which sedation is practiced is important to the safety and comfort of pediatric patients. The child's immediate environment should be inspected for potential hazards (e.g., uncovered electrical outlets and presence of small objects that could be ingested), and policies regarding fall prevention require strict adherence. Room temperature is often kept cool to prevent over-heating of electronic equipment. As a result, younger patients may be at risk for hypothermia (Hall, 2001). Preventive measures can be easily implemented and include the use of blankets, heating blankets, or warming lamps.

PREPROCEDURE ASSESSMENT

The pediatric patient should be assessed by the monitoring RN before the admin-istration of medications for sedation and analgesia. The purpose of the prepro-cedure assessment is to evaluate the patient for any known or unknown risk factors and to determine the appropriateness of RN monitoring for the patient. A relevant history should include age; allergies and previous allergic reactions; current and recent medications, including herbs and dietary supplements; time and type of last oral intake; personal or family history of sedation and/or anes-thesia and any untoward effects previously experienced; history of tobacco, alcohol, or substance abuse; history of co-morbidities, disorders, and hospital-izations; history of snoring or other symptoms that may indicate potential for airway obstruction; and a review of systems.

Of special interest is a history of asthma or other airway disease, cardiac disease, renal or hepatic impairment, or gastroesophageal reflux disease. Chil-dren with asthma should be allowed to continue bronchodilators until the pro-cedure begins, and drugs with histamine release should be avoided. Respiratory depression in children with congenital heart disease can lead to increased pulmonary vascular resistance with progressive cyanosis caused by hypercapnia. Children with renal or hepatic impairment are at risk for delayed metabolism of the drugs used in sedation. A child with gastroesophageal reflux disease may be a candidate for sedation with an anesthesia provider who can supply a protected airway. Neonates and infants require a history of gestational age, current post-conceptual age, and any history of apnea. Adolescents need to be screened for any possibility of pregnancy (Malviya Voepel-Lewis, Tait, et al, 2000).

Physical examination should include weight in kilograms, baseline vital signs including BP, heart rate, respiratory rate, oxygen saturation, cardiac rate and rhythm, and level of consciousness. The physical examination should include an examination of airway, pulmonary, and cardiac status, and observation for loose teeth or dental appliances. Oral and tongue piercings must be removed before the administration of sedation (Marenzi, 2004).

Assessing the airway may be difficult with the very young patient. Any abnor-mal anatomic finding, such as inability to hyperextend the neck or an abnormal airway, such as micrognathia, high arched palate, and macroglossia may indi-cate the necessity for an anesthesia provider and should be reported to the physi-cian. Because of the relatively thin chest wall in pediatric patients, breath sounds may be referred from one lobe to another, necessitating auscultation over all lung fields. Abnormalities in breath sounds (e.g., wheezing, stridor) should be reported to the physician before any sedative medications are administered.

A pain assessment should be conducted for the child and any assessment tools explained to the child and caregiver (Box 8-3). The preparedness of the child for the procedure should be assessed and an appropriate informed consent obtained. See Table 8-1 for other assessments important to the pediatric patient.

The patient's fasting history is important and should be emphasized when gathering the information from both the child and the parent or responsible person. Fasting guidelines include clear liquids up to 2 hours before the procedure (Table 8-2). The patient is at risk for aspiration of gastric contents if an appropriate period of time for gastric emptying has not been allowed.

In an emergency situation, the physician must determine whether the risks of delaying the procedure outweigh the potential risks for aspiration. Although light sedation and local anesthesia may be used, there are other risk factors that may increase the risk for aspiration. These risks include obesity, hiatal hernia, peptic ulcer, old age, diminished pharyngeal reflexes, full stomach, and opioid administration (Mamaril, 2000). In the presence of these risk factors—inadequate preprocedure fasting time and the emergent necessity for a procedure—

Table 8-1 | Preoperative Assessments Important to the Pediatric Patient

Physical

Head circumference
Loose teeth
Skin: rashes, possible signs of communicable disease
Recent exposure to communicable disease
Currency of vaccinations
Recent illness of child or siblings

Social

Parental validation of NPO status
Preferred name to be called
Specific fears
Typical behavior patterns when in pain

Parental

Understanding of preoperative instructions, especially NPO ramifications
Availability of child care assistance for travel
Availability of child car seat and/or appropriate restraint device
Resources for postoperative care of child
Understanding of potential complications: signs and symptoms, when to call for help

---

From Ireland, D. (2000). Pediatric patients and their families. In N. Burden, D.M.D. Quinn, D. O'Brien, & B.S.G. Dawes (Eds.). Ambulatory surgical nursing. Philadelphia: Saunders, p. 620.

Box 8-3   NURSING CARE OF THE CHILD IN PAIN

Focused Assessment

Regardless of setting (inpatient, clinic, or home), the nursing assessment for the child in pain begins in the same way if the child is verbal. The child is questioned to determine what word or words are used for pain. Then the parents are questioned as to cultural or spiritual beliefs or practices that might impact pain issues. The nurse should remember that parents are to be used as the first resource to help assess the child and the child's response to intervention. Then a pain history is taken from child and parent, including physical, emotional, or psychosocial factors that might affect the child in regard to pain.

The current pain is assessed as to onset, duration, location, intensity, and quality. An age-appropriate pain tool is used to assess the intensity of pain. The same tool is used consistently and it becomes a part of the child's chart as a future reference. Behavioral and physiologic changes are noted also. If the child is preverbal or nonverbal, a behavioral assessment is completed along with use of an assessment tool designed for nonverbal children. Response to the interventions, pharmacologic and nonpharmacologic, is assessed again using pain tools, parents' input, and observation of behavioral and physiologic data.

Nursing Diagnosis

Acute pain related to physical or biologic factors: edema, disease process, infection, invasive procedure, surgery, and trauma.

Expected Outcomes

The child will experience a decrease in pain to an acceptable level as evidenced by reduced pain level on an assessment tool, and demonstrate a relaxed body posture, decreased crying, fussiness, restlessness, and facial grimacing. The child will return to the activity level experienced before the onset of pain.

Intervention	Rationale
1. Observe and document behavioral and physiologic signs of pain in the child. Note both verbal and nonverbal responses. Assess vital signs.	1. Assessment of pain in children is based on behavioral and physiologic changes. Children may have difficulty verbalizing pain. The nurse will have to depend on behavioral changes alone to assess infants and other children who are nonverbal or unable to communicate clearly. Physiologic changes vary in response to pain and should be evaluated together with a behavioral assessment.

From James, S.R., Ashwill, J.W., & Droske, S.C. (2002). *Nursing care of children*, 2nd Ed. Philadelphia: Saunders, pp. 434-435.

Continued

Box 8-3   NURSING CARE OF THE CHILD IN PAIN—cont'd

Intervention	Rationale
2. Assess for other factors that might be affecting the child: separation, fear, anxiety, loss of control, and spiritual or cultural beliefs regarding pain.	2. The child's perception of pain and ultimate reaction to pain may be influenced by other factors.
3. Monitor pain based on the child's developmental stage.	3. Infants and children at each developmental level have their own unique way of reacting to and coping with pain.
4. Use a developmentally appropriate pain assessment tool. The tool should be a part of the child's chart for easy reference.	4. Infants and children may have difficulty communicating about their pain. Assessment tools provide more consistent, objective, and quantitative information.
5. Question the child if possible to assess the onset, duration, location, and type of pain and what type of pain relief measures works best.	5. Such factors will influence the choice of analgesic.
6. Note if the child's pain level is different when at rest, ambulating, playing, or during procedures.	6. Pain relief measures can be improved by a thorough understanding of cause and effect.
7. Implement nonpharmacologic pain reduction strategies:	7. Nonpharmacologic pain management strategies can enhance pharmacologic measures and should be implemented before administering analgesics.
a. Distraction	a. Distraction interrupts the transmission of pain.
b. Relaxation techniques	b. Relaxation is also thought to interrupt pain.
c. Cutaneous stimulation, such as massage or warm or cold compresses	c. Cutaneous stimulation blocks pain transmission.
d. Quiet, calm environment	d. A quiet, calm environment is more conducive to rest and sleep, which enhance the effects of analgesia.
e. Repositioning	e. A change in position may relieve pressure or provide for a more relaxed, comfortable body.
f. Decreased environmental noise and light	f. A quiet, comfortable environment can have a soothing, relaxing effect on the child and parent.

Table 8-2 | **Fasting Guidelines**

Food	Minimum Fasting Period
Clear liquids	2 hr
Breast milk	4 hr
Infant formula	6 hr
Nonhuman milk	6 hr
Light meal	6 hr

Data from ASA. (2002). Practice guidelines for sedation and analgesia by non-anesthesiologists. Anesthesiology, 96, 1007.

the possibility of requiring endotracheal intubation increases. As a result, an anesthesia provider is the most appropriate individual to provide patient monitoring under these circumstances.

INTRAPROCEDURE ASSESSMENT

More than 23 nursing specialty organizations support the position statement on the Role of the Registered Nurse (RN) in the Management of Patients Receiving IV Conscious Sedation for Short-Term Therapeutic, Diagnostic, or Surgical Procedures, which states: "The nurse managing the care of the patient should have no other responsibilities that would leave the patient unattended or compromise continuous monitoring" (American Nurses Association, 1991). Nineteen boards of nursing replying to a recent survey (Appendix B) stated specifically that the RN managing the care of the patient should have no other duties that leave the patient unattended (Odom-Forren, 2004). One nurse responsible for monitoring the patient should be provided throughout the procedure. The following monitoring parameters should be obtained and documented throughout the procedure: oxygen saturation, heart rate and rhythm, respiratory rate, adequacy of ventilatory function, BP, level of consciousness, and skin color. Measurement of BP may awaken a child who otherwise would be asleep and cooperative. The frequency of BP monitoring is left to the discretion of the physician based on the condition of the patient and procedure performed (Malviya, Voepel-Lewis, & Tait, et al, 2000).

Because medications administered for sedation and analgesia may result in decreased respirations or respiratory distress, close continuous visual monitoring is critical. The monitoring RN should continuously assess the patient's airway patency. Care should be taken that restraining devices, drapes, and equipment do not block the ability of the RN to visually assess the patient's respiratory and ventilatory status. Table 8-3 identifies five assessment parameters to aid in determining respiratory distress in the pediatric patient. Although the pulse oximeter is used as an aid in providing an early warning of hypoxemia, the RN should also closely monitor chest excursion, ventilatory effort, skin color, and

Table 8-3 | **Signs and Symptoms of Respiratory Distress in the Pediatric Patient**

	Mild Respiratory Distress	*Moderate Respiratory Distress*	*Severe Respiratory Distress*	*Respiratory Failure*
Appearance/ level of consciousness	Alert	Alert or may be confused	Lethargic	Unresponsive
Skin color and color of mucous membranes	Pink	Pink or cyanotic	Cyanotic	Cyanotic
Respiratory rate	Mildly increased	Mildly to moderately increased	Markedly increased	Decreased or apneic
Work of breathing	Subcostal retractions	Subcostal retractions Intercostal and sternal retractions Nasal flaring	Subcostal retractions Intercostal and sternal retractions Nasal flaring Suprasternal retractions	Decreased respiratory effort or none
Heart rate	Mildly increased	Mild to moderately increased	Markedly increased	Decreased

American Academy of Pediatrics, 2002, American Heart Association: Pediatric advanced life support (PALS) provider manual.

the color of mucous membranes. Microstream capnography may be a useful adjunct to the respiratory assessment of the sedated pediatric patient (Vargo et al, 2002 [Tables 8-4 and 8-5]).

The parent who stays in the room during the procedure should be shown where to sit or stand. It is helpful to assign a specific job to the parent, such as holding the child's hand or talking to the child. The parent should not help restrain the child but should be a comfort to the child.

POSTPROCEDURE ASSESSMENT

Some patients become more deeply sedated after the stimulus of the procedure is discontinued. In addition, the pharmacokinetic profile of the sedative medications used may have prolonged effects (AAP, 2002; Malviya Voepel-Lewis,

Table 8-4 | **Normal Respiration and Heart Rates for the Pediatric Patient**

Age	Respiration (Breaths/min)	Heart Rate (Beats/min)
Infant (birth-12 mo)	30-60	120-160
Toddler (1-3 yr)	25-40	90-140
Preschool-age child (4-6 yr)	22-34	80-110
School-age child (6-12 yr)	18-30	75-100
Adolescent (13-18 yr)	12-20	60-100

From Maldonado, S.S. & LeBoeuf, M.B. (2003). Pediatric surgery. In J.C. Rothrock, (Ed.). Alexander's care of the patient in surgery. (12th Ed.). St. Louis: Mosby, p. 1266.

Table 8-5 | **Estimating Blood Pressure for the Pediatric Patient**

Systolic BP (mm Hg) = (2 × age in years) + 80
Diastolic BP (mm Hg) = 2/3 systolic BP

From Maldonado, S.S., & LeBoeuf, M.B. (2003). Pediatric surgery. In J.C. Rothrock, (Ed.). Alexander's care of the patient in surgery. (12th Ed.). St. Louis: Mosby, p. 1266.

Prochaska, et al, 2000). As a result, appropriate recovery and discharge procedures are critical to the safety of pediatric patients undergoing sedation. The patient should be transported to the designated recovery area until the criteria for discharge are met. The same monitoring parameters previously described should be obtained until the patient returns to baseline level of responsiveness (i.e., oxygen saturation, heart rate and rhythm, respiratory rate, BP, level of consciousness, and skin color). Before the patient is discharged, written discharge instructions should be provided to the parent or responsible escort. Discharge instructions should include fluid intake, diet, activity, and any instructions specific to the procedure that was performed. An infant who has been sedated should not ride alone in the back seat in a restraint. One parent or caregiver should ride in the back seat next to the infant to ascertain that the infant does not fall asleep and obstruct the airway.

Developmental Approaches to the Care of the Child Undergoing Sedation and Analgesia

Age-specific and/or developmentally appropriate care of the pediatric patient is essential for positive outcomes in the sedation of children. Anxiety can be minimized by providing care based on a sound knowledge of childhood growth and development. Several theorists have presented their beliefs on social behavior and growth and development. Erik Erikson's theories are the most widely accepted and used in pediatric care (Fox, 2000; Rayhorn, 1998).

Infants

Erikson defines infancy as the age of "trust vs. mistrust." Infants are dependent on adults to meet their needs; therefore they must continue to have their needs met for a successful care plan. Getting acquainted with the child while in the parent's company will help to gain the child's trust. Comfort and security items, such as pacifiers, blankets, or soft toys, should remain with the child. Encouraging parents to stay with their child until the sedative agents have taken effect helps prevent separation anxiety. This is especially true with infants between 6 and 12 months old. During the sedation period it is acceptable to allow infants to be held by their parent. While patients are in the parent's arms, the nurse must pay close attention to the airway of the child. Once the sedation begins to take effect, the infant may be transitioned to the procedure bed from the parent's arms. Parents should be reminded to remain quiet and use subdued vocalizations with their child during this period so as not to interrupt their sedation. If the child uses thumb sucking for comfort, every effort should be made to keep the thumb free. Intravenous access should be obtained on the opposite hand whenever possible.

Toddlers

Erikson defines toddlers as the developmental period of "autonomy vs. shame." This period spans from 1 to 3 years of age. Children in this developmental stage often experience fear of abandonment. For this reason it is important to maintain parenteral presence in the procedure area until the child is sedated to allow for easy separation. Language is developing in this age group and decision-making skills. Toddlers are renowned for wanting to "do it myself." Giving the toddler small tasks, such as allowing them to place an ECG sticker on a doll, can integrate them into their care. Using a papoose in children in this age group allows them security while removing their feelings of shame for not being able to cooperate with the procedure to be done.

Preschool

"Initiative vs. guilt" marks the developmental stage of the preschooler as described by Erikson. In this age group of 3 to 6 years, the preschooler is able to initiate activities. They begin to experience enjoyment from learning; however, their difficulty in mastering tasks may lead to fear of failure and punishment. Interventions in this group include parenteral presence in the induction phase of sedation. The preschooler should be allowed to make simple choices. For example, the child can be allowed to choose which arm to have his BP measured. Care must be taken to set limitations on these choices, however. When performing tasks with children in this developmental group, it is important not to ask for permission, for example, "Can I start your IV now?" Undoubtedly the answer will be "no." Behavioral interventions to encourage and reinforce positive behaviors include praise and rewards, such as stickers. Children of this age group will remember information; therefore it is important to include them in teaching.

School Age

The next developmental level is the school-age child. Erikson describes this phase as "industry vs. inferiority." The age range is 6 to 11 years. Children in this group are moving from concrete to abstract thinking. They have a heightened interest in their environment, resulting in an intense curiosity level. They are beginning to master cognitive and physical skills. They are also developing self-esteem and their sense of humor.

Children in this developmental group can adhere to rules and are able to follow direction. Therefore they may be more involved in their care. Parents may or may not be present during induction of sedation. The child may want to be included in this decision making. All questions that the child asks must be answered truthfully. Incorrect or untruthful answers can lead to mistrust and feelings of betrayal. Since children in the school-age years are developing their self-esteem, care must be taken to maintain their modesty. Privacy while changing and taking care not to expose them unnecessarily is essential. Children in this age group must be involved in teaching. They are inquisitive and need to know and understand what to expect from their procedure.

Adolescence

The final stage of childhood development is adolescence. Erikson defines this period as "identity vs. role confusion." Adolescents are undergoing physical and emotional growth. They need to be involved in their care. Allowing some control of their environment may result in better cooperation from this age group. This can be established by giving the patient choices (i.e., parents in room, music choices, and wearing a hospital gown vs. own clothes). It is important to maintain their modesty by limiting staff in the room and for staff to prevent unnecessary exposure of the patient. Teaching should be directed to adolescents with explanations of what to expect preprocedure, intraprocedure, and postprocedure. Ensuring that the patient understands follow-up care is essential. Including parents in this discussion may be beneficial to ensure proper follow-up is achieved.

MEDICATION ADMINISTRATION

Selection of medications and route of administration are determined by the physician. Many medications administered for sedation and analgesia are not approved for pediatric use as evidenced by the information presented in the *Physicians' Desk Reference (PDR)* and pharmaceutical package insert material. Detailed research involving appropriate clinical trials is required by the Food and Drug Administration before recommended dosages may appear in the *PDR* and pharmaceutical educational materials. However, this does not prevent the administration of such medications to populations for whom little research exists. The physician is responsible for the selection of such medications, and the monitoring RN should be trained and competent in the administration of each medication.

Determination of Dosage

The physician is responsible for selecting and determining the correct dosage to achieve the desirable effects of sedation and analgesia. The RN is responsible for the administration of sedation and analgesia medication(s) under the direction of the physician and for monitoring the patient. The RN must be knowledgeable about the pharmacologic effects of each medication administered, including indications, contraindications, the expected action, duration of action, typical pediatric dosage, possible adverse effects, and available reversal agents.

Although the physician is responsible for determining the dosage, the RN who administers the medication is also legally responsible for understanding the appropriate dosage for the pediatric patient. A variety of formulas may be used to determine pediatric medication dosage. However, formulas determine pediatric dosages in relation to standard adult dosage and are often inaccurate. Sedation dosages must be clearly defined based on the patient's weight. There must be maximum dose ranges identified and appropriate intervals for administration. Institutions that provide care for children undergoing sedation must establish appropriate policies and procedures that address all aspects of caring for these patients.

Route of Administration

Adverse events have been associated with all routes by which sedation can be administered and the use of multiple drugs increases this potential (Fiordalisi, 2003). The ability to titrate the dose to the desired effect is lost with the oral, rectal, and intramuscular (IM) routes, making the IV route more desirable in many situations.

Oral Sedation

Children often exhibit increased anxiety in response to medical interventions. Intravenous sedation and analgesia is an effective method of pediatric sedation. The insertion of the IV catheter for sedation use can cause fear and anxiety in children. Procedures requiring IV sedation may benefit from the use of an oral premedication dose of midazolam.

Oral sedation offers advantages over other routes, because it is essentially painless and is convenient to administer. Disadvantages of oral sedation include the time required to maximize the sedative effect and lack of adequate sedation for invasive or painful procedures. In addition, antagonists (reversal agents) are not available for a significant number of oral sedatives. There have been rare adverse events associated with oral sedation. Most catastrophic events can be attributed to four factors: inadequate preoperative evaluation, lack of knowledge concerning the pharmacology of drugs employed, inadequate monitoring during the procedure, and lack of training in the management of emergencies (Silegy & Jacks, 2003).

Care must be taken to measure the dose accurately. A plastic disposable syringe offers the most accurate method for measuring small pediatric doses. It may also serve as a convenient vehicle for administering the medication. When administering the medication, the RN should place the syringe tip along the side of the mouth and slowly squirt the medicine toward the buccal vestibule, not toward the throat. Medications that are not palatable may be mixed with flavoring to disguise the taste (e.g., flavored syrups and juice).

Intramuscular Sedation

IM sedation is infrequently used because of the discomfort caused to the patient and the lack of predictability of the sedative level. In the absence of intravenous access, the ability to administer opioid or benzodiazepine antagonists in an emergency situation is severely compromised. However, there may be rare instances in which administration of sedative medications via the IM route is indicated. The preferred IM injection sites for children include the vastus lateralis, ventrogluteal, dorsogluteal, and deltoid. Most basic nursing textbooks include information on IM injection techniques for use with pediatric patients. Medications from a glass ampule should be drawn up with a filtered needle to prevent injecting small fragments of glass.

Rectal Sedation

Rectal sedation is often used for the patient who is unable to take medication by mouth. One major disadvantage of this method is that the level of sedation is unpredictable. For example, absorption of the medication is delayed if stool is present.

The suppository is administered by gently inserting it into the rectum beyond the anal sphincter. If the child expels the suppository, it may be reinserted by gently holding the buttocks together until the urge to expel the contents passes. Because of the imprecise measurement of medication that is achieved by cutting or breaking a suppository, a dose of less than one full suppository is not recommended.

Intravenous Administration

Intravenous (IV) administration allows for titration of medication to the desired patient response. The most common sites selected for IV sedation in pediatric patients are the superficial veins in the hand, foot, wrist, or arm. Often the biggest fear of the pediatric patient is the IV insertion. Fear of "the shot" causes increased stress and worry in the child. This fear can span all age groups. A local dermal anesthetic, such as lidocaine plus prilocaine cream (EMLA, Astra

Pharmaceuticals, Wayne, Pa.) or lidocaine plus epinephrine delivered by iontophoresis (Numby, Iomed, Inc., Salt Lake City) can be used to minimize the pain of needle stick (Love, 2000; Squire, Kirchhoff, & Hissong, 2000).

EMLA 5%, a eutectic mixture of local anesthetics, may be applied to the site to provide analgesia before venipuncture. To achieve optimal effects, the EMLA cream should be applied to the potential site(s) 60 minutes before venipuncture and covered with a moisture-proof dressing to prevent the cream from rubbing off. The Numby Stuff system employs two pads: a grounding pad and a medication pad. A hand-sized box is attached to these pads via lead wires. When the device is in place it delivers 2, 3, or 4 milliamperes (mA) of electrical current to administer the medicine quickly into the skin. At 2 mA numbing is achieved in 20 minutes, at 3 mA in 14 minutes, and at 4 mA in just 10 minutes. Another benefit of Numby Stuff is the depth of anesthetic. Topical anesthesia is achieved to a depth of 10 mm (1 cm) as opposed to EMLA, which can only penetrate to 3 to 4 mm. Because venipuncture is frightening for the pediatric patient, distraction techniques, such as stickers, music, and bubbles, should be used.

A variety of IV catheters are available for pediatric use in a wide range of sizes. If IV fluids are administered, caution should be taken to prevent the potential for fluid volume overload. This is most frequently accomplished through the use of a drip control chamber (e.g., Burette). Drip control chambers can be used in conjunction with a mechanical IV pump. Pediatric IV administration sets are calibrated to flow at 60 drops per milliliter. An appropriate period of time should be allowed for full evaluation of the effects of the medication on the patient.

Commonly Administered Medications

Nursing staff should be educated about the proper administration of all medications that are approved by the institution for pediatric sedation. Table 8-6 lists doses of medications commonly used for pediatric sedation. This list is only a guide. Consideration should be given to the type of procedure, age of the child, weight, anxiety level, desired level of sedation, and route options for the particular medication.

CONCLUSION

The RN responsible for the management of the pediatric patient scheduled for sedation and analgesia must be competent in the psychologic, emotional, and physiologic care of the child. He or she must be proficient in pediatric airway management and interventions. Knowledge of the child's age and weight is essential to determine appropriate medication dose ranges before administering any medication. It is recommended that institutions have a separate standard of care for the administration of sedation and analgesia that includes detailed guidelines for the nonanesthesia provider caring for children undergoing diagnostic and therapeutic procedures (see Appendix G).

Table 8-6 | **Drugs Commonly Used for Sedation**

	Dose*	Usual Adult Dose	Onset	Duration	Comments†
Pentobarbital	i.v.: 1-6 mg/kg	100 mg	3-5 min	15-45 min	Give i.v. doses in aliquots of 1-2 mg/kg until desired effect
	i.m.: 2-6 mg/kg	150-200 mg	10-15 min	60-120 min	
	p.r.: <4 y 3-6 mg/kg >4 y 1.5-3 mg/kg	120-200 mg	15-60 min	1-4 h	
Thiopental	i.v.: neonates 3-4 mg/kg infants 5-8 mg/kg children 1-12 y 5-6 mg/kg >12 y 3-5 mg/kg	3-5 mg/kg	30-60 sec	5-30 min	Contraindicated in porphyria i.v.: for induction of anesthesia
	p.r.: 5-10 mg/kg 25 mg/kg (deep sedation)	3-4 g/dose	7-10 min	1-5 h	
Methohexital	i.v.: 0.5-1.5 mg/kg	20-40 mg	1 min	7-10 min	Infants <1 mo: safety not established
	p.r.: 20-35 mg/kg	500 mg	5-15 min	1-1.5 h	p.r.: use 1% solution; avoid in patients with temporal lobe epilepsy or porphyria
Diazepam	i.v./i.m.: 0.04-0.3 mg/kg	5-7.5 mg	i.v.: 1-5 min i.m.: within 20 min	i.v.: 15-60 min i.m.: unknown	
	p.r.: 0.2-0.4 mg/kg		Unknown	4-12 h	
	p.o.: 0.2-0.3 mg/kg	10 mg	30-60 min	Up to 24 h	

From Perkin, R., Swift, J.D., & Newton, D.A. (2003). *Pediatric hospital medicine: Textbook of inpatient management. Philadelphia: Lippincott, Williams & Wilkins*, pp. 767-768.

i.v., Intravenous; *i.m.*, intramuscular; *p.r.*, rectal; *p.o.*, oral.

*Doses are those usually required; smaller doses should be given for higher-risk patients or when given in conjunction with other neurotropic drugs likely to cause sedation (e.g., opiates).

†Comments do not include all adverse effects and contraindications. The reader is referred to *Pediatric Dosage Handbook, 8th ed. Cleveland: Lexi-Comp*, 2001.

Continued

Table 8-6 | Drugs Commonly Used for Sedation—cont'd

	Dose*	Usual Adult Dose	Onset	Duration	Comments†
Lorazepam	i.v., i.m., p.o.: 0.05 mg/kg	2-4 mg	i.v.: within 15-30 min	8-12 h	Use with caution in neonates, congestive heart failure, renal, pulmonary, hepatic disease; full recovery may take up to 24 h
	May use 0.01-0.03 mg/kg every 20 min; titrate to effect		i.m.: within 30-60 min	8-12 h	
			p.o.: within 60 min	8-12 h	
Midazolam	i.v.: 6 mo-5 y: 0.05-0.1 mg/kg up to 0.6 mg/kg or 6 mg (max total dose) 6-12 y: 0.025-0.05 mg/kg up to 4 mg/kg or 10 mg (max total dose) 12-16 y: 1-2 mg/dose Usual total dose 2.5-5 mg	6 mg	1-5 min	20-30 min	
	i.m.: 0.1-0.15 mg/kg up to 0.5 mg/kg or 10 mg (max total dose)		5 min	Up to 6 h	
	p.o.: 6 mo-5 y and less cooperative patients: up to 1 mg/kg may be required ≥6 y or cooperative patients or high-risk patients: 0.25 mg/kg Maximum oral dose: 20 mg	20 mg	10-20 min	*Approximately* 30-60 min	

	Dose	Onset	Duration	Comments
	i.n.: 0.2-0.3 mg/kg May repeat in 5-15 min s.l.: 0.2 mg/kg	Within 5 min	30-60 min	i.n.: use 5 mg/mL concentration; 1/2 dose In each nare s.l.: use 2 mg/ml flavored syrup Emergence reactions, especially in patients >15 y; minimized with concomitant use of midazolam
Ketamine	i.v.: 0.5-1 mg/kg aliquots Usual dose 1-2 mg/kg	1 min	Approximately 30-60 min 5-10 min	Contraindicated in raised intracranial pressure, raised intraocular pressure, hypertension, and similar conditions Excellent analgesic
	i.m.: 2-3 mg/kg aliquots up to 7 mg/kg	7 min	15-25 min	
Chloral hydrate	p.o./p.r. Neonates: 25 mg/kg × 1 dose only	30-100 min	4-8 h	Cannot be easily "titrated" to effect; oversedation and respiratory depression can occur Contraindicated in cardiac, renal, hepatic dysfunction, gastritis/ulcers
	Infants/children: 25-50 mg/kg × 1 dose: may be repeated × 1 in 30 min to max 100 mg/kg or 1 g for infants, 2 g for children	10-100 min		

i.n., Intranasal; *s.l.,* sublingual.

Continued

Table 8-6 | Drugs Commonly Used for Sedation—cont'd

	Dose*	Usual Adult Dose	Onset	Duration	Comments†
Flumazenil	i.v.: 0.01 mg/kg initial dose Maximum dose 0.2 mg over 15 sec; may repeat after 45 sec then every 1 min to max total cumulative dose 0.05 mg/kg or 1 mg, whichever is lower	0.2 mg/dose to maximum 1 mg or 3 mg in 1 h	1-2 min	10-20 min	Reverses sedative effects but does not reliably reverse respiratory depression Should not be used when benzodiazepines have been given to control a serious illness (e.g., status epilepticus) or in tricyclic antidepressant overdose
Propofol	Must be individualized. Initial ≤0.5 mg/kg/dose until desired level of sedation achieved	Continue infusion Initial: 0.3 mg/kg/h; increase by 0.3-0.6 mg/kg/h every 5-10 min until desired level of sedation is achieved	Within 30 sec of bolus infusion	Approximately 3-10 min	Contraindicated in hypersensitivity to any component (e.g., soybean oil, egg phosphatide)

References

Agency for Health Care Policy and Research, Public Health Services, U. S. Department of Health and Human Services. (February 1992). Acute pain management: Operative or medical procedures and trauma: Clinical practice guideline (AHCPR Pub. No. 92-0032). Rockville, MD: Acute Pain Management Guideline Panel.

American Academy of Pediatrics. (1992). Guidelines for monitoring and management of pediatric patients during and after sedation for diagnostic and therapeutic procedures. Pediatrics, 89(6), 1110-1115.

American Academy of Pediatrics. (2002). Guidelines for monitoring and management of pediatric patients during and after sedation for diagnostic and therapeutic procedures: Addendum. Pediatrics, 110(4), 836-838.

American Nurses Association. (1991). Position statement on the role of the registered nurse (RN) in the management of patients receiving IV conscious sedation for short-term therapeutic, diagnostic, or surgical procedures. Kansas City: Author.

American Society of Anesthesiologists. (2002). Practice guidelines for sedation and analgesia: An updated report by the ASA task force on sedation and analgesia by non-anesthesiologists. Anesthesiology, 96, 1004-1017.

Colman, Y., & Krauss, B. (1999). Microstream capnography technology: A new approach to an old problem. Journal of Clinical Monitoring and Computing, 15, 403-409.

Dial, S., Silver, P., Bock, K., & Sagy, M. (2001). Pediatric sedation for procedures titrated to a desired degree of immobility results in unpredictable depth of sedation. Pediatric Emergency Care, 17(6), 414-420.

Fiordalisi, I. (2003). Sedation. In: R.M. Perkin, J.D. Swift, & D.A. Newton (Eds.). Pediatric hospital medicine: Textbook of inpatient management. Philadelphia: Lippincott, Williams and Wilkins, pp. 762-771.

Fox, V.L. (2000). Pediatric endoscopy. Gastrointestinal Endoscopy, 10(1), 175-94.

Hall, S.C. (2001). Sedation and analgesia for diagnostic and therapeutic procedures in children. Anesthesia and Analgesia, 92(3S), 54-59.

Hoffman, G.M., Nowakowski, R., Troshynski, T.J., Berens, R.J., & Weisman, S.J. (2002). Risk reduction in pediatric procedural sedation by application of an American Academy of Pediatrics/American Society of Anesthesiologists process model. Pediatrics, 109, 236-243.

Lawson, G.R. (2000). Sedation of children for magnetic resonance imaging. Archives of Disease in Childhood, 82, 150-152.

Lightdale, J.R., Sethna, N.F., Heard, L.A., Donovan, K.M., & Fox, V.L. (2002). A pilot study of end-tidal carbon dioxide monitoring using microstream capnography in children undergoing endoscopy with conscious sedation. Gastrointestinal Endoscopy, 55, AB145.

Love, G. (2000). Electrifying news about iontophoresis. Nursing, 30(1), 48-49.

Malviya, S., Voepel-Lewis, T., Prochaska, G., & Tait, A.R. (2000). Prolonged recovery and delayed side effects of sedation for diagnostic imaging studies in children. Pediatrics. Retrieved October 2003, from http://www.pediatrics.org/cgi/content/full/105/3/e42.

Malviya, S., Voepel-Lewis, T., Tait, A.R., & Merkel, S. (2000). Sedation/analgesia for diagnostic and therapeutic procedures in children. Journal of PeriAnesthesia Nursing, 15, 415-422.

Marenzi, B. (2004). Body piercing: A patient safety issue. Journal of PeriAnesthesia Nursing, 19, 4-10.

Mamaril, M.E. (2000). Clinical emergencies and preparedness. In N. Burden, D.M.D. Quinn, D. O'Brien, & B.S.G. Dawes (Eds.). Ambulatory surgical nursing (2nd Ed.). Philadelphia: Saunders.

Odom-Forren, J. (2004). Survey of state boards of nursing regarding statements on sedation/analgesia. Unpublished research.

Rayhorn, N. (1998). Sedating and monitoring pediatric patients. Defining the nurse's responsibilities from preparation through recovery. MCN, American Journal of Maternal Child Nursing, 23(2), 76-86.

Shobha, M., Voepel-Lewis, T., & Tait, A.R. (1997). Adverse events and risk factors associated with the sedation of children by nonanesthesiologists. Anesthesia and Analgesia, 85(6), 1207-1213.

Silegy, T., & Jacks, S.T. (2003). Pediatric oral conscious sedation. CDA Journal, 31, 413-418.

Squire, S.J., Kirchhoff, K.T., & Hissong, K. (2000). Comparing two methods of topical anesthesia used before intravenous cannulation in pediatric patients. Journal of Pediatric Health Care, 14(2), 68-72.

Vargo, J.J., Zuccaro Jr, G., Dumot, J.A., Conwell, D.L., Morrow, J.B., & Shay, S.S. (2002). Automated graphic assessment of respiratory activity is superior to pulse oximetry and visual assessment for the detection of early respiratory depression during therapeutic upper endoscopy. Gastrointestinal Endoscopy, 55, 826-831.

9

Geriatric Sedation

Elderly patients have an increased variability of drug response. Elderly patients have a decreased requirement for most anesthetic drugs. Elderly patients have a prolonged redosing interval.

—E. Darling

The term "geriatrics" was introduced into industrial societies at the beginning of the twentieth century. Since that time advances in nutrition, public health, education, and social services have produced major changes in longevity and life expectancy (Barash et al, 2001). Geriatrics is the branch of medicine that deals with the physiologic effects of aging and the diagnosis and treatment of persons who are 65 years of age or older (Naglehout et al, 2001). As a person ages, physiologic function gradually declines. Clinical manifestations may include an increased prevalence of age-related, concomitant diseases, such as hypertension, renal failure, atherosclerosis, chronic obstructive pulmonary disease, myocardial infarction, diabetes, cardiomegaly, liver disease, congestive heart failure, angina, cerebrovascular accident, and more (Naglehout et al, 2001). Approximately 80% of the elderly population has at least one chronic health problem—usually arthritis, heart or respiratory disease, hypertension, or impaired vision or hearing (Mangim & Piano, 2000). These problems often occur simultaneously. When caring for the geriatric patient, it is necessary to take into account the psychosocial, physiologic, and biologic changes that normally occur during the aging process (Mangim & Piano, 2000). It is reasonable to assume that the functional reserve of all organ systems is progressively and significantly decreased in elderly patients (Barash et al, 2001).

Care of the geriatric patient during moderate sedation and/or analgesia is of significance because of the physiologic changes that occur during the later years (Odom, 2000). However, age alone is not a major determinant of morbidity. Age-related diseases and excessive or rapid dosing contribute more to the cardiorespiratory complications of moderate sedation than age itself (American Society for Gastrointestinal Endoscopy, 2000). The disease processes that have afflicted the patient in the past play a critical role in increasing the risk of the elderly patient receiving moderate sedation/analgesia. While administering sedation,

Table 9-1 | Six Principles to Improve Care for Elderly Surgical Patients

Considerations to Use as a Guide to Improve Care for Elderly Surgical Patients:

Clinical presentation—this may be subtle or somewhat different from the general population and may lead to delay in diagnosis.

Lack of reserve—organ system reserve affects the elder's ability to handle severe stress, such as extensive or emergency surgery.

Preoperative preparation—perioperative risk increases when preoperative preparation is decreased or suboptimal. Examples of preoperative preparation include smoking cessation, perioperative antibiotics, treatment of hypertension, anemia, bronchitis, and thromboembolic prophylaxis.

Emergency surgery—elective surgery produces far better outcomes than surgery performed under emergent conditions. Because of the elder's lack of reserve and the inability to do adequate preoperative preparation, the risk of emergency surgery is associated with at least a threefold increase in mortality and morbidity than planned for elective procedures.

Attention to detail—elders respond poorly to complications; therefore vigilance is the key to successful outcomes. Restoring and maintaining homeostasis, lowering the risk of septic complications, preventing anastomotic leaks, and hemodynamic monitoring greatly reduce the surgical risk.

Age is a specific fact—no particular chronological age should be considered a contraindication for surgery.

Data from Felice Meckes, P.G. (2003). Geriatric surgery. In J.C. Rothrock (Ed.). Alexander's care of the patient in surgery, (12th Ed.). St. Louis: Mosby, p. 1296; Katlic, M.R. (2001). Principles of geriatric surgery. In R.A. Rosenthal et al (Eds.). (2001). Principles and practice of geriatric surgery. New York: Springer.

the registered nurse (RN) must recognize how certain drugs affect the elderly patient. See Table 9-1 for six principles of geriatric surgery to be used as a guide to improve care for elderly surgical patients.

PHYSIOLOGIC CHANGES OF AGING

Elderly patients present a unique challenge for the nurse providing moderate sedation and/or analgesia. The physiologic changes of aging combined with pathologic conditions necessitating surgical intervention mandate careful assessment, planning, and implementation of the nursing process (Schick, 2004). A careful plan of care must be developed for each individual patient.

Cardiovascular

Elderly patients experience a variety of cardiovascular changes. These include arteriosclerotic changes, such as loss of large artery elasticity and vessel fragility. Patients will have decreased organ perfusion and decreased compensatory regulation. Myocardial changes include left ventricular hypertrophy, increased myocardial irritability, and calcification of valves. These changes may lead to dysrhythmias, decreased contractility, and valve incompetence. Altered hemodynamics may also be seen in the elderly patient and include decreased cardiac output, decreased stroke volume, increased blood pressure, a slower circulation time, and a decreased cardiac reserve (Schick, 2004). Because of decreased cardiac output and resulting decreases in circulation times in the elderly the onset of intravenous agents is slowed, and there is an increased duration of action (Odom, 2000). The RN monitoring the moderate sedation and/or analgesia patient should be aware of any cardioactive drugs taken by the patient preoperatively, use caution with fluid replacement, expect a slower metabolism of drugs, and allow adequate time for response to medications before redosing. In addition, the nurse should monitor the patient, provide adequate oxygenation, and assess heart and lung sounds for signs of overload or heart failure (Koehle, 2000).

Respiratory

Geriatric patients may have increased secretions and airway resistance because of the effects of aging on the respiratory system (Odom, 2000). The lungs lose elasticity, contributing to an increase in functional residual capacity, residual volume, and dead space. The lungs increase in size and are lighter in weight with aging (Meckes, 2003). Arthritic changes in the rib cage may cause increased chest wall rigidity, and loss of skeletal muscle mass may lead to a wasting of the diaphragm and skeletal muscles (Schick, 2004). The muscles responsible for inhalation and exhalation may be weakened. In addition, as a person ages, oxygen content in the blood decreases. It should also be noted that the loss of teeth, sometimes seen in aged patients, will change the jaw structure and can lead to difficult airway maintenance (Schick, 2004). The RN should elevate the patient's head when possible, position the patient for ease of chest expansion, provide oxygen support as needed, and try to reduce the patient's anxiety, stress, and pain (Koehle, 2000).

Central Nervous System

The elderly patient may have a decrease in neuronal density and nerve conduction secondary to neurogenic atrophy and loss of peripheral nerve fibers (Schick, 2004). The atrophic changes that interfere with the basic neuronal process cause an increased susceptibility of the older patient to central nervous system side effects of drugs (Odom, 2000). Patients may also have slowed or delayed reflexes. In addition, compromised thermoregulation is a common problem in the elderly. It is important to prevent unplanned hypothermia in these patients. Other significant neurologic changes include a loss of position sense in the toes, decreased tactile sense, changes in sleep patterns, and atypical response to pain (Meckes, 2003). The nurse needs to observe the patients for prolonged or toxic effects of medications and be aware of the need for reduced drug doses (Koehle, 2000).

Renal/Genitourinary

The geriatric patient may have decreased renal blood flow and a decreased glomerular filtration rate, causing a decreased drug clearance and an increased drug half-life and duration action (Odom, 2000). Patients may also have a decreased ability to adapt to electrolyte and fluid changes. The nurse should observe for prolonged drug effects and monitor intravenous (IV) infusions and urinary output. Elderly patients may also have a decreased bladder capacity and muscle tone, resulting in incontinence and an increase in residual urine (Schick, 2004). Nurses should offer bedpans and urinals frequently and reassure and support patients emotionally to prevent embarrassment (Koehle, 2000).

Gastrointestinal

Decreased salivation, decreased peristalsis, and decreased hepatic blood flow are commonly seen in the elderly patient (Schick, 2004). It is important for the nurse to observe for toxic or prolonged drug effects and be aware of an increased risk of aspiration caused by delayed gastric emptying. The geriatric patient may also have changes in the esophageal musculature that may lead to reflux or esophageal spasm. It is helpful to position the patient with their head up when possible (Koehle, 2000).

Integumentary

Elderly patients have a loss of subcutaneous fat, leading to an increased risk of hypothermia, a compromise in thermoregulation, and a loss of padding for bony prominences (Schick, 2004). Measures should be taken to prevent heat loss and to prevent hypothermia. Bony prominences should be protected and padded and the patient position changed frequently when possible (Koehle, 2000).

Sensory

Sensory changes in vision, hearing, taste, smell, and touch may occur in the elderly patient and may influence a response to patient care (Meckes, 2003). Visual changes include decreased visual acuity, decreased peripheral vision, decreased accommodation (presbyopia), retinal vascular changes, cataracts, and glaucoma (Schick, 2004). Nurses should provide large-print instructions when indicated and provide constant support, explanation, and discussion about what is being done (Koehle, 2000). It is helpful to allow the patient to keep their eye glasses with them as long as possible.

Auditory changes include decreased sensitivity to sound, loss of high-pitched sound perception, and impairment of sound localization (Schick, 2004). Geriatric patients may be labeled "confused" or "senile" because they respond inappropriately to questions they did not hear (Meckes, 2003). Nurses should let patients wear hearing aids when possible and allow adequate time for feedback to verify patient understanding. It is also important to raise voice volume, but not pitch, and to speak slowly and face the patient when possible (Koehle, 2000).

Some elderly patients may experience a decrease in smell and taste perception and tactile changes, such as decreased sensitivity to touch. The decreased sense of touch may affect the elderly patient's ability to localize stimuli and may also reduce the speed of reaction to tactile stimulation (Meckes, 2003).

PATIENT SELECTION

Selection of patients for moderate sedation/analgesia should be based on established criteria that have been developed by a multidisciplinary team of health care professionals (DeLamar, 2003). Health care facilities must adopt patient selection criteria to assure that only patients suitable for nurse-administered moderate sedation and/or analgesia are selected. The classification system of patient physical status by the American Society of Anesthesiologists (ASA) is frequently used to determine appropriate patient categories for RN-monitored sedation and/or analgesia (see Chapter 2). It is important for health care providers to be aware that there are risks associated with different settings for patients with certain risk profiles. Researchers have identified four factors that place geriatric patients undergoing surgery at an increased risk. These four factors are advanced age, inpatient hospital admission within 6 months before surgery, surgery being performed at a physician's office or outpatient facility, and the invasiveness of the surgery (Fleisher, 2004).

Patients must be thoroughly assessed physiologically and psychologically before the procedure. As described elsewhere in this book (see Chapter 2), the assessment must include a review of physical examination findings, current medications taken, allergies, current medical problems, history of smoking or substance abuse, current chief complaint, baseline vital signs, height and weight, age, emotional state, any communication deficits, and the patient's perception of the procedure and moderate sedation (DeLamar, 2003). Any of these considerations may increase the risk for an undesirable outcome for the patient receiving moderate sedation/analgesia (ASA, 2002). The objective is to avoid any patient with an existing complication that may increase the likelihood of a poor outcome (AORN, 2002). The ASA developed practice guidelines for sedation and analgesia by nonanesthesiologists. In these guidelines, the task force members note that for patients with significant underlying medical conditions (i.e., extremes of age; severe cardiac, pulmonary, hepatic, or renal disease; pregnancy; and drug or alcohol abuse) a preprocedure consultation with an appropriate medical specialist (i.e., cardiologist and pulmonologist) decreases the risk associated with moderate sedation, and they strongly agree that it decreases the risks associated with deep sedation (ASA, 2002). The guidelines go on to say that for patients with significant *sedation-related* risk factors (i.e., uncooperative patients, morbid obesity, potentially difficult airway, and sleep apnea) the task force consultants are equivocal regarding whether preprocedure consultation with an anesthesiologist increases the likelihood of satisfactory moderate sedation, although they do agree that it decreases adverse outcomes (ASA, 2002).

For moderate sedation, the consultants are equivocal regarding whether the immediate availability of an individual with postgraduate training in anesthesiology increases the likelihood of a satisfactory outcome or decreases the associated risks. For deep sedation, the consultants agree that the immediate availability of such an individual improves the likelihood of satisfactory sedation, and that it will decrease the likelihood of adverse outcomes (ASA, 2002).

The ASA guideline consultants recommend that whenever possible appropriate medical specialists be consulted before administration of sedation to patients with significant underlying conditions (ASA, 2002). For significantly compromised or medically unstable patients (i.e., anticipated difficult airway, severe obstructive pulmonary disease, coronary artery disease, or congestive heart failure), or if it appears likely that sedation to the point of unresponsiveness will be necessary to obtain adequate conditions, practitioners who are not trained in the administration of general anesthesia should consult an anesthesiologist (ASA, 2002). If a nurse does not feel comfortable managing the care and monitoring of a particular patient, the attending physician and an anesthesia provider should be consulted (DeLamar, 2003). A joint decision may be necessary to determine who is the most appropriate person to monitor the patient and the appropriate medications and monitoring measurements to use.

CARE OF THE PATIENT

The RN responsible for administering and monitoring the elderly patient receiving moderate sedation should be prepared to use smaller doses of medications, as ordered by the physician. Medications should be titrated very carefully. A decreased clearance rate and an increased duration of the effect of the medication should be expected (Odom, 2000).

Oxygen saturation must be monitored carefully and the head of the bed should be elevated if possible (Odom, 2000). Patients should be encouraged to deep breathe as often as possible. Maintaining normothermia will help to aid in drug clearance. It is important to remember that the elderly patient cools more quickly and rewarms more slowly than the younger adult. Complications with hypothermia can include myocardial or cerebral ischemia, respiratory acidosis, and hypoxia (Odom, 2000). Elderly patients must be monitored for hypertension and hypotension, and the nurse should be prepared to intervene quickly when necessary. The nurse should keep in mind to speak loudly and clearly if the patient has a hearing loss.

AGE-SPECIFIC COMPETENCY

In addition to demonstrating clinical competency in the administration of moderate sedation and/or analgesia (see Chapter 7) and in the use of monitoring

Table 9-2 | **Geriatric Age-Specific Competency**

Perform a Nursing Assessment of the Geriatric Patient.

Obtain a baseline and interval blood pressure and pulse measurement.
Obtain baseline and interval respiratory measurements, including rate, effort, rhythm, and SpO_2.
Determine fluid volume status, fluid intake, and blood/fluid loss.
Perform an assessment of the integumentary system.
Identify sensory norms for the geriatric patient.
Identify cognition/communication norms for the aging patient.
Identify skeletal/neuromuscular status of the geriatric patient.
Recognize signs and symptoms of elder abuse.
Communicate and document all pertinent information per institution/unit specific policy/protocol.

From The American Society of Perianesthesia Nurses' competency based orientation credentialing program, 2002.

equipment and oxygen-delivery systems, resuscitation, and airway management, the RN must illustrate age-specific competency in caring for the geriatric patient. According to the American Society of Perianesthesia Nurses (ASPAN), the nurse must "demonstrate a geriatric assessment, identify specific changes common to the aging process, and identify appropriate nursing interventions related to perianesthesia needs of the geriatric patient" (Godden, 2002). See Table 9-2 for the criteria for the nursing assessment of the geriatric patient.

CONCLUSION

The administration and monitoring of moderate sedation/analgesia in the elderly patient are skills expected of nurses in various settings. Although managing the care of the elderly patient can present a real challenge for nurses administering moderate sedation/analgesia, it can also be a rewarding and satisfying experience. It is necessary that the nurse considers the complex health care needs of the geriatric patient to provide comprehensive patient care. The nurse will find that safe and effective quality care can be provided to the elderly patient who is in the hands of the prepared, educated, and proficient nurse.

REFERENCES

American Society for Gastrointestinal Endoscopy. (2000). Modifications in endoscopic practice for the elderly. Gastrointestinal Endoscopy, 52, 849-851.
American Society of Anesthesiologists. (2002). Practice guidelines for sedation and anesthesia by non-anesthesiologists. Anesthesiology, 96, 1004-1017.

Association of periOperative Registered Nurses. (2002). Recommended practices for managing the patient receiving moderate sedation/analgesia. AORN Journal, 75, 642-652.

Barash, P.G., Cullen, B.F., & Stoelting, R.K. (2001). Handbook of clinical anesthesia (4th Ed.). Philadelphia: Lippincott, Williams & Wilkins, pp. 648-661.

DeLamar, L.M.. (2003). Anesthesia. In J.C. Rothrock (Ed.). Alexander's care of the patient in surgery. (12th Ed.). St. Louis: Mosby, pp. 244-245.

Fleisher, L.A., Pasternak, L.R., Herbert, R., & Anderson, G.F. (2004). Inpatient hospital admission and death after outpatient surgery in elderly patients: Importance of patient and system characteristics and location of care. Archives of Surgery, 139, 67-72.

Meckes, P.G.F. (2003). Geriatric surgery. In J.C. Rothrock (Ed.). Alexander's care of the patient in surgery. (12th Ed.). St. Louis: Mosby, pp. 1295-1315.

Godden, B. (Ed.). (2002). Competency based orientation credentialing program, Cherry Hill, NJ: American Society of PeriAnesthesia Nurses, pp. 337-339.

Koehle, M.M. (2000). Special needs of the older adult. In N. Burden, D.M.D. Quinn, D. O'Brien, B.S.G. Dawes (Eds.). Ambulatory surgical nursing. (2nd Ed). Philadelphia: Saunders, pp. 643-667.

Mangim, E.J., & Piano, L.A. (2000). Geriatric care. In Springhouse (Ed.). Nursing procedures. (3rd Ed.). Springhouse, PA: Springhouse Corporation, pp. 770-787.

Naglehout, J.J., Zaglaniczny, K.L., & Hagulund, V.L. (2001). Handbook of nurse anesthesia. (2nd Ed.). Philadelphia: Saunders, pp. 125-126.

Odom, J.L. (2000). Conscious sedation/analgesia. In N. Burden, D.M.D. Quinn, D. O'Brien, B.S.G. Dawes (Eds.). Ambulatory surgical nursing. (2nd Ed) Philadelphia: Saunders, pp. 309-330.

Schick, L. (2004). The elderly patient. In D.M.D. Quinn & L. Schick (Eds.). Perianesthesia nursing core curriculum: Preoperative, phase I and phase II PACU nursing. Philadelphia: Saunders, pp. 209-225.

10

Sedation in the Mechanically Ventilated Patient

There are many indications for the administration of sedation and analgesia to the critically ill patient. This chapter will focus on the assessment and interventions for agitation and delirium as a means of determining the necessity for and patient outcomes related to sedation and analgesia. The RN will be able to identify risk factors for agitation and delirium, describe interventions aimed at correcting conditions that precipitate agitation and delirium, and address pharmacologic and nonpharmacologic measures that are an integral part of management in the mechanically ventilated patient.

Critically ill patients who require mechanical ventilation often have high levels of anxiety and discomfort. Some studies of intensive care units (ICU) have reported patient symptoms ranging from severe anxiety to excruciating pain. Many patients show signs of restlessness and delirium (Cohen et al, 2002; Jacobi et al, 2002; White et al, 2001) Many critically ill patients are not able to express themselves, making it very difficult and often challenging to assess their levels of pain, anxiety, drug or alcohol withdrawal, or delirium. In caring for these patients, nurses often rely on patient assessments including signs and symptoms of pain, agitation, and delirium (e.g., restlessness, anxiety, and fear). Based on these ongoing individual patient assessments, the plan of care is modified accordingly. There is evidence that morbidity and mortality rates are higher among agitated patients and patients experiencing withdrawal syndromes, so prompt identification and management of agitation are essential for achieving positive patient outcomes (Cohen et al, 2002; Koleff et al, 1998; Kress et al, 2000).

Anxious and agitated patients are often in a state of restlessness and may resist therapeutic interventions, such as positioning, pulmonary toileting, and ventilation. When the sensation of dyspnea, anxiety, or pain is not effectively managed, the symptoms exert a powerful negative impact on several organs. Excess motor activity caused by anxiety can exhaust the patient's already limited ability to deliver adequate oxygen and nutrition to the cells. The agitated patient tends to resist the mechanical ventilation, sometimes to the point of biting the endotracheal tube and occluding it. These patients can be at risk for safety issues as evidenced by attempts to self-extubate, pulling at invasive lines, and resisting treatments and nursing care. The resultant deterioration in oxygen delivery exacerbates the patient's sense of dyspnea and heightens the agitation. Persistent anxiety, pain, and dyspnea coupled with major hemodynamic or metabolic disturbance can cause the patient's agitation to progress to an acute confusional state. This condition affects as many as 50% of all adult ICU patients (Clifford & Buchman, 2002; Luer, 1995; McGaffigan, 2002).

One of the roles of the nurse is to assess for agitation and to relieve the underlying causes by direct intervention. If dyspnea is a result of hypoperfusion states (pump failure, shock, and anemia), the symptoms will not be eliminated until the underlying abnormality is corrected. Unlike other organs, the brain depends on a constant supply of glucose and oxygen. Interruption in the delivery of these vital nutrients quickly disrupts the delicate chemistry of the brain. Many disease processes affecting the critically ill patient impair glucose and oxygen transport to the brain, whereas other abnormalities, such as drug toxicity or high ammonia levels, directly alter neurotransmission.

Because dyspnea and pain are common problems in the ventilated patient, every effort is made to assess for the causes. The dyspneic patient is examined for bilateral breath sounds, signs of bronchial constriction, accumulation of secretions, and proper endotracheal tube placement. The patient should be suctioned to remove secretions and to assess for changes in pulmonary flora and for the presence of blood or frothy sputum, suggesting pulmonary emboli or edema, respectively.

Ventilatory parameters are evaluated for changes in the patient's condition. Rising peak airway pressures may signify pneumothorax, airway plugging, or decreased lung compliance as a result of adult respiratory distress syndrome (ARDS). Decreased expiratory volumes suggest an air leak, which may be caused by improper tube placement, inadequate seal by the balloon, or breaks or loose connections in the tubing, caps, or nebulizer. Increased minute ventilation is a nonspecific sign that the patient is not adequately oxygenating the tissue. It does not pinpoint the cause as pulmonary organ failure but directs attention to impaired gas exchange or delivery. An internal failure of the ventilator itself must also be considered.

If the endotracheal tube is not in the trachea, as evidenced by patient vocalization and air movement from the nose and mouth during mechanically assisted inspiration, the tube should be removed. The patient is manually ventilated with 100% oxygen and an anesthesia provider is paged STAT. Intubation equipment and extra sedation are brought to the bedside in preparation for reintubation. The patient's oxygen saturation, color, and vital signs are closely observed.

Immediate interventions should be aimed at correcting the oxygen deficit and may include selecting the appropriate ventilator mode, adjusting the percentage of delivered oxygen, and administering bronchodilators as necessary. Additional interventions may include the administration of analgesic and anxiolytic medications, assessing their efficacy, and providing nonpharmacologic measures, such as therapeutic touch, patient and family education, and reassurance.

Patient discomfort in the ICU can be expressed in many ways. Intubated patients often experience discomfort related to dyspnea for a variety of reasons. These patients are likely to have varying degrees of dyspnea that may result from impaired gas exchange (e.g., pulmonary disorder) or other disorders that prevent the delivery of oxygen to the cells (impaired perfusion states and severe anemia). If an adequate supply of oxygen is not readily provided to the cells, the acutely dyspneic patient's coping mechanisms may quickly break down to a state of panic. Pain is a noxious sensation that elicits an immediate urge to withdraw from the source. There are multiple causes of pain that the patient may experience (e.g., surgical incision site, chest tubes, arterial-venous punctures, and ischemia to limbs or internal organs). Pain, whether continual, intermittent, or episodic, elicits a fear response, which exacerbates the patient's underlying anxiety. Pain can also stimulate sympathetic nervous system activation, which can lead to tachycardia, hypotension or hypertension, and increases in oxygen consumption, potentially worsening symptoms of dyspnea.

Delirium, sometimes called ICU psychosis, is now understood to be a reversible organic syndrome. Current research suggests that when a critically ill patient becomes agitated and confused, the condition is due primarily to dysfunction of brain metabolism related to abnormal neurotransmission, and it has a broad range of unwanted consequences (Cohen et al, 2002; Ely, Siegel, & Inouye, 2001; Jacobi et al, 2002). There is a newly developed CAM-ICU scale (confusion assessment method for ICU) that has been validated for assessing delirium in the critically ill adult (Ely et al, 2001; Ely et al, 2002; Truman & Ely, 2003; Tullman, 2001).

When an adult patient who complains of chest pain is encountered, the nurse may initially entertain a diagnosis of acute myocardial infarction. In the same manner, the nurse in the ICU must learn to consider a diagnosis of acute brain dysfunction when the patient becomes agitated or delirious. This interpretation of agitation encourages the nurse to assess for deteriorating organ systems and to appraise the patient's level of discomfort and confusion.

PATHOPHYSIOLOGIC MECHANISMS OF AGITATION AND DELIRIUM

Excessive, uncontrolled, or irrational motor activity, heightened autonomic discharge, and internal tension characterize agitation in the critically ill patient (Cohen et al, 2002; Clifford & Buchman, 2002; Ely, Siegel, & Inouye, 2001; Truman & Ely, 2003). Agitation manifests itself in the patient pulling on tubes, side rails, or bed sheets, thrashing in the bed, and fighting against the ventilator rather than breathing with it. Delirium by definition is "a mental disorder characterized by confusion, disordered speech, and hallucinations" (Miriam Webster Dictionary, 2004). Cohen et al (2002) further defined delirium as "an acute, reversible organic mental syndrome with disorders of attention and cognitive function, increased or decreased psychomotor activity, and a disordered sleep wake cycle." Delirium is becoming more prevalent with the advanced age and increased acuity of ICU patients, with estimates of occurrence between 15% and 40% of ICU patients. Delirium causes increased morbidity and is associated with a mortality rate up to 30% (Riker & Fraser, 2002).

Agitation

In the early stages, characteristics of anxiety and agitation include restlessness, difficulty sleeping, and a short attention span. Patients are expected to lie quietly when they are bombarded by the sounds of technology in the critical care arena. It is often necessary to restrain patients to prevent dislodgment of lines and tubes. This often leads to a state of increased agitation as patients try to escape from the restraining forces. Increases in motor activity during this time lead to increased metabolic demands at a time when these supplies may be limited (Crippen, 2002). Psychologic coping mechanisms are eroded, and the patient exhibits a diminished tolerance for uncomfortable procedures. Often the patient is unable to lie still or sleep unless given sedatives or neuroleptics. The patient may heed a command to "Lie still!" for a time but moments later may strain to reach the endotracheal tube despite clear, firm instructions to the contrary.

Patients who are mechanically ventilated may have cognitive dysfunctions caused by sedation or frustrations experienced by lack of ability to comprehend their surroundings or to communicate with care providers. If the agitation progresses, neurologic assessment reveals symptoms of global cognitive impairment. The patient becomes unable to process information rationally or to retain information for more than a few minutes. The patient may require vigorous verbal and tactile stimulation to get his or her attention and is likely to soon forget instructions or information. Other neurologic abnormalities associated with agitation include alternating periods of hyperalertness and lethargy, which are virtually diagnostic (Cohen et al, 2002; Crippen, 1994; Ely, Siegel, & Inouye, 2001).

Delirium

Delirium has been categorized into three clinical subtypes. Hypoactive delirium is when the patient demonstrates flat affect, lethargy, apathy, decreased mobility, and signs of decreased responsiveness to obtundation, and carries the worst prognosis. Hyperactive delirium is characterized by symptoms of agitation; emotional instability; pulling at catheters and tubes; combativeness, including lashing out at care providers; and restlessness. Patients exhibiting hyperactive delirium may have a progression of symptoms after sedative therapy is initiated. Patients are assessed as mixed delirium when there are concurrent assessments revealing features of hypoactive and hyperactive delirium at the same time (Jacobi et al, 2002).

Patients must first be assessed for levels of sedation before performing an assessment for delirium. Patients who are not able to respond or are very sedated cannot be assessed for delirium. If the level of sedation allows the patient to respond to verbal stimuli or if the patient is minimally responsive, he or she should be assessed for cognitive function and delirium. The CAM-ICU scale assesses the patient using four features. Feature 1 assesses for acute onset of mental status changes or for patients who have fluctuating mental status changes. Feature 2 assesses for the patient's inattentiveness. Feature 3 assesses for disorganized thinking, and feature 4 assesses for altered level of consciousness. The CAM-ICU scale, which has been validated, states that the assessment must include both category 1 and 2, plus either 3 or 4 to establish a diagnosis of delirium (Ely et al, 2001; Truman & Ely, 2003). The characteristics of agitation and delirium are summarized in the CAM-ICU scale, available at www.icudelirium.org (Ely, 2002).

With poor coordination and short-term memory deficit, the patient may have difficulty writing a complete sentence in answer to questioning. Sometimes the patient cannot write his or her full name, faltering after making the first few letters and then losing track of the goal. Agitation was once considered a psychologic response to the stress of major illness and admission to the ICU. It is now known to be a reversible organic syndrome related to dysfunction of the brain. It differs from true psychosis in several ways. First, a functional psychosis is not known to have an organic cause (American Psychiatric Association [APA], 1996; Justic, 2000). Secondly, functional psychosis usually has an internal consistency, whereas those with delirium exhibit fragmented thoughts. The psychotic individual may have bizarre ideas, but the ideas are for the most part consistent and logical within that frame of reference. Psychotic and delirious patients may have hallucinations and paranoid ideas, and both may have delusions, which are fixed, illogical beliefs that are not responsive to conflicting evidence.[1] Third, the delirium of the patient with impaired brain metabolism is more global than that of the functional psychotic. Memory and attention span are diminished, and there is disruption of the sleep-wake cycle. In some cases the excessive release of neurotransmitters will prevent the ICU patient from sleeping for several days.

Some researchers suggest that preexisting personality disorders can contribute to the ICU patient's agitation and delirium (Clifford & Buchman, 2002; Justic, 2000; Tullman, 2001). Individuals who have obsessive-compulsive disorders may have high levels of anxiety because of their restricted movements. Patients who have a strong need to control others may decompensate in the ICU environment, where caregivers take charge of the patient's every function.

Perhaps the most striking symptoms that set the delirious, critically ill patient apart from the functional psychotic one are the musculoskeletal abnormalities seen in critical care. These patients exhibit tremors, rigidity, hyperreflexia, uncoordinated movements, and disequilibrium. These signs are not commonly associated with the outpatient schizophrenic or delusional person.

Two mechanisms produce neurologic abnormalities in the critically ill patient. The first is the impact of prolonged states of apprehension and discomfort, especially dyspnea and pain, on the brain. The second mechanism involves the hemodynamic and metabolic disorders that affect critically ill patients (Box 10-1).

Box 10-1   FACTORS THAT IMPAIR BRAIN FUNCTION

Subjective Factors

Dyspnea
Pain
Anxiety
Nausea, thirst, hunger
Diarrhea, urinary incontinence
Preexisting psychopathology
Intense sensory input
Sleep deprivation

Objective Factors

Increased production of:
   Norepinephrine
   Dopamine
   β-Endorphins
   Corticotropin-releasing factor
Decreased production of:
   Intraneural enzymes that return transmitters to producing neurons

Hemodynamic and Metabolic Disorders

Intrinsic to brain
   Stroke
   Increased intracranial pressure caused by trauma
   Space-occupying lesions
   Meningitis
   Toxoplasmosis
   Withdrawal from addictive substances
Extrinsic to brain
   Hypoxemia
   Hypercapnia
   Hypotension/shock
   Hypoglycemia
   Electrolyte imbalance
   Acid-base imbalance
   Drug toxicity
   Renal or liver failure

Neurologic Signs/Symptoms of Brain Dysfunction

Global mental impairment
Alternating hyperalertness and lethargy
Loss of short-term memory
Uncontrolled motor activity
Tremulousness, musculoskeletal rigidity
Disorientation
Delusions and hallucinations
Paranoid ideation
Coma

Brain Function

In addition to its autonomic regulatory functions, the central nervous system processes sensory input and channels it to higher regions of the brain, where it is interpreted against past experience (Cohen et al, 2002; Clifford & Buchman, 2002). At the same time the brain supplies emotional response to the data, which affects the intensity of the experience and the response.

The brain disregards 99% of the sensory input it receives. It selects significant input and channels it through neuronal circuits to the appropriate motor and cognitive centers in the cortex. These centers then send out appropriate responses through the motor axis and cerebellum, producing purposeful, coordinated actions.

The emotional response to the sensory input depends on its comparison with previous experience. For example, the sight of a snake in the grass usually elicits an immediate fear response. The brain releases a surge of catecholamines and corticotrophin-releasing factor, which prepare the body for fight or flight. If the perceiver decides that the snake is harmless, the emotional response abates with the release of other inhibiting transmitters, such as γ-aminobutyric acid (GABA), and emotional equilibrium is restored.

Prolonged periods of apprehension elicit an increased production of norepinephrine from central structures, principally the locus caeruleus. High levels of norepinephrine produce anxiety, restlessness, and the inability to sleep and impair the brain's ability to filter out unwanted sensory input. As a result, ICU patients lose their ability to discriminate, which heightens anxiety or agitation (Clifford & Buchman, 2002).

The patient's subjective state is similar to the condition that follows ingesting a cold remedy containing ephedrine, a sympathomimetic, at bedtime. The resulting state of restlessness, palpitations, and inability to sleep is due to the stimulating effects of the catecholamine analog and is similar to the experience of the ICU patient. Unrelieved pain and hypoxia elicit similar outflows of catecholamines and produce even more pronounced stress on cerebral metabolism.

In response to the continued sympathetic discharge, the cerebral cortex becomes exhausted (Crippen, 1994; Ely, Siegel, & Inouye, 2001; White et al, 2001). The brain's resources, which are likely to be already compromised, are further taxed, and its ability to metabolize nutrients is impaired. It is important to remember that an anxious patient who becomes restless, irritable, and unable to sleep may be demonstrating the early warning signs of impending brain dysfunction. This condition warrants immediate assessment of all organ systems and laboratory values to determine the causative agent.

Metabolic Disturbances

Brain metabolism is also impaired by hemodynamic and metabolic disorders, which commonly affect critically ill patients. Disorders that are intrinsic to the brain may include stroke, space-occupying lesions, and swelling resulting from trauma, hydrocephalus, or infection (Box 10-2).

Box 10-2 HEMODYNAMIC AND METABOLIC CAUSES OF AGITATION
AND CONFUSION

Hemodynamic

Impaired cerebral perfusion caused by cerebrovascular accident, tumor, increased
intracranial pressure
Meningitis, toxoplasmosis
Anoxic encephalopathy
Hypotension caused by sepsis or cardiogenic, anaphylactic, or hemorrhagic shock

Metabolic

Hypoglycemia
Acidosis
Hyponatremia
Elevated blood urea nitrogen and creatinine levels
Elevated serum ammonia levels
Myxedema
Corticosteroid insufficiency

Drug Effects

Antihistamines
Anticholinergics
Corticosteroids
Digitalis
H_2 antagonists
Imipenem, penicillin, amphotericin B, cephalosporins
Lidocaine, procainamide, quinidine, propranolol
Nitroprusside
Metoclopramide
Nonsteroidal antiinflammatory drugs
Theophylline

Drug Withdrawal

Opiates, cocaine, alcohol
Exogenous steroids
Tranquilizers
Antidepressants
Amphetamines

*Data from Crippen, D. (1994). Critical Care Nurse Quarterly, 16(4), 80-95; Geary, S. (1994).
Critical Care Nursing Quarterly, 17(1), 51-63; Harvey, M. (1996). American Journal of Critical Care,
5(1), 7-15.*

A number of hemodynamic and metabolic disease processes extrinsic to the
brain alter its metabolism. Common examples are hypoxemia, hypotension, and
hypoglycemia. Hypoxemia, a state of low partial pressure of oxygen in the blood,
may develop from pulmonary disorders, such as bronchospasm, pneumonia,
pulmonary effusions, or pulmonary emboli (Cohen et al, 2002; McGaffigan,
2002). Disorders such as chronic obstructive pulmonary disease (COPD),

asthma, or cancer of the lung may also lead to decreased gas exchange and lowered blood oxygen levels.

Mechanical problems with the ventilator or endotracheal tube may impede oxygen delivery. An inadequately inflated endotracheal balloon or dislodgment of the endotracheal tube will compromise oxygen delivery. A decrease in peak airway pressure may also stem from leaks in the ventilator tubing or an improperly sealed cap or nebulizer. The increased respiratory rate of an agitated patient who is not adequately sedated can lead to ventilator dysynchrony. Any of these problems may make the patient severely agitated as a result of a rapidly falling blood oxygen level. Any persistent low-oxygen state impedes brain metabolism and disrupts neurotransmission.

Hypotension caused by pump failure, sepsis, anaphylaxis, or hemorrhage impairs the delivery of oxygen to and removal of carbon dioxide from the brain. Even if the lung is able to exchange gases at the alveolar-capillary interface, there is inadequate delivery of oxygen at the cellular level. The acidosis that results from this ventilation and/or perfusion mismatch further impairs brain metabolism caused by decreased cardiac output. Persistent hypotension causing cellular hypoxia can lead to a cycle of cellular ischemia and death. This can then progress to multiple organ dysfunction.

Hypoglycemia rapidly disrupts brain metabolism, setting off a cascade of injury that alters neurotransmission and the rediffusion of transmitters back into the producing cells. Dopamine surges from the limbic system, causing widespread disruption of cerebral and lower regions of the brain.

Other metabolic disorders that disrupt brain function include metabolic acidosis, elevated blood urea nitrogen (BUN), creatinine, ammonia levels, and hyponatremia. Reaction to one of many medications commonly administered in the ICU may contribute to agitation. Steroids are a well-known cause of confusion. H_2 blockers, antibiotics, bronchodilators, and antihistamines have also been linked to agitation and confusion (Cohen, 2002; Crippen, 1994; Luer, 1995).

Withdrawal—Alcohol and Substance

Withdrawal from opiates, sedatives, antidepressants, alcohol, or tobacco can cause agitation and confusion. Forms of substance abuse may be overlooked in the ICU when the focus is on major organ failure. Not infrequently, tobacco addiction contributes to a patient's anxiety and agitation. Use of a nicotine patch often alleviates a significant part of the patient's discomfort and allows for lower doses of anxiolytics.

Alcohol withdrawal, a familiar syndrome to ICU nurses, is sometimes missed if the patient's history of drinking is not known to the family or acknowledged in the admission interview. Even heavy coffee drinkers, who are dependent on large doses of caffeine, can show signs of withdrawal that contribute to agitation. By interviewing family members and reviewing the documented history and physical examination, the nurse may often determine the factors that are contributing to the patient's agitation.

Drug effects and hemodynamic and metabolic disturbances alter neurotransmission in the motor axis, reticular substance, basal ganglia, cerebellum, and motor cortex (Cohen et al, 2002; Jacobi et al, 2002). The brain can no longer channel information to the cortical regions and interpret it on the basis of past memories. Instead the input is mischanneled to lower regions of the brain—the basal ganglia, reticular formation, vestibular nuclei, and extrapyramidal system. These regions respond with uncoordinated, nonpurposeful movements, tremors, musculoskeletal rigidity, and repetitive motion. Reactions may be highly emotional because of the dominance of lower, more primitive centers in the brain over higher regions, which would normally provide rational control.

Agitation then is a disturbance of brain function with behavioral and psychologic characteristics that presents as globally impaired cognitive function, restlessness, rigidity and tremors, and alternating periods of hyperalertness and lethargy. Agitation is caused by impaired brain metabolism brought on by impaired delivery of oxygen and glucose to the brain or by metabolic disturbances, including drug toxicity or withdrawal. Psychologic stresses, such as dyspnea, pain, and anxiety, contribute to agitation, but they are not the primary cause of a reversible organic syndrome.

Because impaired brain metabolism is the primary cause of agitation and confusion in critically ill patients, treatment is aimed at restoring normal brain function. After the assessment eliminates basic contributing factors, such as hypoxia, metabolic and electrolyte disturbances, alcohol withdrawal and delirium tremens, then appropriate steps should be taken to correct the underlying hemodynamic and metabolic disturbance. At the same time, pharmacologic agents are administered to restore equilibrium in neurotransmission and to suppress behaviors that are taxing the patient's reserves and jeopardizing care.

PHARMACOLOGIC MEASURES

The level and type of sedation used in the ICU have changed over the last two decades. Deep sedation in which the patient was completely detached from the environment was considered the ideal in the past. Neuromuscular blocking agents were also frequently administered. The effects from these agents resulted in prolonged immobility and contributed to developing decubitus, congestive heart failure, pulmonary congestion, and aspiration of feeding material. By 1990 only 16% of ICUs used paralyzing agents (Koleff et al, 1998; Kress et al, 2000; Shelly, 1994).

Today the goal of pharmacologic intervention is to relieve pain, anxiety, and other discomforts; to facilitate mechanical ventilation and other treatment modalities; and to provide amnesia for the more unpleasant aspects of critical illness. The preferred level of sedation is one in which the patient is asleep but easily aroused and able to cooperate with care. This level also allows for patient mobility, including chair rest and turning side to side. The ideally sedated patient is calm, cooperative, and cognitively intact enough to broadly comprehend what is happening to and expected of the patient (Roberts, 2001).

While doing all that can be done to alleviate the source of the anxiety and discomfort, the RN may also administer one or more medications. If the discomfort is mild, the doses are similar to the moderate sedation protocols used in short-procedure units (e.g., endoscopy, surgery, or radiology). However, because of their abnormal brain chemistry, ICU patients frequently require larger doses of medication than are customarily administered to non-ICU patients. Unless the patient is on a weaning mode, such as intermittent mandatory ventilation (IMV) or pressure support, mechanically ventilated patients are not in danger of respiratory arrest. Because anxiety and pain could impair synchrony with the ventilator, sedatives and analgesics improve oxygen exchange by slowing the respiratory rate, by allowing the patient to breathe with the ventilator, and by permitting the patient to cooperate with pulmonary toilet functions, such as chest physiotherapy and coughing.

For several reasons, the preferred route of administration in critical care is intravenous. First, oral medications are usually difficult to administer to the intubated patient, although some patients with tracheostomies are able to swallow pills, water, and even food. Absorption across the gastrointestinal (GI) tract is not always certain in these patients because of edematous bowel and decreased gastric motility. Also, as much as 90% of a sedative's bioavailability may be lost in passing through the GI tract and the liver (Koleff et al, 1998; Kress et al, 2000; Physicians' Desk Reference [PDR], 2003; White et al, 2001).

The intravenous route offers improved efficacy and more accurate blood levels. Patients who may be hypothermic or hypoperfused have decreased blood flow to peripheral tissue, leading to delayed and unpredictable absorption of medications administered intramuscularly. IV administration also provides a more rapid onset and allows for titration of administration, which is extremely useful for critically ill patients, whose condition may change abruptly. The intravenous route also prevents the local irritation to muscle produced by intramuscular or subcutaneous administration for several of the medications.

In the past, pain and sedation agents were administered as a continuous infusion. Recent literature supports use of lower dose continuous infusions with intermittent bolus injections to achieve satisfactory states of sedation (Koleff et al, 1998). Many institutions have developed guidelines for sedation that must be individualized for each patient. Patients who are mechanically ventilated experience different levels and types of agitation and will respond differently to pharmacologic agents administered.

Koleff and colleagues (1998) studied patients in the ICU who were being mechanically ventilated. They studied patients who were sedated by continuous infusions, intermittent bolus, or no sedation. The results of their study revealed that the group receiving continuous IV sedation had notably longer duration of mechanical ventilation, increased length of stay in the ICU, and overall longer hospital stay. This study shows that outcomes can be impacted by methods of sedation delivery.

The consensus statement from the Society of Critical Care Medicine, American College of Chest Physicians, and American Society of Hospital Pharmacists led to development of guidelines for sedation of critically ill patients. The goal of this statement is to provide adequate sedation for comfort and safety of the critically ill patient. Sedation medications should be initiated after attempts have been made to achieve adequate pain control (Jacobi et al, 2002).

On-request sedation may lead to periods when the patient does not receive medication, and it is likely to produce even greater variations in blood levels than a regularly scheduled individual dose. This gap in treatment can contribute to recurrent agitation with negative consequences to the patient. Regularly scheduled sedatives and analgesics provide a steady state only after repeated scheduled doses. A bolus plus a continuous infusion of sedation that is supplemented by occasional miniboluses provides less variation in serum drug levels (i.e., a better steady state) than the bolus administration alone does. However, the future practice for sedation administration is moving toward maintaining sedation control with the use of intermittent bolus dosing and using low dose continuous infusion only if adequate sedation control is not achieved with intermittent dosing schedules (Koleff et al, 1998).

Currently there is no definitive evidence that continuous infusion of sedation yields a more effective relief of agitation than regularly scheduled bolus dosing. Bolus doses take four to five elimination half-lives to achieve a steady state. Advocates of the infusion method point out that bolus administration may not achieve a constant blood level of the medication for 24 hours or longer. The peak levels can cause oversedation and hemodynamic side effects. Trough levels can lead to new outbreaks of agitation, which puts the patient at risk of self-extubation (Shelly, 1994).

There is theoretic evidence that the patient can reach a steady state more quickly with a loading dose followed by a continuous infusion than with bolus dosing alone. The infusion can be supplemented with miniboluses, and the titration increased depending on the patient's level of sedation. Some clinicians believe it is possible to reach a steady state more quickly with the infusion and/or minibolus method (Koleff et al, 1998; Luer, 1995).

The patient with a mild degree of anxiety or pain is given low to moderate doses of sedatives or analgesics, either in single doses or in a loading dose and an infusion. If discomfort is severe enough to cause agitation, higher doses are required (Tables 10-1 and 10-2). The continuous infusion can be titrated up or down depending on the patient's level of sedation. If the patient shows signs of delirium, a neuroleptic may be added. It is important to keep in mind that, in addition to treating the patient's subjective state, the RN must continually seek the causes of the agitation and confusion and treat those causes.

Frequently the combination of a benzodiazepine and opiate establishes calm and comfort in the ICU patient. To treat confusion, a neuroleptic and a benzodi-

Table 10-1 | **Loading Dose, Infusion Rate, and Titration for Low to Moderate Signs/Symptoms of Anxiety and Discomfort***

Drug	Load	Infuse	Titrate
Morphine	1-5 mg	1-5 mg/hr	1 mg
Fentanyl	50-100 mcg	50-250 mcg/hr	50 mcg
Dilaudid	0.5-2mg	0.5 mg/hr-2 mg	0.5
Diazepam	2-5 mg	2-5 mg/hr	2 mg
Lorazepam	1-2 mg	1-4 mg/hr	1 mg
Midazolam	0.5-1.5 mg	1-5 mg/hr	0.5 mg
Propofol	50-150 mg	50-150 mg/hr	50 mg
Haloperidol	2-10 mg	2-10 mg/hr†	1-2 mg

Patient weighs 70 kg.

†*If no improvement in patient condition after 20 to 30 minutes, double dose. Check intravenous infusion over time.* NOTE: *Literature supports administration of haloperidol in slowly increasing doses.*

Table 10-2 | **Loading Dose, Infusion Rate, and Titration for Moderate to Severe Signs/Symptoms of Anxiety and Discomfort***

Drug	Load	Infuse	Titrate
Morphine	5-15 mg	5-10 mg/hr	2 mg
Fentanyl	100-200 mcg	100 mcg	75-1200 mcg
Dilaudid	0.5-2 mg	0.5-2 mg	0.5 mg/hr
Diazepam	5-10 mg	5-10 mg/hr	3-5 mg
Lorazepam	2-10 mg	2-10 mg/hr	2 mg
Midazolam	1.5-3 mg	5-7 mg	1 mg
Precedex	1 mcg/kg over 10 minutes	0.2-0.7 mcg/kg/hr	0.2-0.7 mcg/kg/hr for 24 hrs max
Propofol	150-300 mg	150-300 mg/hr	75-100 mg
Haloperidol	10-100 mg	10-50 mg/hr†	5 mg

Patient weighs 70 kg.

†*If no improvement in patient condition after 20 to 30 minutes, double dose. Check intravenous infusion over time.* NOTE: *Literature supports administration of haloperidol in slowly increasing doses.*

azepine are often combined. Because the drugs are synergistic, combination therapy allows for lower doses of each drug, thereby reducing risk for unwanted side effects. Results are better because anxiety, discomfort, and confusion are relieved.

Analgesics

Opiates are the mainstay of pain control in critical care. Their efficacy has been well established, and their side effects are known and in most cases controlled by adjusting the dose and rate of administration or by taking countermeasures, such as intravenous fluids for transient hypotension. No other class of drugs has the efficacy of opiates. Opiates bind to several discrete receptor sites in the brain and spinal cord. They decrease postsynaptic membrane response to excitatory transmitters, such as norepinephrine and epinephrine, thereby decreasing the transmission of pain signals.

Despite the availability of opiates, many patients report that they received inadequate pain relief during their ICU stays (Jacobi et al, 2002). Patients' perceptions of pain vary related to disease process and can be influenced by the presence of an endotracheal tube, surgical procedures, treatments, and routine nursing care. Prior experiences with pain, ability for comprehension and cognition regarding their environment, and psychologic and emotional well-being can influence individual response to pain. Past concerns about inducing addiction have proved unfounded; however, adjustments must be made for patients with a prior history of substance abuse. The persistence of apparent undertreatment of pain argues strongly for the use of pain assessment scales and the development of more accurate and comprehensive measuring devices.

Among the opiates, meperidine is used less often than in the past because of its side effects (i.e., confusion, nausea, vomiting, and a potential to lower seizure thresholds). Ketorolac tromethamine (Toradol), a nonopiate prostaglandin inhibitor, is becoming more popular for the relief of short-term pain, especially in the emergency department. However, ketorolac does not have the potency or beneficial secondary effects of the opiates and is not approved for continuous intravenous infusion. Morphine and fentanyl are currently the most commonly prescribed opiates in critical care.

An opiate's undesirable effects on the cardiovascular system are particularly advantageous for the pulmonary system in a mechanically ventilated patient. The reduced preload decreases congestion in the pulmonary capillary bed, increasing pulmonary compliance. This enhances alveolar expansion and gas exchange, a phenomenon that is often seen when administering morphine intravenously to patients with flash pulmonary edema. Symptoms are reduced quickly and dramatically, peak airway pressures are lowered, and chest x-ray films demonstrate improvement in pulmonary congestion.

Opiates decrease gastric motility, leading to constipation and a potential small bowel ileus. Gastric emptying may be slowed; nausea and vomiting create a risk for aspiration pneumonia, even with an inflated cuff balloon. Patients receiving enteric support should be assessed frequently (i.e., every 2 to 4 hours) for abdominal distention and residual gastric feeding. The frequency, amount, and quality of bowel movements should be documented so that constipation can be identified and treated early.

With good pain relief, the patient is able to relax, allowing for easier chest excursion and improving thoracic compliance. The patient is able to better tolerate mechanical ventilation and cooperate with suctioning and chest physiotherapy. The actions, advantages, disadvantages, and unwanted side effects of analgesics are summarized in Table 10-3.

Table 10-3 | Summary of Medications Used in Treatment of Agitation and Delirium

Medication	Actions/Advantages	Side Effects/Disadvantages
Fentanyl	Crosses blood-brain barrier more readily than morphine sulfate More rapid onset when given in low to moderate dose Produces less hypotension than morphine sulfate	Respiratory depression Hypotension May cause glottic rigidity if given rapidly, complicating intubation May cause sleep deprivation
Ketorolac	Sustained pain relief Does not cause hypotension	Less effective than opiates
Diazepam	Rapid onset Effective anxiolysis Easily and quickly reversed Good musculoskeletal relaxation	Irritates small veins Precipitates in intravenous lines and solutions Hypotension Active metabolite extends elimination half-life Respiratory depressant
Lorazepam	Rapid onset Effective anxiolysis No active metabolites Inexpensive	Precipitates in intravenous lines and solution Solution must be changed every 12 hours Respiratory depression Hypotension Slower onset than midazolam
Midazolam	Rapid onset Effective anxiolysis Not irritating to veins Does not precipitate in solution	Respiratory depression Hypotension Expensive Has active metabolite
Propofol	Rapid onset Effective sedation Rapid clearance shortens wake-up time Effective for patient with opiate tolerance/addiction	Hypotension Respiratory depression Potential for bacterial contamination No reversing agent available
Haloperidol	Blocks dopamine at postsynaptic receptor sites Relieves confusion, tremors	Extrapyramidal symptoms Prolongs Q-T interval May induce torsades de pointes May cause neuroleptic malignant syndrome Exacerbates symptoms of Parkinson's disease

Continued

Table 10-3 | **Summary of Medications Used in Treatment of Agitation and Delirium—cont'd**

Medication	Actions/Advantages	Side Effects/Disadvantages
Clonidine	Inhibits norepinephrine release centrally Reduces anxiety, restlessness Synergy allows lower doses of opiates and benzodiazepines	Hypotension Bradycardia, conduction blocks
Morphine	Quickly reversed Short half-life makes it rapidly titratable	May cause hypotension due to decreased preload (vasodilation) Decreases gastric motility and may induce ileus or vomiting May cause histamine release and decreased broncho-constriction
Dilaudid	Rapid onset More potent than morphine Potent analgesic without hypnotic effects	Nausea and vomiting, less frequent than morphine Hypotension Respiratory depression
Precedex	Rapid onset Sedation and analgesia properties without respiratory depression	Hypotension and bradycardia, more pronounced in hypovolemic patients Recommended 24 hour infusion only

On administration of intravenous opiates, there is a rapid rise in blood levels. The serum level drops off as the drug diffuses into the third space, soft tissue, and bone marrow. A second dose yields a higher serum drug level because the medication has already become bound to receptor sites and been distributed throughout the body. A higher serum level results in a higher rate of elimination, assuming a normal liver and renal function.

The distribution of opiates is altered as a result of fluid retention, a common problem in critically ill patients. Mechanical ventilation causes a decrease in blood return to the heart, which promotes increased antidiuretic hormone (ADH) production, and a resultant sodium and water retention. Because opiates must diffuse into a relatively large extracellular volume, the patient may require higher doses than those given for the ideal weight.

If microcirculation is compromised, as in shock states, ischemic processes, or sepsis, opiates may be sequestered in poorly perfused tissue for prolonged periods of time. This may lead to reabsorption and resedation several hours or even days after opiates have been discontinued. This mechanism of poor distribution supports IV administration of the drug, regardless of whether the bolus or infusion method is used.

The abnormal brain function of agitated, critically ill patients further contributes to the need for higher doses of opiates. The excessive production of norepinephrine antagonizes the effects of opiates. Dopamine surges induce restlessness, sleeplessness, and musculoskeletal rigidity. These symptoms may not resolve unless relatively high doses of opiates are administered.

Opiates given to the ICU patient have been shown to undergo an unusually prolonged elimination half-life. This prolongation of half-life may be due to liver failure, which metabolizes the opiate, or renal failure, which excretes the active metabolite. The change in the drug's pharmacokinetics has also been attributed to low serum albumin levels and sequestration of active metabolites in poorly perfused tissue. Shock states may dramatically decrease elimination times. Exact mechanisms that affect drug elimination in the critically ill patient are not known. Prolonged elimination times can produce abnormally high serum drug levels. If the dose is not titrated downward, oversedation and unwanted side effects can occur. These can be prevented by careful patient assessment, by the use of a sedation scale, and by considering the patient's age and liver and renal function. Any patient who is hypotensive or who receives a continuous opioid infusion should be assessed frequently (e.g., hourly neurologic assessment) for increased opiate effects (Cohen et al, 2002; Jacobi et al, 2002; McGaffigan, 2002; PDR, 2003).

Morphine

Morphine is a pure opiate agonist that binds to opiate receptor sites in the central and peripheral nervous system. Morphine blocks the transmission and perception of pain. Morphine is given intravenously to prevent local irritation of intramuscular or subcutaneous injections. Because it is not lipophilic, morphine has a slower onset than fentanyl. Once a therapeutic blood level has been established, it provides relief for 2 to 4 hours.

Morphine's actions can affect the cardiac, pulmonary, GI, and neurohormonal systems. It is known to stimulate histamine release, which causes hypotension because of peripheral vasodilation. The decreased preload lowers filling pressures in the right side of the heart. Hypotension is more common and more pronounced in patients with hypovolemia or decreased left ventricular function. Patients with a reduced peripheral vasoconstrictive response, which may be the result of paralysis, diabetic neuropathy, or administration of alpha-blocking medication, are vulnerable to opiate-induced hypotension. These patients should receive lower doses of morphine that are administered slowly.

Morphine has the active metabolite M6G, which can remain in the serum for several hours. Even when the parent drug—morphine—is broken down by the liver and excreted, the psychoactive metabolite can notably extend the wake-up time. Because morphine is not lipophilic, it is relatively slow to cross the lipid-rich blood-brain barrier. The drug becomes distributed in the third space and internal organs and enters bone marrow. It is metabolized by the liver and excreted by the kidneys and in bile salts.

An initial dose of morphine, 1 to 5 mg given by slow intravenous injection, is given for mild to moderate pain; 5 to 10 mg is given for moderate to severe pain. By diluting 10 mg/cc of morphine in 9 ml of sterile water or normal saline, the drug can be administered in 1 to 5 mg bolus doses every 5 to 10 minutes until the patient is comfortable. A slow administration minimizes cardiac side effects. The loading dose may be followed by an infusion of 2 to 10 mg/hr, with additional small boluses for breakthrough pain. The dose is titrated until the patient is comfortable, provided cardiac parameters are within acceptable limits. Patients who receive up to 20 mg/hr of morphine infusion for a week or longer should be weaned slowly and monitored for signs and symptoms of opioid withdrawal (Gahart & Nazareno, 2003; PDR, 2003).

Fentanyl

Fentanyl (Sublimaze) is an opiate agonist that is widely used in the ICU because of its rapid onset. A highly lipophilic drug, fentanyl readily crosses the blood-brain barrier and binds with receptor sites in the brain and spinal cord.

Like morphine, fentanyl can cause hypotension and a decreased respiratory rate as a result of lowered sensitivity to carbon dioxide receptors in the brain. Constipation, nausea and vomiting, and decreased gastric emptying may also occur. A large loading dose may induce glottal rigidity, complicating intubation. If fentanyl is chosen before intubation for its rapid onset, it should be given in low to moderate amounts.

Even with its rapid onset, fentanyl has a longer elimination half-life than morphine does. This longer half-life is more likely to occur in patients who have received prolonged fentanyl infusions or who have liver or renal failure. Its lipophilicity causes fentanyl to be stored in fatty tissue, from which it is slowly released into the blood. This may lead to oversedation after several days of administration or to resedation after the medication is discontinued.

Because of its potential for slow elimination, fentanyl infusions should be stopped if the patient shows signs of oversedation or hypotension. The gradual drop off of drug levels after bolus and intravenous infusions suggests that merely lowering the infusion rate will not produce a rapid decline in blood levels because the infusion continues to administer the drug. Stopping the opiate until the unwanted side effects have resolved and restarting at a lower rate produce a more rapid resolution of the problem. Weaning must be done more slowly than in patients receiving short-term analgesia or sedation.

For low to moderate discomfort, 50 to 100 mcg is administered intravenously over 1 to 2 minutes. This may be followed by an infusion of 50 to 250 mcg/hr. If the patient remains uncomfortable and if hemodynamic parameters are within acceptable limits, a minibolus of 50 mcg may be given to control breakthrough pain. This regimen is repeated until the patient is comfortable or at goal per pain scale (Gahart & Nazareno, 2003; PDR, 2003).

Dilaudid

Dilaudid (hydromorphone) is an opium derivative narcotic and analgesic closely related to morphine, with six times greater potency. The exact mechanism of action is not known, but specific receptors in the central nervous system (CNS) have been identified. Dilaudid provides potent analgesia without hypnotic effects. Indications for use of Dilaudid are for control of moderate to severe pain. Dilaudid is used in the postoperative population and for patients who fail to respond to or are allergic to morphine.

Suppression of the cough reflex and respiratory depression occurs by effect on the medulla oblongata in the brain stem. Hypotension occurs as a result of peripheral vasodilation. Histamine may also be released, which causes vascular dilation that can also contribute to hypotension. The usual assessments, monitoring, and precautions used for morphine administration should be applied to patients receiving Dilaudid as described above.

Onset of action is in 15 to 20 minutes. The drug effect lasts 4 to 6 hours, with a half-life of 2.6 hours. Dilaudid is metabolized by the liver and excreted in the urine. Dilaudid is contraindicated in patients with known hypersensitivity asthma, and in pregnancy.

Dosing is 0.5 to 2 mg of Dilaudid IVP over 2 to 5 minutes, every 3 to 4 hours. The drug may be administered orally but note that oral doses are less than 50% as effective as parenteral doses. Continuous infusion of hydromorphone is generally via a patient-controlled analgesia (PCA) pump device, and infusion dosing is 0.5 to 2 mg/hr. Terminally ill patients may tolerate doses up to 2 to 9 mg/hr by infusion (Gahart & Nazareno, 2003; PDR, 2003).

Anxiolytics and Hypnotics

The benzodiazepines are the agents most commonly used in the ICU to relieve anxiety, restore normal sleep, provide amnesia, and relax skeletal muscles. No other class of medications provides the efficacy and low risk of complications as the benzodiazepines. They are often used concomitantly with opiates or neuroleptics, creating a synergy that affords improved comfort and allows for lower doses of each agent.

These agents appear to bind with benzodiazepine receptor sites in the CNS, where they potentiate or mimic the inhibitory neurotransmitter GABA and glycine. They reduce anxiety, produce dose-dependent amnesia, and relax skeletal muscles. The three most commonly administered benzodiazepines in the ICU include diazepam, lorazepam, and midazolam (Gahart & Nazareno, 2003; PDR, 2003).

Diazepam

Diazepam (Valium) was the most commonly prescribed intravenous benzodiazepine in the 1980s (Shelly, 1994). It is a long-acting sedative that has become less frequently used in the ICU because of its prolonged duration and undesirable side effects. Diazepam has the advantage of a rapid onset of 1 to 5 minutes because of its high lipid solubility. It provides effective relief of anxiety and muscle rigidity and is often effective for acute cessation of seizures. Diazepam is metabolized by the liver and excreted by the kidneys.

Phlebitis in a peripheral vein may result from the propylene glycol used as the vehicle for intravenous diazepam. When mixed in a solution for continuous administration, diazepam easily precipitates. The solution must be checked frequently for signs of precipitation and discarded if such signs are visible.

Diazepam may produce respiratory depression by suppressing carbon dioxide sensitivity in the brain, and it may cause hypotension because of peripheral vascular dilatation. Its major disadvantage is its prolonged effect. This is due in part to diazepam's long elimination half-life of 24 to 72 hours. Its active metabolite, N-desmethyl diazepam, has an elimination half-life of up to 96 hours. Even when the parent drug, diazepam, has been metabolized in the liver, the metabolite's CNS-depressing effects continue.

For mild to moderate agitation, diazepam is given slowly in a 2- to 5-mg dose. For moderate to severe agitation, a 5- to 10-mg dose may be used. Infusion rates of 2 to 10 mg/hr are common. If diazepam alone does not relieve the patient's agitation, administration in combination with an opiate is very effective. When combination therapy is used, smaller doses of each medication are indicated to prevent excessive side effects (Gahart & Nazareno, 2003; PDR, 2003).

Lorazepam

Lorazepam (Ativan) is an intermediate-acting sedative with a slower onset than diazepam or midazolam. Because it does not have an active metabolite, its sedating effects are removed as it is metabolized by the liver. Lorazepam is distributed in body fluids.

One disadvantage of lorazepam is that it, like diazepam, precipitates easily. For this reason, it should be mixed in a glass bottle, and the bottle and tubing should be changed every 12 hours. Nephrotoxicity and/or osmolar gap metabolic acidosis may occur with lorazepam infusions exceeding 8 mg/hr as a result of the polyethylene glycol and propylene glycol solvents contained in solution (Laine et al, 1995). As with any benzodiazepine, lorazepam may cause respiratory depression or hypotension.

Onset of action is 15 to 30 minutes, and effects last 6 to 8 hours and may last up to 24 hours. Average half-life is 9.5 to 19 hours. A 1- to 2-mg intravenous dose is administered to the patient with mild to moderate agitation. This may be followed by regularly scheduled intravenous boluses or by a continuous infusion of 1 to 2 mg/hr. The more severely agitated patient may require a 2- to 10-mg bolus followed by a 2 to 10 mg/hr drip as necessary. As with all benzodiazepines, patients with a history of benzodiazepine use, such as alprazolam (Xanax), require higher doses of this sedative or combination with an opiate or propofol (Gahart & Nazareno, 2003; PDR, 2003).

Midazolam

Midazolam (Versed) is a short-acting benzodiazepine with good sedating and amnesic properties. A water-soluble preparation, midazolam does not irritate peripheral veins, nor does it precipitate in solutions or intravenous lines.

It has a rapid onset, and when used for fewer than 3 to 5 days, has an elimination half-life of 2 to 4 hours. However, after long-term use midazolam's elimination half-life may be extended to 5 to 26 hours. This occurs when the drug is sequestered in poorly perfused fatty tissue, metabolism is slowed because of liver failure, or elimination is diminished because of renal failure. These conditions cause midazolam to act more like an intermediate-acting rather than a short-acting drug in critically ill patients. Its active metabolite has an elimination half-life of 1 hour.

An intravenous dose of 0.5 to 1.5 mg is given over 1 minute. Patients more than 65 years old or with COPD are initially given the lowest dose to prevent respiratory depression. Peak effect occurs in 2 to 3 minutes. Repeat doses of 0.5 mg may be given after 4 to 5 minutes until the patient is adequately sedated. Patients receiving opiates should be given one third to one fifth the normal dose of midazolam. Hypotension and respiratory depression are possible side effects. Infusions of 1 to 7 mg/hr may be used to control agitation (Gahart & Nazareno, 2003; PDR, 2003).

Propofol

Propofol (Diprivan), a nonbenzodiazepine, nonopiate anesthetic provides excellent sedation in the ICU for mechanically ventilated patients. Because of its rapid onset and short half-life, propofol is widely used in the critical care setting for patients requiring frequent neurologic assessment.

Propofol is suspended in a 10% lipid solution, which may have unwanted side effects. When lipids are metabolized they break down to carbon dioxide and water. Elevations of arterial carbon dioxide of 5% to 10% have been documented in patients with COPD who have received propofol. Elevated serum triglyceride and glucose levels have been found in patients with a restricted ability to metabolize fat. Patients receiving intravenous hyperalimentation should have their caloric intakes adjusted if they are to receive long-term propofol infusions.

The most serious unwanted side effect reported in the literature is bacteremia. There have been documented cases of patients having bacterial infection because of contamination of the propofol solute. This danger can be prevented with the use of a scrupulous aseptic technique when handling the medication. Some hospital protocols require that the intravenous solution containing propofol and the tubing be changed every 12 hours to prevent contamination. The site must be carefully checked for signs of local infection, and any sign of bacterial colonization warrants discontinuing the drug and changing the intravenous site.

Propofol is also an aphrodisiac and is known to cause vivid sexual dreams. Patients and families should be cautioned before propofol sedation is initiated that the patient may experience sexual dreams, and they are not to be confused with real experience. Currently, there is no reversal agent for this drug.

The patient does not receive a loading dose, as is common with opiates and benzodiazepines. Some anesthesiologists administer a very small test dose to be sure there is no allergic reaction. Because it can be irritating to the vein, the infusion is initiated slowly and gradually increased as the patient becomes somnolent.

The normal elimination half-life is 4 to 9 hours, but this does not correlate with the normal wake-up time, which is 10 to 30 minutes. As with opiates and benzodiazepines, the elimination half-life in the critically ill patient has been found to extend to 24 to 30 hours for the same reasons as the other sedating drugs. This may extend wake-up times, although clinical experience has not confirmed this.

An infusion of 50 to 150 mg/hr provides light to moderate sedation in a 70-kg adult. The infusion may be increased by 50 mg up to a dose of 300 mg/hr. The most common side effect is hypotension from peripheral vasodilation, which is more likely in the patient who is hypovolemic or elderly or who has decreased left ventricular function (Gahart & Nazareno, 2003; PDR, 2003).

ANTAGONISTS

Antagonists for opiates and benzodiazepines are available for emergency interventions. They are not approved for routine use to accelerate weaning from the sedating medication and must be used with caution because they can precipitate acute withdrawal signs.

Narcan

Narcan (naloxone) is a competitive opiate antagonist. It binds readily with opiate receptors in the CNS and spinal cord, driving out opiates. The opiates are then metabolized by the liver and excreted. When therapeutic blood levels of naloxone are maintained, opiates will not affect the nervous system.

The therapeutic dose of naloxone is 0.4 to 1 mg titrated intravenously. It has a rapid onset, producing reversal in 1 minute or less, depending on blood transit times. Because the half-life of opiates in the critically ill patient may be prolonged, the reversing agent may have to be repeated at 0.5- to 1-hour intervals if signs of resedation appear (Gahart & Nazareno, 2003; PDR, 2003).

Flumazenil

Flumazenil (Romazicon) is a benzodiazepine-reversing agent. It has a rapid onset, producing reversal in 1 minute or less. A dose of 0.2 to 1 mg is given by a slow intravenous route. The dose should not exceed 0.2 mg/min. Onset is in 1 to 3 minutes, and peak drug levels occur in 6 to 10 minutes.

Flumazenil may be repeated every 20 minutes, with the total dose not exceeding 3 mg/hr. Its serum half-life is 0.6 to 1.3 hours. As with the opiates, the elimination times of benzodiazepines may be prolonged in the ICU. The patient is monitored for resedation, and flumazenil may be repeated as necessary. Patients with a history of seizures should be watched closely because flumazenil can lower seizure thresholds (Gahart & Nazareno, 2003; PDR, 2003).

NEUROLEPTICS AND SYMPATHETIC INHIBITING AGENTS

Delirium in the critically ill patient is caused by a reversible organic syndrome caused by impaired brain metabolism and can occur in up to 60% of older patients who are hospitalized. Abnormal neurotransmission results in loss of cognitive function, restlessness and tremulousness, uncontrolled motor activity, and musculoskeletal rigidity. This syndrome is often a sign that one or more organ systems are deteriorating and should elicit an immediate assessment of all patient parameters. These include vital signs, arterial oxygen, pH and carbon dioxide levels, liver and renal function, and glucose levels. All medications should be reviewed for possible toxicity, and the patient's history of medication or drug abuse should be scrutinized.

Although treatment of the underlying causes of delirium is the primary focus of care, the confusional state may continue for hours or even days. In these cases medications are administered to restore a more normal neurotransmission.

Chlorpromazine hydrochloride (Thorazine) was one of the early antipsychotic medications. Its use has been curtailed by unwanted side effects, including leukopenia, extrapyramidal symptoms, and electrocardiographic changes, including widened QRS and QT intervals, and constipation. Chlorpromazine use has been generally replaced by haloperidol, which has fewer unwanted side effects and provides better relief of symptoms.

Haloperidol

Haloperidol (Haldol) is the drug of choice for delirium in the ICU (Cohen et al, 2002; Jacobi et al, 2002). It has no analgesic or sedating properties, but it may help the patient achieve a calm state when confusion is frightening.

Haloperidol acts by blocking surges of dopamine from several regions of the brain, including the limbic system. By suppressing the effects of this neurotransmitter, haloperidol relieves restlessness, tremors and uncontrolled muscle movements, and disorientation. It helps restore organized thinking, which enables the patient to better comprehend what is happening.

Side effects of haloperidol include extrapyramidal symptoms, laryngospasm, and bronchospasm. Rarely a neuromalignant syndrome has been reported. Its symptoms include high fever, tachycardia, hypotension, muscle stiffness, diaphoresis, and autonomic instability. The drug must be discontinued immediately if these signs occur, and interventions must be aimed at specific abnormalities. Fever is corrected; fluid resuscitation, cooling therapies, and a dopamine agonist (amantadine hydrochloride) may be used.

The QT interval should be measured every shift and documented because haloperidol has been associated with widening a QT and torsades de pointes, a potentially fatal dysrhythmia. If the QT interval is prolonged more than 450 msecs or by more than 25% from the baseline, haloperidol should be stopped, the physician notified, and all serum electrolyte levels checked. Low serum potassium and magnesium have been associated with increased risk of torsades de pointes. Serum electrolyte levels should be brought to a high normal level in the face of this electrocardiographic change. QT is measured from an electrocardiographic tracing, from the beginning of the Q wave to the end of the T wave. Measure the QT in a lead where it appears to be the longest. When the patient's heart rate is less than 100 bpm, the normal QT measurement should be less than half the R to R interval. The QT is considered to be borderline prolonged if it measures half the R to R interval. The QT is prolonged if it is more than half the R to R interval. When patients have irregular heart rates, tachycardia, or bradycardia, the QT must be corrected for the rate. The formula for QTc : QT / √ R to R. This calculation is used for rates less than 60 and more than 100 bpm. The normal measurement is 0.36 to 0.44 msecs. The QT or QTc should be measured before initiation of any drug that is known to prolong the QT interval.

Haloperidol is contraindicated for patients with a history of Parkinson's disease, a disease of decreased dopamine production in the brain. Because haloperidol blocks dopamine, it can worsen signs and symptoms of this disease.

Intravenous administration is the most effective route. The recommended dose is 2 to 10 mg intravenously. If symptoms are not improved in 20 to 30 minutes, the dose can be doubled. If symptoms are not improved in 30 minutes, the dose can be doubled again. This regimen is continued until the patient improves, or until the dose exceeds hospital protocols.

If haloperidol alone does not resolve signs of delirium, combination with a benzodiazepine has been shown to be efficacious. As with any combination, the amount of each medication should be reduced because of the synergy. Adding a benzodiazepine also reduces the incidence of side effects from haloperidol (Gahart & Nazareno, 2003; PDR, 2003).

Clonidine

Clonidine (Catapres) is an alpha-adrenergic agonist that inhibits the release of norepinephrine from central and peripheral presynaptic junctions by a negative feedback mechanism. Excessive production of catecholamines is thought to be linked to ICU delirium, especially to hyperalertness, sleep intolerance, and tremulousness. By blocking this potent neurotransmitter, clonidine reduces signs and symptoms of agitation.

Prolonged administration of opiates has been implicated with excessive norepinephrine release. Clonidine is especially helpful for these patients. It enables the use of lower doses of opiates to achieve comfort, thereby reducing the risk of hypotension or respiratory depression. Clonidine is also thought to have analgesic properties, although the mechanism of action is not known.

Clonidine also acts synergistically with benzodiazepines and with haloperidol. It helps to relieve confusion and agitation and allows for lower doses of both drugs.

The loading dose is 0.1 to 1 mg orally twice daily, depending on the severity of symptoms. A transdermal patch releasing 0.1 to 0.3 mg/hr can be added after the loading dose is given orally. An intravenous preparation has been used in Europe and is currently undergoing clinical trials in the United States. When it is approved, intravenous clonidine is likely to become an important adjunct treatment for agitation in the ICU (PDR, 2003).

Dexmedetomidine

Dexmedetomidine (Precedex) is a selective alpha$_2$-adrenergic receptor agonist that has sedative and analgesic effects. Presynaptic activation of alpha$_2$-adrenoreceptors hinders the release of the catecholamine norepinephrine. Postsynaptic activation of alpha$_2$-adrenoreceptors in the CNS causes the inhibition of sympathetic activity and a decrease in blood pressure and heart rate, resulting in sedation and anxiolysis.

Dexmedetomidine has an advantage for the agitated, mechanically ventilated patient in that it does not cause respiratory depression. Patients can be weaned from mechanical ventilation and extubated while on low dose dexmedetomidine. It has a rapid distribution with a half-life of 2 hours. Elimination is via the hepatic system and should be decreased in patients with hepatic dysfunction. Response to the drug may be altered in patients with hepatic or renal dysfunction.

Dexmedetomidine is given by IV infusion using an infusion pump and may be administered peripherally. The loading dose is 1 mcg/kg over 10 minutes followed by an infusion dose of 0.2 to 0.7 mcg/kg/hr, adjusted to desired level of sedation and patient response. Dexmedetomidine is not recommended for infusions lasting longer than 24 hours. The use of dexmedetomidine is not recommended in patients who are experiencing bradycardia, hemodynamic instability, or hypovolemia because adverse effects may include hypotension or bradycardia (Gahart & Nazareno, 2003; PDR, 2003).

COMBINATION THERAPY

Many clinicians obtain improved effects by combining opiates, benzodiazepines, neuroleptics, and propofol in varying combinations. The choice of agents depends on the specific disorder being treated and on how well the patient tolerates each class of medication. If raising the dose of a single medication does not resolve the patient's discomfort or agitation, adding a second drug often yields improved results.

Each class of drugs works synergistically with the others. For this reason it is important to lower the dose of each one. Continuous infusions may be run concomitantly. Bolus administrations may be alternated, so that the patient receives a medication frequently.

An example of a combination therapy is lorazepam, 4 mg intravenously every 4 hours around the clock, and haloperidol, 10 mg intravenously every 4 hours to alternate with lorazepam. With this regimen, the patient receives a sedating or calming medication every 2 hours.

Propofol can be combined with opiates. The propofol infusion is given in a lower infusion rate because the hypotensive effects can be magnified by the combined drug effects. Combination therapy is particularly advantageous in preventing tolerance and when weaning a patient. There are reports that after 5 to 7 days of intravenous sedation, prolonged elimination half-lives of the drug develop (Cohen et al, 2002; Gahart & Nazareno, 2003; PDR, 2003, Jacobi et al, 2002).

Tolerance and Extended Elimination Half-Lives

Tolerance is the phenomenon of requiring progressively higher doses of a medication to obtain the same results. It is why a heroin addict requires increasing amounts of an opiate to experience positive effects. In the ICU, patients who have no history of drug addiction may begin to show signs of opiate tolerance in 5 to 7 days. They may report inadequate pain relief after receiving the previously effective dose.

This tolerance results from the body's natural tendency to respond to a continuous CNS-depressing effect. Opiates and benzodiazepines dull sensation. After receiving repeated doses, the body produces increasing amounts of excitatory neurotransmitters. In response to chronic opiate use, the brain produces large amounts of norepinephrine in the locus caeruleus. The brain also increases the sensitivity of norepinephrine receptors, almost as if it were trying to rouse itself from a forced slumber.

The stimulatory effects of excitatory transmitters counteract the sedating effects of opiates and benzodiazepines. The RN is forced to administer higher doses of medication to achieve a satisfactory level of comfort for the patient. One way to prevent or reduce tolerance is to use combination drug therapy. Benzodiazepines, which reduce the anxiety that contributes to pain, work synergistically with opiates, allowing for lower dosing of the analgesic. This combination slows the development of opiate tolerance. For patients who require high doses of benzodiazepines, the addition of haloperidol allows better control of agitation and confusion and lowers the necessary dose of the sedative.

Several theories have been brought forth to explain the extended half-life of opiates and sedatives. Liver failure slows the metabolism of these medications and plays an important role. Renal insufficiency or failure impairs elimination of the active metabolites, which contributes to the drugs' sedating properties. With low serum albumin levels, a common finding in the ICU patient, analgesics and sedatives are less able to bind to protein for transport to the brain.

Compromised microcirculation plays a role in prolonging drug half-lives. Poorly perfused tissue stores drugs for prolonged periods. After the serum level has dropped, stores of the drug slowly diffuse into the bloodstream and are transported to the brain and spinal cord, causing resedation and unwanted side effects. A sedation scale may also be continued after a sedative is discontinued as a way to monitor the patient's level of consciousness and comfort.

NONPHARMACOLOGIC MEASURES

Direct interventions to relieve the patient's discomfort are an essential part of nursing care. The goal is to correct the condition that is causing the discomfort and to initiate interventions that promote comfort and a sense of well being.

Pain can originate from sources that are sometimes overlooked. Because the patient has difficulty communicating information, it may be difficult to ascertain the precise location and type of pain. A patient who points to the upper abdomen or lower chest may be indicating chest pain, abdominal pain, inferior pleuritic pain, pancreatic pain, or gall bladder pain. Often only a complete physical assessment and thorough review of laboratory values will reveal the probable source of the discomfort.

Other physical discomforts afflicting the patient may be nausea and the urge to vomit, which can be terrifying to the intubated patient who cannot easily turn and expectorate gastric material. An itch that cannot be scratched, a sensation of cold or fever, a need to urinate or defecate, or the desire to change position and relieve stiffened joints may be extremely disquieting to the patient. The patient's inability to communicate these needs can further heighten the discomfort and lead to agitation.

Anxiety arises from many sources that are not always apparent. Identifying the source often requires effort and imagination. Patients are often extremely troubled by the fear of painful procedures, the loss of control over activities of daily living, and the dependence on strangers to provide the necessities of life. These necessities include a constant supply of oxygen, nutrition, fluids, and the elimination of urine and feces, activities of daily living that the healthy individual may take for granted. The patient's abrupt change from independent to dependent person can be deeply disturbing to the patient and to the family.

Critical illness presents a family with a major crisis. Issues related to employment and income, responsibility and leadership in the family, and other personal issues stress the patient. Frequently the patient is separated from significant others at a time when the patient has a heightened need for their emotional support. Spouses of many years may find forced separation frightening or depressing. Early involvement of social services and case managers may alleviate patient and family fears and concerns.

Some ICUs have introduced liberal visiting hours. Others maintain strict limits on the number of visitors allowed and the length of the visit. There is a growing trend to allow more liberal visitations as hospitals recognize the impact of isolation on the critically ill patient, but practices vary widely among institutions and at times even among critical care units within an institution.

Communication for the mechanically ventilated patient is difficult. In addition, it is sometimes complicated by a language barrier. Hospitals may maintain a list of bilingual employees to provide translators who assist in taking a history and providing information and reassurance to the patient and family. Communication devices such as alphabet boards may be useful in improving communication.

Cards with phrases and translations can help relieve a patient's anxiety. Basic needs are expressed, and broad information about the patient's prognosis, probable length of stay, and the need for further diagnostic tests and treatments can be conveyed to the patient.

Confusion can cause a patient much anxiety, especially if accompanied by hallucinations or delusions, which are difficult to assess in this patient population. The RN must make every effort to reorient the patient while at the same time validating the patient's feelings. Phrases such as, "I'm sure you feel frightened, Mr. Smith. I would feel the same way, but I can assure you that you are in a hospital, I am your nurse, and we are treating you for pneumonia. Do you understand?" support the patient's emotions and redirect the patient toward a more realistic appraisal of reality.

Many institutions try to soften the harsh environment with soft lighting, restful music, and pleasant interior designs. Attempts to restore a normal sleep cycle can be hampered by excessive auditory and tactile stimuli. Efforts should be taken to prevent false alarms (e.g., secure electrocardiograph electrode placement) and unnecessary noise.

Orientation to time and place may be enhanced by the use of large clocks and calendars and by reading highlights from a daily newspaper, including the weather report. Pictures from home not only help the patient recall loved ones but remind caregivers of the patient's identity before becoming critically ill, nonverbal because of the endotracheal tube, and possibly disoriented. Orientation can be facilitated by using a television if present in the patient's room. Having the family identify the patient's favorite shows (news, sports, games, and entertainment) may help with orientation by offering distraction.

Other means of nonpharmacologic therapy can be used to offer distraction. These include music therapy, guided imagery, therapeutic touch, aromatherapy, and pet therapy.

SEDATION SCALE AND OTHER MEASURES OF SEDATION

In the past decade the use of sedation scales has increased for the patient receiving intravenous sedation. Sedation scales serve two basic functions: (1) they measure the patient's subjective state (e.g., pain, anxiety, confusion, or other discomforts) and (2) they measure the objective behaviors that usually accompany internal tension (e.g., restlessness, hyperreflexia, inability to sleep, tremulousness, and musculoskeletal rigidity). Many sedation scales are found in the literature; most are numerical and evaluate patients' responses to pain or stimuli. Although the scales are different, they are similar in what they are measuring. Regardless of the scale used, use of a sedation scale to evaluate the effect of medication administration in the mechanically ventilated patient is vital.

Sedation scales also provide a means to define the goal, which is the desired level of sedation. This measures the efficacy of treatment and tells the practitioner whether the interventions have been successful. Sedation scales may help the practitioner avoid undersedation or oversedation. Studies have shown that by using a sedation scale the RN is able to establish the desired sedation level more quickly and safely (Weinart, Chlan, & Gross, 2001).

Some institutions have adopted an algorithm approach to managing the uncomfortable patient. This method begins by assessing for anxiety, pain, dyspnea, or delirium. The nurse then identifies probable causes for each problem. The algorithm then suggests treatments specific to each type of problem. Although the algorithm does not measure level of sedation as such, it does address the need to identify specific problems that produce agitation or confusion.

One widely used sedation scale in the ICU setting is the Ramsay scale. It is a simple six-point sedation score that focuses on the agitated patient requiring sedation. The Ramsay scale measures three levels of waking and three levels of sleep (Table 10-4) showing different levels of variable responses to loud noise, verbal communication, and glabellar tapping. When used as a guide for sedating the patient, the physician orders medication to be given to achieve a specific Ramsay score. The medication may be ordered to be given as necessary, in which case the RN administers medication until the desired level of sedation is reached. Or the medication dose may be variable, within preprescribed limits, which the RN adjusts in line with the patient's level of agitation and discomfort.

The preferred depth of sedation has changed considerably in the last 15 years. In the past a deep level of sleep, which would today be measured as a 5 or 6 on the Ramsay scale, was frequently the goal. Today, most practitioners aim for a lighter level of sedation, usually a Ramsay score of 2 to 3, or a Riker score of 3 to 4. Patients with severe pulmonary disease who require high levels of positive end-expiratory pressure or who experience persistent, marked degrees of dyspnea often require a deeper level of sedation. The higher doses promote muscle relaxation and improve pulmonary compliance.

One major limitation of the Ramsay scale is that it was never validated by objective measures (Jacobi et al, 2002; McGaffigan, 2002). There is ambiguity and overlap in some of the categories. For example, a patient who is intermittently sleeping and who awakens to verbal stimuli (level 4) may be anxious and restless (level 1). Also, different raters who simultaneously observe the same patient have been known to assign different Ramsay scores to the patient. Other limitations of the Ramsay scale include the lack of focus on the specific type of discomfort causing the agitation or confusion. Because this scale does not

Table 10-4 | Comparison of Different Sedation Scales

Patient Condition	Frequency of Assessment/ Medication	Score
Ramsay Scale		
Level 1 Patient awake; anxious and agitated or restless (or both)		
Level 2 Patient awake; cooperative, oriented, and tranquil		
Level 3 Patient awake; responds to commands only		
Level 4 Patient asleep; brisk response to light glabellar tap or loud auditory stimulus		
Level 5 Patient asleep; sluggish response to light glabellar tap or loud auditory stimulus		
Level 6 Patient asleep; no response to light glabellar tap or loud auditory stimulus		
Luer Scale (abridged)		
Combative; interferes with care; severe potential for self-harm	Every 30 minutes Repeat loading dose	1
Anxious, agitated, fearful; moderate potential for self-harm	Every hour Repeat loading dose	2
Restless; mild potential for self-harm/ objective parameter (e.g., asynchronous breathing, low oxygen saturation)	Every 2 hours Give 50% loading dose	3
Awake, calm, and cooperative; follows commands	Every 4 hours Maintain infusion, consider titrating down after 24 hours	4
Asleep but arousable	Every 4 hours	5
Difficult to arouse by verbal stimuli	Every hour	6
Minimal or no response to tactile stimuli	Every hour; decrease infusion 1 mg; notify physician	7
No response to painful stimuli	Call physician	8
Shelly Scale		
Eyes open		
Spontaneously		4
To speech		3
To pain		2
None		1
Response to nursing procedures		
Obeys commands		4
Purposeful movements		3
Nonpurposeful movement		2
None		1
Cough		
Spontaneous, strong		4
Spontaneous, weak		3
On suction only		2
None		1

Table 10-4 | Comparison of Different Sedation Scales—cont'd

Patient Condition	Frequency of Assessment/ Medication	Score
Shelly Scale—cont'd		
Respirations		
Extubated		5
Spontaneous, intubated		4
IMV-triggered respiration		3
Respiration against ventilator		2
No respiratory effort		1
Riker Sedation-Agitation Scale (SAS)		
Dangerously agitated, tried to remove catheters/ET tube, tries to get out of bed, requires restraints		7
Very agitated, does not calm down even with verbal reminders, requires restraints		6
Agitated, tries to sit up, calms down in response to verbal commands		5
Calm and cooperative		4
Sedated, follows simple commands		3
Very sedated, arousable but does not follow commands		2
Unarousable, no response to noxious stimuli		1

identify levels of pain, dyspnea, or anxiety, it is difficult to use the score to evaluate the efficacy of specific treatments.

Luer (1995) developed an eight-point scale that addresses specific sources of agitation in the mechanically ventilated patient (see Table 10-4). The categories include problems such as asynchrony with the ventilator, decreased oxygen saturation, and increased heart rate. The score ranges include the following: score 1, the combative patient who interferes with care and has a severe potential for self-harm; score 2, the anxious, agitated, or fearful patient who is moderately at risk; score 3, the restless patient with a mild potential for harm; score 4, the awake, calm, cooperative patient; score 5, the sleeping but arousable patient; score 6, the patient who is difficult to arouse by verbal stimuli; score 7, the minimally responsive patient; and score 8, the unresponsive patient.

Luer's categories include recommendations for the frequency of drug administration. For example, the combative patient receives a sedative every 30 minutes; the less agitated, an hourly sedation; the restless patient, a sedative every 2 hours; and so on. For the unresponsive patient, the sedation is stopped and the physician notified. The eight-point scale offers a more comprehensive neurologic assessment than the Ramsay scale does. It also suggests problem-oriented interventions, somewhat like the algorithm. Luer's scale appears to have some advantages over the others and warrants further clinical study.

The Riker Sedation-Agitation Scale (SAS) was the first scale to be formally tested for reliability and validity in the ICU (Cohen et al, 2002; Roberts, 2001). The SAS identifies 7 levels of sedation and agitation ranging from dangerous agitation to deep sedation (see Table 10-4). This scale provides descriptions of patient behavior in varying levels that assist the bedside practitioner in distinguishing between the levels of sedation. The score ranges include the following: 1, unarousable; 2, very sedated; 3, sedated; 4, calm and cooperative; 5, agitated; 6, very agitated; 7, dangerous agitation.

The Motor Activity Assessment Scale (MAAS) is similar to the SAS and uses patient behavior in response to stimulation to describe the different levels of agitation. The MAAS identifies seven levels ranging from unresponsive to dangerously agitated, much like the Riker, but can be applied to patients with altered cognitive function (Clemmer et al, 2000; Jacobi et al, 2002).

A somewhat different approach taken by Shelly identifies four problems that can cause agitation and impair mechanical ventilation. The four problems identified include level of consciousness, ability to cooperate with nursing procedures, ability to assist with pulmonary toilet, and the degree of ventilatory support required (see Table 10-4). This scale is a useful way to categorize problems because it is goal directed. Improvement in patient outcomes can be discerned by noting specific scores and the patient's overall level of comfort and respiratory status. Although it does not identify degree of confusion, it is useful in defining salient end points and linking treatment to those end points. Shelly's scale also warrants additional clinical trials (Shelly, 1994).

Most critical care flow sheets include a basic Glasgow Score of level of consciousness: motor activity and confusion based on verbal ability. It might be useful to replace the Glasgow Score on the nursing flow sheet with a scale that more accurately assesses the patient's type and degree of discomfort. By introducing a scale similar to Luer, Shelly, Riker SAS, or MAAS, the flow sheet would offer a way to compare the patient's discomfort and/or confusion with the infusion of sedation, vital signs, ventilatory status, and urinary output. Integrating a sedation scale into the flow sheet could simplify documentation and analysis of the sedation strategy.

The development of noninvasive, objective monitors of brain function using electroencephalogram (EEG) signals may lead to a more standardized assessment of agitation and sedation. One example, the Bispectral Index (BIS) monitor, is a measurement based on EEG and provides the practitioner a more objective analysis of the level of sedation. A digital readout of 0 to 100 is obtained from a sensor that is placed on the forehead. This number correlates with the patient's level of sedation and will fluctuate with sedation dosing and stimulation. Completely awake patients have scores from 90 to 100 on the BIS monitor; moderately sedated patients 70 to 89; patients undergoing general anesthesia 50 to 69; deep hypnotic state or comatose patients 0 to 49. The BIS monitor is useful while titrating sedation medication to maintain optimal levels of sedation and preventing episodes of oversedating or undersedating the patient. This monitoring

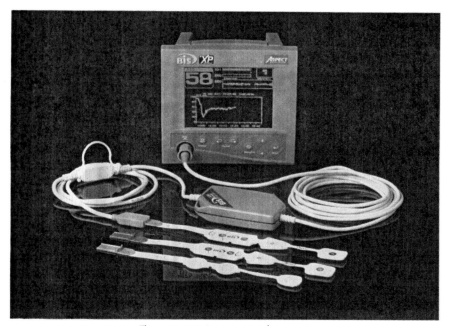

Figure 10-1 BIS monitor and sensors.

system is also useful for identifying breakthrough agitation during procedures or routine care that may necessitate bolus dosing, instead of increasing medication infusions, to regain adequate levels of sedation and comfort. The BIS monitor has been validated as an assessment tool for sedation. Preventing episodes of oversedation or undersedation helps to maintain optimal comfort and reduce potential for traumatic experiences and memories in the ventilated and sedated patient. Early studies comparing objective and subjective assessments of sedation show that they do correlate highly (McGaffigan, 2002; Roberts, 2001) (Figures 10-1 and 10-2).

Daily Wake Up

Continuous IV infusion of sedatives is often used to provide a more constant level of sedation and increase patient comfort. However, sedating agents depress neurologic function, making it impossible to accurately assess the patient's neurologic status to ensure that a neurologic insult has not occurred. Infusion of sedating agents should be interrupted daily to perform a thorough neurologic assessment. The sedation is decreased slowly until the patient is responsive to stimuli and is ideally calm and cooperative. The nurse then assesses the patient's neurologic status and facilitates orientation to their environment. This also enables the nurse to assess other physiologic parameters including resting heart

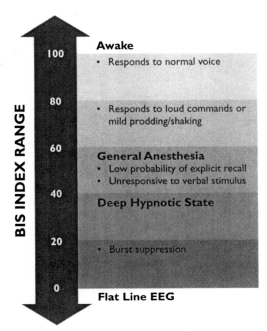

Figure 10-2 BIS range guidelines.

rate, respiratory rate, and effort. Patients should be evaluated for the appropriateness of daily wake ups every AM, and sedation medication titrated down or weaned per protocol. Situations in which the patient is not stable, and weaning medication may be detrimental include: hemodynamic instability, respiratory instability, increased intracranial pressure, or need for patient immobilization. The decision for daily wake up is a joint decision of the patient care team but driven by the expert nurse clinician providing direct care to the patient.

Daily wake ups also enable the nurse to determine the minimum dose required to provide sedation. The medication is increased slowly until the defined end point, the goal of sedation therapy, is reached. If the patient reaches this level with a lower dose than was formerly used, there is less risk of unwanted side effects. Since continuous IV sedation has been identified as an independent predictor of longer duration of mechanical ventilation and increased ICU days, the goal should be to wean continuous IV sedation as soon as possible, provided the patient can be managed with intermittent bolus dosing (Kress et al, 2000).

A study by Kress et al (2000) showed that daily interruption of the infusion of sedatives is a safe and practical approach to treating patients who are receiving mechanical ventilation. This practice has been shown to decrease the duration of mechanical ventilation, length of stay in the ICU, and doses of benzodiazepines used. It also allowed clinicians to perform daily neurologic examinations and reduced the necessity for diagnostic studies to evaluate unexplained alterations in mental status.

Family visits may be timed to coincide with the daily wake up to promote communication within the family. If the patient shows renewed signs of discomfort, agitation, or confusion, the sedation is increased. A minibolus may be administered to rapidly raise serum blood levels and reach a steady state more rapidly (White et al, 2001).

SEDATION AND WEANING PROTOCOL

Sedation medications should be titrated on a daily basis to reach safe and comfortable goals. Using a nurse-driven sedation protocol enhances patient outcomes. Patients should be assessed daily for their ability to be weaned from the ventilator and sedation medications. Use of protocols not only standardizes care on all patients, but has been shown to decrease ventilator days, complications of ventilation, and ICU length of stay. Sedation administered via accepted protocol results in more consistent medication administration based on adopted sedation scales, decreased use of sedation medications, early mechanical ventilator weaning, and decreased overall costs (Brook et al, 1999; Koleff et al, 1998).

DRUG TOLERANCE AND WEANING FROM VENTILATOR

When pulmonary and other organ systems improve to the point that the patient can be weaned from ventilatory support, the level and type of sedation in use must be carefully considered. The ideal weaning practice is to slowly decrease sedation at the same time that ventilatory support is decreased. Because this is a period of increased risk of self-extubation, sedation must be decreased cautiously, and the patient must be observed closely for signs of renewed agitation. As the patient becomes more awake, the patient's inherent respiratory rate and effort can be measured, and progress toward extubation is made with reliable indicators of respiratory muscle strength.

Protocols for weaning vary among institutions and among practitioners. Often the ventilatory mode is changed to an IMV, CPAP, or pressure support so that the patient's inherent expired tidal volume, minute ventilation, and peak flow can be measured. The patient must have a positive gag reflex to protect the airway. The patient should be awake enough to cooperate with instructions related to pulmonary toilet, such as coughing, deep breathing, and use of incentive spirometry. The patient must also be able to generate a negative inspiratory pressure great enough to ensure an acceptable spontaneous tidal volume and minute ventilation. Arterial blood gases confirming adequate oxygenation during the ventilatory weaning are standards of practice.

Five drug-related factors can complicate the gradual withdrawal of mechanical ventilation, including (1) tolerance, (2) prolonged elimination half-life, (3) drug withdrawal, (4) persistence of confusion or agitation, and (5) nutritional deficit.

Tolerance, as discussed earlier in the chapter, is the brain's response to sedation. The dose of medication is slowly decreased in preparation for weaning from the ventilator while maintaining acceptable comfort levels. In some cases the patient can be treated with an opiate agonist-antagonist, such as nalbuphine hydrochloride (Nubain). These agents have fewer sedating and respiratory depressant effects. However, because they possess agonist and antagonist effects affecting different opiate receptors, they cannot be administered in conjunction with pure opiate agonists, such as morphine, or they may precipitate signs of opiate withdrawal.

The second factor complicating weaning from the ventilator is a prolonged half-life of any medication the patient is currently taking. Because critically ill patients are less able to metabolize and excrete sedating medications, the parent drugs and their active metabolites accumulate in the blood, fatty tissue, and receptor sites. Morphine's half-life can be extended from 4 to 13 hours, that of fentanyl from 5 to 25 hours, and that of propofol from 3 to 30 hours (Gahart & Nazareno, 2003; McGaffigan, 2002; PDR, 2003).

There is evidence that morphine concentrations in the brain are increased because of hypercapnia and the resulting respiratory acidosis. Because carbon dioxide retention can occur during the weaning process, it is particularly important to watch for signs of increased opiate binding to brain receptor sites, manifested by increasing lethargy and hypoventilation.

As medications are titrated down, stores in fat, muscle, and bone are redistributed to the blood and brain, causing resedation. This has been found in patients up to 24 hours after the medication was discontinued. The lingering respiratory depressant effects of the drugs can decrease pulmonary parameters, which slow the weaning process (Riker & Fraser, 2002).

Sedation scales are particularly important during this period. Usually the physician asks that the patient be brought to a lighter level of sedation. Neurologic assessments document the lightening of sedation, which indicates that respiratory depression is also decreased. If the patient has received long-term sedation with a benzodiazepine, some clinicians prefer to switch the patient to propofol for the final weaning and extubation. The opiates and benzodiazepines are discontinued, and a propofol infusion is initiated. The propofol is gradually decreased until the patient is awake, comfortable, and able to follow commands. There should be no signs of hypoventilation. When all extubation criteria are met, the propofol is discontinued. Ten to 15 minutes later, the patient is extubated. Vital signs, especially oxygen saturation and respiratory rate, are watched carefully for 24 hours for signs of resedation (Jacobi et al, 2002; Koleff et al, 1998; McGaffigan, 2002).

The third factor complicating weaning from the ventilator is the possibility of withdrawal symptoms emerging. Patients who receive intravenous sedation for more than 5 to 7 days are at risk of development of signs of withdrawal. If opiates are withdrawn too quickly, signs of acute opiate withdrawal may appear. These can include anxiety, restlessness, and sleeplessness; nausea, vomiting, and watery diarrhea; piloerection; and gross large muscle spasms (Cohen et al, 2002; Shelly, 1994; White et al, 2001).

Rapid withdrawal of benzodiazepines can cause anxiety, insomnia, elevated blood pressure, tremors, and diaphoresis. Abruptly discontinuing these medications from the elderly patient leads to hallucinations and agitation. Rapidly discontinuing propofol after an infusion of more than 5 to 7 days can lead to agitation, confusion, and convulsions. Longer periods of infusion require a more gradual rate of decrease. Rapid withdrawal of benzodiazepines can elicit acute withdrawal symptoms that include anxiety and confusion, seizures, and hallucinations.

To prevent opiate or benzodiazepine withdrawal, the dose can be decreased by 10% to 25% per day. Thus if a patient received a total of 480 mcg of fentanyl over 24 hours (20 mcg/hr) the previous day, then a 10% decrease of dose would equal 432 mcg/24 hr (18 mcg/hr) and a 25% decrease would equal 360 mcg/24 hr (15 mcg/hr) (Jacobi et al, 2002; Koleff et al, 1998; White et al, 2001).

The fourth factor complicating ventilatory weaning is the persistence of delirium after the pulmonary disorder has been resolved. The organic syndrome, which causes delirium, is slow to resolve. Abnormal brain function often lasts well after the patient's oxygen transfer has been normalized and will require administration of neuroleptic medications after the patient is weaned. But because haloperidol is not a respiratory or CNS depressant, it will not complicate extubation. Decreasing the dose of a benzodiazepine or an opiate may be necessary to ward against resedation, but continuing haloperidol should not present a problem (Ely et al, 2001; Ely, Siegel, & Inouye, 2001; Koleff et al, 1998).

It is important not to discount the effects of poor nutritional status on the patient's ability to be weaned off the ventilator. Critically ill patients frequently have low serum albumin levels. Their caloric intake may have been decreased as the result of persistent symptoms, such as dyspnea, weakness, fatigue, nausea, or pain. Many critical illnesses impair the ability of the GI tract to absorb nutrients. Intubated patients often have diarrhea, which further impedes intake of calories and vitamins.

Malnourished patients tire more easily when switched to a weaning mode. It is important to begin optimizing the patient's nutritional state from the beginning of the ICU stay. That way, when the pulmonary disorders have improved sufficiently to allow for extubation, the patient will have enough strength to move sufficient air. After the patient is extubated, dosing regimens are adjusted to a level of comfort where the patient is responsive or functioning at the neurologic baseline.

For the patient undergoing moderate sedation, medication is administered per the institution's sedation protocol for the nonintubated patient. Hemodynamic parameters must still be monitored, and the sedation scale must still be used. The possibility of resedation, even days after extubation, must be borne in mind. Please refer to previous chapters for sedation in the nonintubated patient. See Figure 10-3 for an example of an institutional protocol.

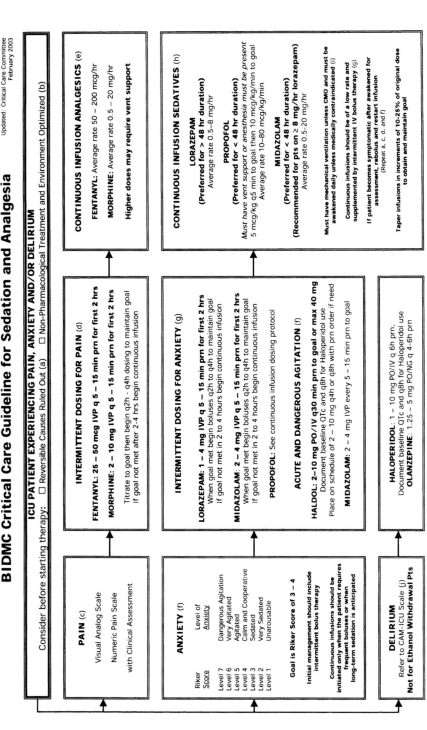

Figure 10-3 BIDMC sedation protocol. (*With permission of Beth Israel Deaconess Medical Center, Boston, MA.*)

CONCLUSION

The administration of sedation and analgesia to the critically ill patient involves unique forms of pathophysiologic mechanisms, pharmacokinetics, and modes of drug delivery. The nurse must employ constant vigilance while caring for the sedated mechanically ventilated patient. This assessment includes evaluating for anxiety, discomfort, or confusion, and identifying causes. Once identified, appropriate interventions can then be initiated. Additional nursing responsibilities include monitoring hemodynamic parameters, observing for unwanted side effects, and assessing the effectiveness of the interventions. When administering sedation and analgesia, the RN must observe for signs and symptoms of drug accumulation and tolerance. During weaning from mechanical ventilation and sedation medications, the nurse must evaluate the patient's need for continued medications, while simultaneously observing for signs of drug withdrawal. The recommendations in this chapter will assist the RN managing the care of the critically ill mechanically ventilated patient receiving sedation and analgesia.

REFERENCES

American Psychiatric Association. (1996). Diagnostic and statistical manual of mental disorders. (3rd Ed.). Washington, DC: Author.

Brook, A.D., Ahrens, T.S., Schaiff, R., Prentice, D., Sherman, G., Shannon, W., & Kollef, M.H. (1999). Effect of a nursing-implemented sedation protocol on the duration of mechanical ventilation. Critical Care Medicine, 27(12), 2609-2615.

Cohen, I.L., Gallagher, T.J., Pohlman, A.S., Dasta, J.F., Abraham, E., & Papadokos, P.J. (2002). Management of the agitated intensive care unit patient. Critical Care Medicine, 30(1), S97-S123.

Clemmer, T.P., Wallace, J.C., Spuhler, V.J., & Bailey, P.P. (2000). Origins of the Motor Activity Assessment Scale Score: A multi-institutional process. Critical Care Medicine, 28(8), 3124-3132.

Clifford, J.O. & Buchman, T.G. (2002). Sedation modulates recognition of novel stimuli and adaptation to regular stimuli in critically ill adults. Critical Care Medicine, 30(3), 609-616.

Crippen, D. (1994). Brain failure in critical care medicine. Critical Care Nurse Quarterly, 16(4), 80-95.

Crippen, D. (2002). High-tech assessment of patient comfort in the intensive care unit: Time for a new look. Critical Care Medicine, 30(8), 1919-1920.

Ely, E.W. (2002). CAM-ICU worksheet. Retrieved May 28, 2004 from http://www.icu-delirium.org/delirium/training-pages/worksheet.pdf.

Ely, E.W., Inouye, S., Bernard, G.R., Gordon, S., Francis, J., May, L., et al. (2001). Delirium in mechanically ventilated patients: validity and reliability of the confusion assessment method for the intensive care unit. JAMA, (286), 2703-2710.

Ely, E.W., Siegel, M.D., & Inouye, S. (2001). Delirium in the intensive care unit: An under-recognized syndrome of organ dysfunction. Seminars in Respiratory and Critical Care Medicine (22), 115-126.

Gahart, B.L., & Nazareno, A.R. (2003). Intravenous Medications. (19th Ed.). St. Louis: Mosby,.

Jacobi, J., Fraser, G.L., Coursin, D.B., Riker, R.R., Fontaine, D., Wittbrodt, E.T., et al. (2002). Clinical practice guidelines for the sustained use of sedatives and analgesics in the critically ill adult. Critical Care Medicine, 30(1), 119-141.

Justic, M. (2000). Does "ICU Psychosis" really exist? Critical Care Nurse, 20(3), 28-37.

Koleff, M.H., Levy, N., Ahrens, T.A., Schaiff, R., Prentice, D., & Sherman, G. (1998). The use of continuous IV sedation is associated with prolongation of mechanical ventilation. Chest, 114(2), 541-548.

Kress, J.P., Pohlman, A.S., O'Conner, M.F., & Hall, J.B. (2000). Daily interruption of sedative infusions in critically ill patients undergoing mechanical ventilation. New England Journal of Medicine, 342, 1471-1477.

Laine, G.A., Hossain, S.M., Solis, R.T., & Adams, S.C. (1995). Polyethylene glycol nephrotoxicity secondary to prolonged high-dose intravenous lorazepam. The Annals of Pharmacotherapy, 29, 1110-1114.

Luer, J. (1995). Sedation and chemical relaxation in critical pulmonary illness: Suggestions for patient assessment and drug monitoring. AACN Clinical Issues, 6(2), 333-343.

McGaffigan, P.A. (2002). Advancing sedation assessment to promote patient comfort. Critical Care Nurse, 22, S29-S36.

Physicians' Desk Reference (2003). (57th Ed.). Montvale, NJ: Medical Economics Company.

Riker, R.R., & Fraser, G.L. (2002). Sedation in the intensive care unit: Refining the models and defining the questions. Critical Care Medicine, 30, 1661-1663.

Roberts, B.L. (2001). Managing delirium in adult intensive care patients. Critical Care Nurse, 21(1), 48-54.

Shelly, M. (1994). Assessing sedation. Care of the Critically Ill, 10(3), 118-121.

Truman, B., & Ely, E.W. (2003). Monitoring delirium in critically ill patients: Using the confusion assessment method for the intensive care unit. Critical Care Nurse (23), 25-38.

Tullman, D.F. (2001). Assessment of delirium: another step forward. Critical Care Medicine, 29, 1481-1483.

Miriam Webster Dictionary on line, (2004). Retrieved 5/27/04 from www.m-w.com.

Weinert, C.R., Chlan, L., & Gross, C. (2001). Sedating critically ill adults: factors affecting nurses' delivery of sedative therapy. American Journal of Critical Care, 10(3), 156-167.

White, S.K., Hollett, J.K., Kress, J.P., & Zellinger, M. (2001). Technological advances and sedation strategies. Critical Care Nurse, 21, S1-14.

11

Risk Management/Legal Issues

There are risks inherent in any expanded function that a nurse provides, even though registered nurses (RNs) have been providing sedation and analgesia for procedural sedation for more than a decade. The nurse must know limitations and function within approved practice parameters. In an ever-evolving practice, such as moderate sedation and analgesia, the nurse must stay abreast of all current issues and controversies. The nurse must also know common causes of liability associated with sedation and analgesia and promote prevention.

Risk management endeavors to prevent injuries and minimize losses when those injuries occur (Odom, 2000). The process for risk management is identification, analysis, treatment, and evaluation of any risks related to the process of sedation and evaluation. The process is very similar to what nurses easily recognize as the nursing process: assessment, diagnosis and planning, intervention, and evaluation.

Risk identification (assessment) involves identifying those areas that are associated with the service. The American Society of Anesthesiologists (ASA) has identified patients who receive sedation and analgesia as being at risk for respiratory depression. ASA also identified those persons more at risk during sedation and analgesia as those at extremes of age or with severe cardiac, pulmonary, hepatic, or renal disease; pregnancy; or drug or alcohol abuse (ASA, 2002). Risk for a population might be identified through the process of incident reports and/or adverse events in a health care organization.

Risk analysis (diagnosis and planning) entails addressing those risks that have been identified. When we know that all patients who undergo sedation and analgesia are at risk for respiratory depression, we plan the means to reduce those risks. Risk treatment (intervention) involves controlling the risks by eliminating them entirely (e.g., refusing to allow nurse-monitored sedation) and preventing those risks from occurring or reducing the chance they will occur (proper monitoring of patients during the procedure). A hospital policy and procedure that requires monitoring the patient's ventilatory status according to published guidelines would be a step toward risk reduction.

Risk evaluation is the process of looking at patient outcomes. Evaluating those patient outcomes in all areas where moderate sedation occurs can aid in determining whether the risks have actually been reduced or prevented. This part of the risk management cycle is linked very closely with the quality component of care (Brent, 2001).

LEGAL CONCEPTS

There are four essential elements of professional negligence or malpractice: duty, breach of duty, causation, and damages. In any negligence case, the plaintiff (person who claims the harm) must prove all four elements for the cause of action to succeed (Odom-Forren, 2004; Higginbotham & McCarthy, 2001; Brent, 2001).

Duty

A duty must exist between the person injured and the one who allegedly caused the injury. When the RN assumes responsibility for the patient who is receiving moderate sedation, she or he has established a duty to that patient. That duty means that the nurse will adhere to standards, guidelines, facility policy, and procedure and is educated and competent to perform the task.

Breach of Duty

Breach of duty means that the nurse did something he or she should not have done or did not do something that should have been done. To prove this particular element, the standard of care must be defined for that particular circumstance—what a reasonable nurse would or would not have done (Higginbotham & McCarthy, 2001). A breach of duty could be a nurse who does not monitor vital signs during the procedure or a nurse who administers an incorrect amount of medication.

Causation

Causation is the most difficult element to prove in a negligence case. The element of causation requires that the breach of duty actually caused the injuries incurred by the patient. If the same injury would have occurred without the breach of duty, then that breach of duty may not be the actual cause of the injury (Higginbotham & McCarthy, 2001). For example, a nurse administers a medication during the sedation process that is noted as a patient allergy. The patient has an allergic reaction but recovers with a dose of diphenhydramine. Later in the procedure the patient codes and dies of what is determined to be a cerebral hemorrhage. The nurse actually incurred a breach of duty, but the breach of duty did not cause the cerebral hemorrhage. On the other hand, if the nurse injects a bolus of 5 mg of midazolam and the patient has a respiratory arrest and subsequently dies, the nurse could be held responsible, because the drug literature and published literature all discuss the necessity of titrating the sedative medications.

Box 11-1   Common Causes of Liability for the RN

Failure to monitor
Failure to communicate
Errors in the use of equipment
Errors in medication or treatment
Patient falls
Operating room errors
Mix-up during patient transfers
Failure to report deviations from practice
Failure to follow a physician's orders
Failure to follow hospital procedure
Discharge teaching
Emergencies

From Odom-Forren, J. (2004a). Legal issues. In D.M.D. Quinn & L. Schick (Eds.). Perianesthesia nursing core curriculum: preoperative, phase I and phase II nursing. St. Louis: Saunders.

Damages or Injuries

The patient must prove that damages or injury occurred for the fourth element to be in place. There are several types of injuries that are compensated with a monetary award: pain and suffering, disfigurement, disability, past and future medical expenses, lost wages, and future earning capacity (Higginbotham & McCarthy, 2001). See Box 11-1 for common causes of liability.

MANAGEMENT OF RISKS AND LIABILITY IN THE PATIENT RECEIVING MODERATE SEDATION

The Institute of Medicine's (1999) report on health care safety emphasized the issue of patient safety when it stated that at least 44,000 persons and perhaps as many as 98,000 persons die in hospitals each year as a result of medical errors that could have been prevented. That does not take into account the patients who have bad outcomes that are not attributed to error. There are several risk factors associated with the practice of sedation and analgesia. RNs who administer sedation and monitor the patient receiving sedation need to examine those risks and then determine the best way to avoid or prevent negative outcomes.

Fortunately, in the health care setting today, the emphasis is on the cause of errors and not on the person who actually was responsible, such as a nurse who administers the wrong medication. The system that allowed that error to occur is analyzed with every effort made to improve that system. Standards and guidelines that apply to sedation and analgesia can help decrease those risks.

Practice Issues

The RN responsible for administering sedation and analgesia should know what the state board of nursing's position is on the practice. As noted in Appendix A, some state boards of nursing have very specific standards or guidelines and expect adherence. The nurse should also be aware of any standards and guidelines issued by appropriate specialty organizations.

Policies and Procedures

Each health care facility should have a policy and procedure concerning sedation and analgesia of patients. The policy and procedure should be consistent throughout the facility, the same in every unit. The best policies and procedures are written with a multidisciplinary approach. This includes not only nurses from every area that is involved in sedation and analgesia but also all specialties involved (e.g., anesthesia department, pharmacy, surgeon, and gastroenterologist.) The policy and procedure should be based on the guidelines of the state board of nursing if applicable and organizational standards. The RN must also know the policy and procedure and adhere to the practices outlined.

Education and Competence

The nurse must be educated in all aspects of the practice of sedation and analgesia and competent to perform the task. Box 11-2 lists the learning objectives from the ANA position statement that was endorsed by 23 nursing organizations

---

Box 11-2 REQUIRED COMPETENCIES

The RN managing the care of the patient receiving sedation is able to:

Demonstrate the acquired knowledge of anatomy, physiology, pharmacology, cardiac dysrhythmia recognition, and complications related to intravenous conscious sedation and medications.

Assess total patient care requirements during intravenous sedation and recovery. Physiologic measurements should include—but not be limited to—respiratory rate, oxygen saturation, blood pressure, cardiac rate and rhythm, and patient's level of consciousness.

Understand the principles of oxygen delivery, respiratory physiology, transport and uptake, and demonstrate the ability to use oxygen delivery devices.

Anticipate and recognize potential complications of intravenous sedation in relation to the type of medication being administered.

Possess the requisite knowledge and skills to assess, diagnose, and intervene in the event of complications or undesired outcome and to institute nursing interventions in compliance with orders (including standing orders) or institutional protocols or guidelines.

Demonstrate skill in airway management resuscitation.

Demonstrate knowledge of the legal ramifications of administering intravenous sedation and/or monitoring patients receiving intravenous sedation, including the RN's responsibility and liability in the event of an untoward reaction or life-threatening complication.

From American Nurses Association. (1991). Position statement on the role of the registered nurse (RN) in the management of patients receiving intravenous conscious sedation for short-term therapeutic, diagnostic, or surgical procedures. Retrieved 6/4/04 from http://nursingworld.org/readroom/position/joint/jtsedate.htm.

as early as 1991. Most boards of nursing have language requiring education and competence whether stated specifically for sedation and analgesia or more broadly, as in any expanded function.

Registered nurses do not learn the practice of sedation and analgesia in basic nursing school. This is an expanded practice that requires further education on the part of the nurse to meet the objectives listed in Box 11-2. The nurse should attend workshops or learn the information in other self-learning forms, such as modules or films. Most facilities require mentoring to determine competence. Education and competence should be documented in the nurse's personnel file. See Chapter 7.

Basic Life Support (BLS) is a requirement that must be met by anyone who is involved with sedation. At this point, there is no guideline that requires advanced cardiac life support (ACLS) certification for moderate sedation and analgesia. AORN (2002) is one organization that has recommended ACLS certification for the nurse who is practicing sedation and analgesia. ASA (2002) states that the nurse who is performing deep sedation should have ACLS certification but does not make that same statement for moderate sedation. Some state boards of nursing and some health care facilities require ACLS. The advantage of ACLS certification is that the nurse is better prepared to handle emergencies that can occur during sedation and aid in bringing those events to a positive conclusion.

However, the ACLS curriculum does not contain all information required by a nurse performing sedation and analgesia (e.g., specific medications and preprocedure assessment), so it is not a substitute for a workshop specific to the needs of those nurses. Patient safety is at the forefront of all educational opportunities.

Preprocedure Care

The preprocedure care of the patient is important to risk assessment. One of the goals of preprocedure assessment is to determine illnesses or conditions that render nurse-monitored sedation inappropriate. A thorough nursing assessment can contribute to this goal. The patient's classification status aids in assigning risk. Objective criteria should be available to determine appropriate patient selection. Consultation with anesthesia providers or other specialties should occur whenever there is any question about the appropriateness of nurse-monitored sedation based on the patient's condition. Although it is a legal responsibility of the physician to obtain informed consent, the nurse has the responsibility to ensure that the patient understands the procedure and the essentials of the sedation process.

Medication Administration

Administration of the medication adds to the risk factors for the patient undergoing sedation. The additive effects of combinations of sedatives and opioids increase the risk for untoward effects, such as hypoxemia, hypercapnia, airway obstruction, apnea, and other complications. It is important to know the sedation continuum and titrate the medication to keep the patient at moderate sedation. The Joint Commission on Accreditation of Healthcare Organizations (JCAHO, 2004) requires that the individual monitoring the patient is capable of rescuing the patient at a deeper-than-expected level of sedation.

To prevent negative patient outcomes, the nurse should titrate the medication to prevent deep sedation. Antagonists should be immediately available for reversal if necessary. The patient requires constant monitoring to prevent and/or quickly treat respiratory depression.

Monitoring of Patient

The most important monitor for the patient is the nurse. There is no substitute for nursing vigilance. The electronic monitors aid the nurse and give the nurse information to base decisions about patient conditions. See Chapter 2 for appropriate monitoring. To prevent poor patient outcomes, the nurse should use all monitoring equipment required in the facility guideline. The equipment should work, and the nurse should know how to interpret the data. Alarms should be on and working. Monitors must be carefully observed and believed. Numerous bad outcomes have occurred when poor monitor readings were not acknowledged or believed and acted upon (Riley, 2003).

Monitoring level of consciousness is of importance to ensure that the patient does not move into deep sedation. Vigilance will ensure that any problems are identified rapidly, and intervention is immediate.

Communication

Communication is vital during the process of sedation and analgesia. Communication with patients occurs during the procedure to assess verbal response. It also allows the nurse to act as patient advocate for any needs the patient may communicate to the nurse. Communication at any point during the procedure demonstrates competence and an attitude of caring to the patient.

Communication with the physician is of importance. The process of sedation should be one of collegiality and teamwork. Of most importance is the communication of any change in the patient's condition to the physician, such as decreased saturation level or blood pressure.

Emergencies

Should a crisis occur, an immediate response can prevent a negative patient outcome. First, the staff should be competent and educated to respond to emergencies quickly. In the case of respiratory depression with hypoxemia, it is vital that one team member oxygenate the patient with a positive pressure breathing device and supplemental oxygen, while another team member administers reversal agents if appropriate and calls for back-up from experts in airway management if necessary. Any emergency equipment should be immediately available and in working condition.

Documentation

All nursing care during the course of the sedation and analgesia should be documented. This documentation should give an accurate picture of the total process of sedation and analgesia from preprocedure to postprocedure. The patient's response to any medication administration should be documented. Vital signs, including oxygen saturation, should be documented at regular intervals. The patient's level of consciousness is also an important piece of documentation. Appropriate, accurate, and thorough documentation can be the nurse's best ally in the event of a negative outcome with a liability issue.

Wrong Site Surgery

The JCAHO (2003) created a universal protocol intended to prevent wrong site, wrong procedure, and wrong person surgery. Implementing this protocol in the facility can decrease risks associated with any error in terms of wrong person and wrong procedure. This protocol should also be implemented in all settings that perform invasive procedures that can cause the patient harm (e.g., for example, endoscopy, emergency department, and radiology). See Box 11-3 for the protocol.

Box 11-3   UNIVERSAL PROTOCOL FOR PREVENTING WRONG SITE, WRONG PROCEDURE, WRONG PERSON SURGERY

Wrong site, wrong procedure, wrong person surgery can be prevented. This universal protocol is intended to achieve that goal. It is based on the consensus of experts from the relevant clinical specialties and professional disciplines and is endorsed by more than 40 professional medical associations and organizations. In developing this protocol, consensus was reached on the following principles:

Wrong site, wrong procedure, wrong person surgery can and must be prevented.

A robust approach—using multiple, complementary strategies—is necessary to achieve the goal of eliminating wrong site, wrong procedure, wrong person surgery.

Active involvement and effective communication among all members of the surgical team is important for success.

To the extent possible, the patient (or legally designated representative) should be involved in the process.

Consistent implementation of a standardized approach using a universal, consensus-based protocol will be most effective.

The protocol should be flexible enough to allow for implementation with appropriate adaptation when required to meet specific patient needs.

A requirement for site marking should focus on cases involving right and/or left distinction, multiple structures (fingers and toes), or levels (spine).

The universal protocol should be applicable or adaptable to all operative and other invasive procedures that expose patients to harm, including procedures done in settings other than the operating room.

Continued

Box 11-3 Universal Protocol for Preventing Wrong Site, Wrong Procedure, Wrong Person Surgery—cont'd

In concert with these principles, the following steps taken together comprise the universal protocol for eliminating wrong site, wrong procedure, and wrong person surgery:

Preoperative Verification Process

Purpose: To ensure that all the relevant documents and studies are available before the start of the procedure, and that they have been reviewed and are consistent with each other and with the patient's expectations and with the team's understanding of the intended patient, procedure, site and as applicable any implants. Missing information or discrepancies must be addressed before starting the procedure.

Process: An ongoing process of information gathering and verification, beginning with the determination to do the procedure, continuing through all settings and interventions involved in the preoperative preparation of the patient, up to and including the "time out" just before the start of the procedure.

Marking the Operative Site

Purpose: To identify unambiguously the intended site of incision or insertion.

Process: For procedures involving right and/or left distinction, multiple structures (such as fingers and toes), or multiple levels (as in spinal procedures), the intended site must be marked such that the mark will be visible after the patient has been prepped and draped.

"Time Out" Immediately Before Starting the Procedure

Purpose: To conduct a final verification of the correct patient, procedure, site and, as applicable, implants.

Process: Active communication among all members of the surgical and/or procedure team, consistently initiated by a designated member of the team, conducted in a "fail-safe" mode (i.e., the procedure is not started until any questions or concerns are resolved).

Data taken from Joint Commission on Accreditation of Healthcare Organizations. (2004). Reprinted with permission. Universal protocol for preventing wrong site, wrong procedure, wrong person surgery. Retrieved 6/23/04 from http://www.jcaho.org/accredited+organizations/ patient+safety/universal+protocol/universal+protocol.pdf

Administration of Anesthetic Agents

At the present time, the controversy surrounding administration of anesthetic agents by the nurse for moderate or deep sedation puts the nurse at risk if not well informed. Propofol moves the patient quickly from moderate to deep sedation and could quickly move the patient to general anesthesia on the sedation continuum. The deeper the level of sedation, the more at risk the patient is for respiratory and cardiovascular emergencies.

Box 11-4 Risk and/or Liability Issues and Methods of Prevention

Appropriate Patient Selection

Titration of drugs to prevent deep sedation
Availability of antagonists for reversal if necessary
Constant monitoring to prevent and/or quickly treat respiratory depression

Communication

With Patient

Assessment of response to verbal communication
Demonstrate an attitude of care and competence

With Physician

Any change in patient's condition

Discharge Criteria

Objective assessment parameters
Verbal and/or written instructions

Documentation

Of all nursing care during course of sedation and/or analgesia
Best ally in event of suit–can decrease costs of adverse event should it occur
Consider documenting every 5 minutes during the procedure

Emergencies

Immediate availability of emergency equipment
Equipment must be maintained in good, working condition
Immediate availability of competent, educated staff to respond
Oxygenate patient first—stimulate, supplemental oxygen, positive-pressure breathing device
Intravenous access

Medication Administration

Titration of drugs to prevent deep sedation
Availability of antagonists for reversal if necessary
Constant monitoring to prevent and/or quickly treat respiratory depression

Monitoring of Patients

Nursing vigilance—strict attention to the patient with no other demands
Constantly reassess patient
Early identification or problems
Rapid intervention in event of crisis
Education and competence—consider ACLS certification

Policies and Procedures

Written with multidisciplinary approach
Nurse knows and follows policy and procedure for sedation and/or analgesia
Are consistently applied throughout facility
Follow policy of state board of nursing

From Odom, J. (2000). Conscious sedation/analgesia. In N. Burden, D.M.D. Quinn, D. O'Brien, & B.S.G. Dawes (Eds.). Ambulatory surgical nursing. (2nd Ed.). Philadelphia: Saunders; Odom-Forren, J. (2004b). RN oversight of moderate sedation: Seven tips for playing it safe. Outpatient Surgery, 4(10), 34-38; Riley, G.P. (2003). Intravenous conscious sedation: Pearls and perils. Nursing risk management 2003. Retrieved 6/3/04 from http://www.afip.org/Departments/legalmed/jnrm2003/riley.htm.

The nurse who administers an anesthetic agent, such as propofol, in a state that has a position stating that it is not within the scope of practice for an RN, is open for liability. As noted in Chapter 1, some medical organizations have issued statements supporting the practice (AGA, 2004), and other organizations have issued statements opposing the issue (ASA, AANA, 2004). To decrease risks associated with this practice, some facilities have determined it is in their best interest for only anesthesia providers to administer any anesthetic agent. Other facilities believe they have minimized the risk by instituting rigid guidelines. Either way, the nurse must be informed about the state board of nursing's position, organizational statements, support or lack of support from the institution, and the nurse's own education and competence to deliver the care.

CONCLUSION

The registered nurse who administers moderate sedation and analgesia can do much to decrease the risks involved in the practice. The issue of patient safety should always be at the forefront of any decisions made. Key to any management of risks is the nurse's education, competence, and knowledge of practice parameters (see Box 11-4).

REFERENCES

American Association of Nurse Anesthetists. (2004). In the news: AANA-ASA joint statement regarding propofol administration. Retrieved 5/19/04 from www.aana.com/news/2004/news050504_joint.asp.

American Gastroenterological Association. (March 8, 2004). AGA News Release: Three gastroenterology specialty groups issue joint statement on sedation in endoscopy. Accessed 5/19/04 from www.gastro.org/media/newsRelease04/statement-Sedation-Endoscopy.html.

American Nurses Association. (1991). Position statement on the role of the registered nurse (RN) in the management of patients receiving intravenous conscious sedation for short-term therapeutic, diagnostic, or surgical procedures. Retrieved 6/4/04 from http://nursingworld.org/readroom/position/joint/jtsedate.htm.

Brent, N.J. (2001). Nurses and the law: A guide to principles and applications. Philadelphia: Saunders.

Higginbotham, E.L., & McCarthy, R.C. (2001). Elements of nursing negligence. In M.E. O'Keefe (Ed.). Nursing practice and the law: Avoiding malpractice and other legal risks. Philadelphia: F.A. Davis, pp. 118-131.

Institute of Medicine. (1999). To err is human: Building a safer health system. Retrieved 6/3/04 from http://www.iom.edu/file.asp?id=4117.

Odom, J.: (2000). Conscious sedation/analgesia. In N. Burden, D.M.D. Quinn, D. O'Brien, & B.S.G. Dawes (Eds.). Ambulatory surgical nursing. (2nd Ed.). Philadelphia: Saunders, pp.327-329.

Odom-Forren, J. (2004a). Legal issues. In D.M.D. Quinn & L. Schick (Eds.). Perianesthesia nursing core curriculum: Preoperative, phase I and phase II nursing. St. Louis: Saunders, pp. 62-69.

Odom-Forren, J. (2004b). RN oversight of moderate sedation: Seven tips for playing it safe. Outpatient Surgery, 4(10), 34-38.

Riley, G.P. (2003). Intravenous conscious sedation: Pearls and perils. Nursing Risk Management 2003. Retrieved 6/3/04 from http://www.afip.org/Departments/legalmed/jnrm2003/riley.htm.

Appendix A

ASA Standards for Basic Anesthetic Monitoring*

(Approved by House of Delegates on October 21, 1986, and last affirmed on October 15, 2003)

These standards apply to all anesthesia care although, in emergency circumstances, appropriate life support measures take precedence. These standards may be exceeded at any time based on the judgment of the responsible anesthesiologist. They are intended to encourage quality patient care, but observing them cannot guarantee any specific patient outcome. They are subject to revision from time to time, as warranted by the evolution of technology and practice. They apply to all general anesthetics, regional anesthetics and monitored anesthesia care. This set of standards addresses only the issue of basic anesthetic monitoring, which is one component of anesthesia care. In certain rare or unusual circumstances, 1) some of these methods of monitoring may be clinically impractical, and 2) appropriate use of the described monitoring may fail to detect untoward clinical developments. Brief interruptions of continual† monitoring may be unavoidable. *Under extenuating circumstances, the responsible anesthesiologist may waive the requirements marked with an asterisk (*); it is recommended that when this is done, it should be so stated (including the reasons) in a note in the patient's medical record.* These standards are not intended for application to the care of the obstetrical patient in labor or in the conduct of pain management.

STANDARD I

Qualified anesthesia personnel shall be present in the room throughout the conduct of all general anesthetics, regional anesthetics and monitored anesthesia care.

---

*ASA Standards for Basic Anesthetic Monitoring, October 15, 2003, is reprinted with permission of the American Society of Anesthesiologists, 520 N. Northwest Highway, Park Ridge, Illinois 60068-2573.
†Note that "continual" is defined as "repeated regularly and frequently in steady rapid succession" whereas "continuous" means "prolonged without any interruption at any time."

238

Objective

Because of the rapid changes in patient status during anesthesia, qualified anesthesia personnel shall be continuously present to monitor the patient and provide anesthesia care. In the event there is a direct known hazard, e.g., radiation, to the anesthesia personnel which might require intermittent remote observation of the patient, some provision for monitoring the patient must be made. In the event that an emergency requires the temporary absence of the person primarily responsible for the anesthetic, the best judgment of the anesthesiologist will be exercised in comparing the emergency with the anesthetized patient's condition and in the selection of the person left responsible for the anesthetic during the temporary absence.

STANDARD II

During all anesthetics, the patient's oxygenation, ventilation, circulation and temperature shall be continually evaluated.

OXYGENATION

Objective

To ensure adequate oxygen concentration in the inspired gas and the blood during all anesthetics.

Methods

1) Inspired gas: During every administration of general anesthesia using an anesthesia machine, the concentration of oxygen in the patient breathing system shall be measured by an oxygen analyzer with a low oxygen concentration limit alarm in use*
2) Blood oxygenation: During all anesthetics, a quantitative method of assessing oxygenation such as pulse oximetry shall be employed.* Adequate illumination and exposure of the patient are necessary to assess color.*

VENTILATION

Objective

To ensure adequate ventilation of the patient during all anesthetics.

Methods

1) Every patient receiving general anesthesia shall have the adequacy of ventilation continually evaluated. Qualitative clinical signs such as chest excursion, observation of the reservoir breathing bag and auscultation of

breath sounds are useful. Continual monitoring for the presence of expired carbon dioxide shall be performed unless invalidated by the nature of the patient, procedure or equipment. Quantitative monitoring of the volume of expired gas is strongly encouraged.*

2) When an endotracheal tube or laryngeal mask is inserted, its correct positioning must be verified by clinical assessment and by identification of carbon dioxide in the expired gas. Continual end-tidal carbon dioxide analysis, in use from the time of endotracheal tube/laryngeal mask placement, until extubation/removal or initiating transfer to a postoperative care location, shall be performed using a quantitative method such as capnography, capnometry or mass spectroscopy.

3) When ventilation is controlled by a mechanical ventilator, there shall be in continuous use a device that is capable of detecting disconnection of components of the breathing system. The device must give an audible signal when its alarm threshold is exceeded.

4) During regional anesthesia and monitored anesthesia care, the adequacy of ventilation shall be evaluated, at least by continual observation of qualitative clinical signs.

CIRCULATION

Objective

To ensure the adequacy of the patient's circulatory function during all anesthetics.

Methods

1) Every patient receiving anesthesia shall have the electrocardiogram continuously displayed from the beginning of anesthesia until preparing to leave the anesthetizing location.*

2) Every patient receiving anesthesia shall have arterial blood pressure and heart rate determined and evaluated at least every five minutes.*

3) Every patient receiving general anesthesia shall have, in addition to the above, circulatory function continually evaluated by at least one of the following: palpation of a pulse, auscultation of heart sounds, monitoring of a tracing of intra-arterial pressure, ultrasound peripheral pulse monitoring, or pulse plethysmography or oximetry.

BODY TEMPERATURE

Objective

To aid in the maintenance of appropriate body temperature during all anesthetics.

Methods

Every patient receiving anesthesia shall have temperature monitored when clinically significant changes in body temperature are intended, anticipated or suspected.

Appendix B

State Boards of Nursing Positions on Moderate Sedation and Administration of Anesthetic Agents*

Data from Odom-Forren, J. (2004). Unpublished research.
*Disclaimer: State Boards of Nursing Rulings are dynamic and in a constant state of change. Please contact your state BON for up-to-date information.

State	Type Statement on Sedation	Anesthetic Agents Addressed Regarding Sedation	Limitations	Additional Information
Alabama	No formal rulings	Not addressed	Administrative code states that RN or LPN shall not administer medications for anesthetic purpose or to render an individual unconscious without meeting requirements of practice as CRNA	Activities beyond basic nursing education must be identified in procedure approved by hospital and include organized program of study, supervised clinical practice, and demonstrated competence. http://www.abn.state.al.us/
Alaska	Position statement	Administration of ketamine and propofol not within RN scope of practice		www.dced.state.ak.us/occ/pnur.htm
Arizona	Advisory opinion	RNs may assist a licensed provider by administering anesthetic agents in situations where the provider is present but unable to personally inject the anesthetic agent because the provider is performing airway management or placement of a peripheral nerve block requiring use of both hands.	May administer for purpose of anesthesia only if the nurse has completed a nationally accredited program in the science of anesthesia	May administer medications to provide deep sedation for ventilator patients in the intensive care setting, but not to provide an anesthetic. Must complete defined educational course; be certified in advanced life support; have no other duties while administering sedation. www.azboardofnursing.org

RN, *Registered nurse;* LPN, *licensed practical nurse;* cRNA, *certified registered nurse anesthetist.*

State	Type Statement on Sedation	Anesthetic Agents Addressed Regarding Sedation	Limitations	Additional Information
Arkansas	Position statement	Not addressed	May administer pharmacologic agents via IV route to produce conscious sedation	Educational/competency requirement; RN managing care should have no other responsibilities; adopted ANA position statement in its entirety. www.arsbn.org
California	Advisory	Not addressed	May administer medications for the purpose of induction of conscious sedation; act as advocate by refusing to administer medications which would render deep sedation and/or loss of consciousness	Knowledge and skills of medications required; shall not leave patient unattended; education and competency required. www.rn.ca.gov
Colorado	No formal ruling	Not addressed		Colorado does not address specific nursing practice issues. Their statute is broadly written so that it allows for judgment of the RN with knowledge and skills regarding new procedures/practices. www.dora.state.co.us/nursing/
Connecticut	Guidelines	Propofol should be administered only by persons trained in the administration	Within scope of practice for RN to manage care of patients receiving IV conscious sedation	Competency validation of knowledge, skills, and abilities related to management of patients receiving IV conscious sedation; RN will continuously monitor the patient

State				
Delaware	Position statement	of general anesthesia unless used as a sedative for already intubated and ventilated patients.		throughout the procedure. www.dph.state.ct.us
District of Columbia	No formal rulings	Not addressed	Not addressed	Endorsed the ANA position statement http://professionallicensing.state.de.us/boards/nursing/index.shtml http://dchealth.dc.gov/prof_license/services/boards_main_action.asp?strAppId=11
Florida	No formal rulings	Declaratory rulings on propofol and ketamine	In answer to specific questions	RN may not administer propofol with anesthesiologist in room or inject additional doses through an IV port. RN may not monitor a patient who has received propofol, even if the anesthesiologist remains in the room; when an RN has administered the medication pursuant to a verbal or written order given by anesthesiologist who remains in the room; administered by an anesthesiologist who leaves the patient in preop while patient is unresponsive. The appropriately educated RN may administer propofol and monitor the patient in ICU who is monitored, intubated, and mechanically ventilated. RN may not administer ketamine. http://www.doh.state.fl.us/Mqa/nursing/nur_home.html

IV, *Intravenous;* ANA, *American Nurses Association;* ICU, *intensive care unit.*

State	Type Statement on Sedation	Anesthetic Agents Addressed Regarding Sedation	Limitations	Additional Information
Georgia	No formal rulings	Not addressed		Refer to decision tree. http://www.sos.state.ga.us/plb/rn/
Hawaii	No formal rulings	Not addressed		Laws are silent. No policy. http://www.state.hi.us/dcca/pvl/ areas_nurse.html
Idaho	No formal rulings	Not addressed		Refer RNs to decision-making model for scope of practice. See Web site. http://www2.state.id.us/ibn/nursing. htm#office
Illinois	No formal rulings	Not addressed		RN allowed to administer medications at direction of physician. However, RNs must practice within their scope of practice. http://www.ildpr.com/WHO/ar/rn/ asp
Indiana	No formal rulings	Not addressed		http://www.in.gov/hpb/boards/isbn/ index.html
Iowa	Declaratory ruling	Not addressed	Refers only to IV administration of Versed	May administer IV Versed in hospital setting. Monitor for underventilation and apnea. http://www.state.ia.ua/nursing/

Kansas	Position statement	Not addressed	Decline orders for additional medications that may cause the patient to reach a deeper level of sedation or analgesia	Education and competency required. Accessibility of physician or CRNA to assume care should deep analgesia/sedation inadvertently occur www.ksbn.org
Kentucky	Advisory opinion	Administration of propofol is not within the scope of RN practice; qualified RN may assist in monitoring and assessing the patient	IV administration of medications for purpose of anesthesia is not within the scope of RN practice	Competency and education required. Right and obligation to refuse to administer and/or continue to administer medication(s) in amounts that may induce deep sedation and/or loss of consciousness. Also state that it is not within scope of ARNP who is not educationally prepared as nurse anesthetist. http://kbn/ky.gov
Louisiana	Declaratory statement	Not within scope of practice for RN to administer anesthetic agent for any level of sedation or monitor anesthesia	Administration of anesthetic agents is reserved for authorized anesthesia providers	Nurse may monitor patient who has received anesthetic agents for purpose of analgesia/sedation. RN may administer nonanesthetic medications and monitor patients in minimal, moderate, and deep sedation. Education and competency required. ACLS or PALS required. RN monitoring patient should have no other responsibility. RN may not monitor adult patient with ASA classification higher than Class III and pediatric patient higher than Class II. May not monitor patient in position that may compromise ability to assess the patient's airway, e.g., prone position. www.lsbn.state.la.us

ARNP, Advanced Registered Nurse Practitioner; ACLS, advanced cardiac life support; PALS, pediatric advanced life support; ASA, American Society of Anesthesiologists.

State	Type Statement on Sedation	Anesthetic Agents Addressed Regarding Sedation	Limitations	Additional Information
Maine	No formal rulings on moderate sedation; practice question regarding propofol administration answered on Web site.	May administer anesthetic agents, such as propofol, for the purpose of analgesia, muscle relaxation, or sedation–provided appropriate training documented based on facility's established policies and procedures	Registered professional nurse may not administer anesthetic medications for purposed of anesthesia unless CRNA	http://www.state.me.us/boardofnursing/
Maryland	Declaratory ruling	The RN may administer propofol by IV infusion to intubated ventilator-dependent adult patient in critical care setting; the RN may NOT administer propofol for a client who is not intubated or for	RN has responsibility to refuse to administer any medications that may produce a state of deep sedation	Very detailed and specific ruling. Education and competency required. Physician giving orders for sedation credentialed by facility. May not leave patient unattended or engage in uninterruptible tasks. Patients continuously monitored throughout procedure. Dosing parameters required. The RN may not administer procedural sedation using medications classified as anesthetic agents, including propofol, ketamine, or inhalation anesthetics.

State				
			nonemergent intubation	Exception: Separate detailed section for pediatric patient, including use of nitrous oxide 50% or less and ketamine in critical care settings. http://www.mbon.org/main.php
Massachusetts	Position statement	Not addressed		RN must be competent and educated. Written protocols including dosing parameters. http://www.state.ma.us/reg/boards/rn
Michigan	No formal rulings	Not addressed		http://www.michigan.gov/cis/0,1607,7-154-10568_17671_17682---,00.html
Minnesota	No formal rulings	No formal ruling, but the board is advising that because propofol is classified as an anesthetic agent and administration of anesthetic drugs is CRNA practice, it is not within RN scope of practice; board is looking at the issue		From statutes, each medical and nursing function is classified as independent nursing function or as a delegated medical function. Administering sedation is medical function that must be delegated by physician to nurse. Nurse must have adequate training and competence. http://www.state.mn.us/cgi-bin/portal/mn/jsp/home.do?agency=NursingBoard
Mississippi	Position statement	Not specifically addressed; see limitations.	States that the appropriately prepared RN may administer IV "non-anesthetic agents" for purpose of conscious sedation	RN must no have additional responsibilities that would interfere with patient monitoring activities; institutional policy must address maximum initial dose that may be administered by RN for conscious sedation. Competency and education required. http://www.msbn.state.ms.us/

State	Type Statement on Sedation	Anesthetic Agents Addressed Regarding Sedation	Limitations	Additional Information
Missouri	No formal rulings	Speaks only to RN administering/ monitoring propofol in the ICU on intubated and mechanically ventilated patients or for rapid sequence intubation		http://pr.mo.gov/nursing.asp
Montana	Declaratory ruling	Not addressed		Within scope of practice for RN to administer IV conscious sedation medication. Competence and instruction are required. http://www.discoveringmontana. com/dli/bsd/license/bsd_boards/ nur_board/board_page.asp
Nebraska	Advisory opinion	Not addressed	Anesthesia can be provided only by qualified anesthesia providers.	RNs may administer medications via catheter routes for purpose of analgesia and conscious sedation; competence and accountability required. List of supported position papers supplied in advisory opinion. http://www.hhs.state.ne.us/crl/ nursing/nursingindex.htm
Nevada	Advisory opinion	May administer anesthetic agents for pain management or moderate sedation	May administer anesthetic agents only at dose levels designed to achieve analgesia, not anesthesia	Knowledge of medication required. May not leave patient unattended nor engage in activities that compromise continuous monitoring of patient. http://www.nursingboard.state.nv.us/

State				
New Hampshire	FAQ on Web site	In answer to question regarding RN scope of practice and administration of propofol for conscious sedation, said drugs used for conscious sedation are within the RN scope of practice	Administration of anesthesia solely within purview of anesthesia department with exception of intradermal administration	Competencies must be met along with guidelines of institution. http://www.state.nh.us/nursing/
New Jersey	No formal rulings by BON	Not addressed		"Conscious" sedation addressed by NJ Administrative Code 13:35-4A.1-4A.10. States sedation may be administered by RN trained and experienced in use and monitoring of anesthetic agents. Defines "anesthetic agents" as "any drug or combination of drugs administered with the purpose of creating conscious sedation, regional anesthesia, or general anesthesia." NJ hospital licensing standards are the same (Chapter 43G; Subchapter 6) http://www.state.nj.us/lps/ca/medical/nursing.htm http://www.state.nj.us/lps/ca/bme/amendregs.pdf http://www.state.nj.us/health/hcsa/njac843g.pdf

BON, *Board of Nursing.*

State	Type Statement on Sedation	Anesthetic Agents Addressed Regarding Sedation	Limitations	Additional Information
New Mexico	No formal rulings	Not addressed		http://www.state.nm.us/clients/nursing/
New York	Position statement	Not addressed	Speaks only to conscious sedation	Uses the ANA position statement, which requires competence and education and that the RN monitoring the patient has no other duties. http://www.op.nysed.gov/nurse.htm
North Carolina	FAQ on Web site	Not addressed	Speaks only to conscious sedation	Competence and education required. RN cannot assume other responsibilities that would leave the client unattended. Refer to ANA position statement and AANA guidelines. http://www.ncbon.com/
North Dakota	Position statement	Drugs classified as anesthetic agents used for moderate/deep sedation for therapeutic, diagnostic, and surgical procedures can be administered by the RN if the patient is in a controlled environment with a secure airway		Education and competence required. Should have no other responsibilities that would leave the patient unattended. http://www.ndbon.org/

State				
Ohio	No formal rulings	Not addressed	State medical board law allows for only CRNAs to administer anesthesia	BON has no authority to issue positions and/or practice statements. According to BON, if medication is an anesthetic that at lower doses may be used as a sedative, hypnotic, or analgesic, the RN may administer the medication at those doses and monitor the patient accordingly. It is the responsibility of the RN to know which medications are within the scope of practice for the nurse to administer. Education, competence would be required. http://www.nursing.ohio.gov/
Oklahoma	Guideline	Not addressed	States that these guidelines do not apply to deep sedation	Requires education and competence. RN should have no other duties during procedure that would leave patient unattended or compromise continuous monitoring. Also have guidelines that address role of LPN during conscious sedation. http://www.youroklahoma.com/nursing/
Oregon	Nursing policy statement	Last sentence reads, "The administration of anesthetic agents by the RN for deep sedation may be appropriate."	Administer only "non-anesthetic" drugs for conscious sedation	Requires education, competence, ACLS, PALs, or equivalent. RN should have no other responsibility that would leave the patient unattended or compromise continuous monitoring. http://www.osbn.state.or.us/

AANA, American Association of Nurse Anesthetists.

State	Type Statement on Sedation	Anesthetic Agents Addressed Regarding Sedation	Limitations	Additional Information
Pennsylvania	Regulations	Not specifically addressed; refer to Nursing Practice Guide to determine specific practice	Must be CRNA to administer anesthesia	RN must be certified in ACLS. Requires education and competence. RN managing care of the patient may not have other responsibilities during the procedure and may not leave the patient unattended or engage in tasks that would compromise continuous monitoring. http://www.dos.state.pa.us/bpoa/cwp/view.asp?a=1104&q=432883 http://www.healthri.org/hsr/professions/nurses.htm
Rhode Island	No formal rulings	Not addressed		
South Carolina	Advisory opinion and position statement	Advisory opinion states that RNs who are not qualified anesthesia providers may not administer agents used primarily as anesthetics, including, but not limited to, ketamine and propofol	RN may not be authorized to manage deep sedation or anesthesia for short-term diagnostic, therapeutic, or surgical procedures	Adopted ANA position statement. RN managing care of patient shall have no other responsibilities that would leave patient unattended or compromise continuous monitoring. Requires education and competence. http://www.llr.state.sc.us/POL/Nursing/INDEX.ASP
South Dakota	Position statement	Not addressed	Applies to moderate sedation only	RN must be ACLS certified. Requires education and competence. RN should have no other responsibilities that would leave the client unattended or compromise

Tennessee	Policy statement and guidelines	RN who is not CRNA is prohibited from administering general anesthetic agents except to secure airway in emergency and provide muscle relaxation and sedation for patient with secured airway	RNs who are not qualified anesthesia providers should not administer agents classified as anesthetics, including propofol	continuous monitoring. Individuals administering moderate sedation should be able to rescue clients who enter a state of deep sedation. http://www.state.sd.us/doh/nursing/ Requires education and competence. Must be ACLS or PCLS certified. RN should have no other responsibilities during the procedure. Task force appointed to update policy and expect significant revisions. http://www2.state.tn.us/health/Boards/Nursing/
Texas	Position statement	States that because of danger of unintended deep sedation and/or general anesthesia with pharmacologic agents classified as "anesthetic" agents, board advises caution for RNs who are not qualified anesthesia providers in administering such agents to nonintubated patients	Says that loss of consciousness should not be the goal and pharmacologic agents used should render this result unlikely; deep sedation is generally beyond the scope of practice for the RN	Employing facilities should have policies and procedures to guide the RN. Refers RN to guidelines from several professional nursing organizations. http://www.bne.state.tx.us/

State	Type Statement on Sedation	Anesthetic Agents Addressed Regarding Sedation	Limitations	Additional Information
Utah	No formal rulings	Not addressed		Utah law and rules are silent on this issue and no practice statements have been made. http://www.dopl.utah.gov/licensing/nurse.html
Vermont	Position statement	Not addressed		Endorses the position statement of ANA. http://vtprofessionals.org/opr1/nurses/
Virginia	No formal rulings	Not addressed		http://www.dhp.virginia.gov/nursing/default.htm
Washington	Policy statement	Does not include specific agents (older opinions did); BON representative stated that the procedural sedation position statement will guide the use of any appropriately used anesthetic agents for conscious sedation	May not administer general anesthesia	Require competence and education. Providers and institutions should have policies and procedures in place. https://fortress.wa.gov/doh/hpqa1/HPS6/Nursing/default.htm

State				
West Virginia	No formal rulings	Not addressed	May not administer for purpose of anesthesia unless anesthesia provider	Refers RN to "Criteria for Determining Scope of Practice for Licensed Nurses." This document assists RNs in determining what activities or tasks are within their individual scope of practice. westvirginiarn@ncsbn.org http://drl.wi.gov/boards/nur/index.htm
Wisconsin	No formal rulings	Not addressed		
Wyoming	Advisory opinion	Opinion states that it is not within scope of practice for RN to administer propofol for conscious sedation	Nurse administering anesthesia must have advanced certification and be recognized as CRNA	Nurse administering analgesia does not require advanced certification and does not need to be recognized as CRNA. Nurse is directed to hospital policy and insurance carrier for the hospital for guidance and direction. http://nursing.state.wy.us/

Appendix C

Position Statement on the Role of the RN in the Management of Patients Receiving IV Moderate Sedation for Short-Term Therapeutic, Diagnostic, or Surgical Procedures

DEFINITION OF INTRAVENOUS CONSCIOUS SEDATION

Intravenous conscious sedation is produced by the administration of pharmacologic agents. A patient under conscious sedation has a depressed level of consciousness but retains the ability to independently and continuously maintain a patent airway and respond appropriately to physical stimulation and/or verbal command.

Management and Monitoring

It is within the scope of practice of a registered nurse to manage the care of patients receiving intravenous conscious sedation during therapeutic, diagnostic, or surgical procedures provided the following criteria are met:

1. Administration of intravenous conscious sedation medications by nonanesthetist RNs is allowed by state laws and institutional policy, procedures, and protocol.
2. A qualified anesthesia provider or attending physician selects and orders the medications to achieve intravenous conscious sedation.
3. Guidelines for patient monitoring, drug administration, and protocols for dealing with potential complications or emergency situations are available and have been developed in accordance with accepted standards of anesthesia practice.
4. The RN managing the care of the patient receiving intravenous conscious sedation shall have no other responsibilities that would leave the patient unattended or compromise continuous monitoring.

5. The RN managing the care of patients receiving intravenous conscious sedation is able to:
   a. Demonstrate the acquired knowledge of anatomy, physiology, pharmacology, cardiac arrhythmia recognition, and complications related to intravenous conscious sedation and medications.
   b. Assess total patient care requirements during intravenous conscious sedation and recovery. Physiologic measurements should include, but not be limited to, respiratory rate, oxygen saturation, blood pressure, cardiac rate and rhythm, and patient's level of consciousness.
   c. Understand the principles of oxygen delivery, respiratory physiology, transport and uptake, and demonstrate the ability to use oxygen delivery devices.
   d. Anticipate and recognize potential complications of intravenous conscious sedation in relation to the type of medication being administered.
   e. Possess the requisite knowledge and skills to assess, diagnose, and intervene in the event of complications or undesired outcomes and to institute nursing interventions in compliance with orders (including standing orders) or institutional protocols or guidelines.
   f. Demonstrate skill in airway management resuscitation.
   g. Demonstrate knowledge of the legal ramifications of administering intravenous conscious sedation and/or monitoring patients receiving intravenous conscious sedation, including the RN's responsibility and liability in the event of an untoward reaction or life-threatening complication.
6. The institution or practice setting has in place an educational/competency validation mechanism that includes a process for evaluating and documenting the individual's demonstration of the knowledge, skills, and abilities related to the management of patients receiving intravenous conscious sedation. Evaluation and documentation of competence occur on a periodic basis according to institutional policy.

ADDITIONAL GUIDELINES

1. Intravenous access must be continuously maintained in the patient receiving intravenous conscious sedation.
2. All patients receiving intravenous conscious sedation will be continuously monitored throughout the procedure as well as the recovery phase by physiologic measurements including, but not limited to, respiratory rate, oxygen saturation, blood pressure, cardiac rate and rhythm, and patient's level of consciousness.
3. Supplemental oxygen will be immediately available to all patients receiving intravenous conscious sedation and administered per order (including standing orders).

4. An emergency cart with a defibrillator must be immediately accessible to every location where intravenous conscious sedation is administered. Suction and a positive pressure breathing device, oxygen, and appropriate airways must be in each room where intravenous conscious sedation is administered.
5. Provisions must be in place for backup personnel who are experts in airway management, emergency intubation, and advanced cardiopulmonary resuscitation if complications arise.

Endorsed by:

American Association of Critical-Care Nurses
American Association of Neuroscience Nurses
American Association of Nurse Anesthetists
American Association of Spinal Cord Injury Nurses
American Association of Occupational Health Nurses
American Nephrology Nurses Association
American Nurses Association
American Radiological Nurses Association
American Society of Pain Management Nurses
American Society of Plastic and Reconstructive Surgical Nurses
American Society of Post Anesthesia Nurses
American Urological Association, Allied
Association of Operating Room Nurses
Association of Pediatric Oncology Nurses
Association of Rehabilitation Nurses
Dermatology Nurses Association
NAACOG, The Organization for Obstetric, Gynecologic, and Neonatal Nurses
National Association of Orthopaedic Nurses
National Flight Nurses Association
National Student Nurses Association
Nurse Consultants Association, Inc.
Nurses Organization of Veterans Affairs
Nursing Pain Association

Appendix D

ASA Practice Guidelines for Sedation and Analgesia by Non-Anesthesiologists*

(Approved by the House of Delegates on October 25, 1995, and last amended on October 17, 2001)

AN UPDATED REPORT BY THE AMERICAN SOCIETY OF ANESTHESIOLOGISTS TASK FORCE ON SEDATION AND ANALGESIA BY NON-ANESTHESIOLOGISTS

Developed by the American Society of Anesthesiologists Task Force on Sedation and Analgesia by Non-Anesthesiologists:

Jeffrey B. Gross, M.D. (Chair) Farmington, CT
Burton S. Epstein, M.D. Washington, DC
Peter L. Bailey, M.D. Rochester, NY
Lesley Gilbertson, M.D. Boston, MA
Richard T. Connis, Ph.D. Woodinville, W A
David G. Nickinovich, Ph.D. Bellevue, W A
Charles J. Cote, M.D. Chicago, IL
John M. Zerwas, M.D. Houston, TX
Fred G. Davis, M.D. Burlington, MA
Gregory Zuccaro, Jr., M.D. Cleveland, OH

Correspondence to:
Jeffrey B. Gross, M.D.
Department of Anesthesiology (M/C 2015) University of Connecticut School of Medicine Fannington, CT 06030-2015
Supported by the American Society of Anesthesiologists under the direction of James F. Arens, M.D., Chairman, Committee on Practice Parameters.

*Readers with special interest in the statistical analyses used in establishing these Guidelines can receive further information by writing to the American Society of Anesthesiologists: 520 North Northwest Highway, Park Ridge, Illinois 60068-2573.

Approved by the House of Delegates, October 17, 2001. A list of the references used to develop these guidelines is available by writing to the American Society of Anesthesiologists.

Reprint Requests to: American Society of Anesthesiologists, 520 N. Northwest Highway, Park Ridge, IL 60068-2573

Key Words: Conscious sedation; deep sedation; analgesia; practice guidelines; propofol; ketamine

Abbreviated Title: Practice Guidelines for Sedation and Analgesia

Introduction

Anesthesiologists possess specific expertise in the pharmacology, physiology, and clinical management of patients receiving sedation and analgesia. F or this reason, they are frequently called upon to participate in the development of institutional policies and procedures for sedation and analgesia for diagnostic and therapeutic procedures. To assist in this process, the American Society of Anesthesiologists has developed these **Guidelines for Sedation and Analgesia by NonAnesthesiologists**.

Practice guidelines are systematically developed recommendations that assist the practitioner and patient in making decisions about health care. These recommendations may be adopted, modified, or rejected according to clinical needs and constraints. Practice guidelines are not intended as standards or absolute requirements. The use of practice guidelines cannot guarantee any specific outcome. Practice guidelines are subject to revision as warranted by the evolution of medical knowledge, technology, and practice. The guidelines provide basic recommendations that are supported by analysis of the current literature and by a synthesis of expert opinion, open forum commentary, and clinical feasibility data.

This revision includes data published since the Guidelines for Sedation and Analgesia by NonAnesthesiologists were adopted by the American Society of Anesthesiologists in 1995; it also includes data and recommendations for a wider range of sedation levels than was previously addressed.

A. Definitions

"Sedation and analgesia" comprise a continuum of states ranging from **Minimal Sedation (Anxiolysis)** through **General Anesthesia**. Definitions of levels of sedation / analgesia, as developed and adopted by the American Society of Anesthesiologists, are given in Table 1. These guidelines specifically apply to levels of sedation corresponding to **Moderate Sedation (frequently called "Conscious Sedation")** and **Deep Sedation**, as defined in Table 1.

B. Focus

These guidelines are designed to be applicable to procedures performed in a variety of settings (e.g., hospitals, freestanding clinics, physician, dentist, and other offices) by practitioners who are not specialists in anesthesiology. Because **Minimal Sedation ("Anxiolysis")** entails minimal risk, the guidelines specifically

Table 1 | **Continuum of Depth of Sedation**

Definition of General Anesthesia and Levels of Sedation/Analgesia
(Developed by the American Society of Anesthesiologists)
(Approved by ASA House of Delegates on October 13, 1999)

	Minimal Sedation ("Anxiolysis")	*Moderate Sedation/ Analgesia ("Conscious Sedation")*	*Deep Sedation/ Analgesia*	*General Anesthesia*
Responsiveness	Normal response to verbal stimulation	Purposeful* response to verbal or tactile stimulation	Purposeful* response following repeated or painful stimulation	Unarousable, even with painful stimulus
Airway	Unaffected	No intervention required	Intervention may be required	Intervention often required
Spontaneous Ventilation	Unaffected	Adequate	May be inadequate	Frequently inadequate
Cardiovascular Function	Unaffected	Usually maintained	Usually maintained	May be impaired

Minimal Sedation (Anxiolysis) *is a drug-induced state during which patients respond normally to verbal commands. Although cognitive function and coordination may be impaired, ventilatory and cardiovascular functions are unaffected.*

Moderate Sedation/Analgesia ("Conscious Sedation") *is a drug-induced depression of consciousness during which patients respond purposefully* to verbal commands, either alone or accompanied by light tactile stimulation. No interventions are required to maintain a patent airway, and spontaneous ventilation is adequate. Cardiovascular function is usually maintained.*

Deep Sedation/Analgesia *is a drug-induced depression of consciousness during which patients cannot be easily aroused but respond purposefully* following repeated or painful stimulation. The ability to independently maintain ventilatory function may be impaired. Patients may require assistance in maintaining a patent airway, and spontaneous ventilation may be inadequate. Cardiovascular function is usually maintained.*

General Anesthesia *is a drug-induced loss of consciousness during which patients are not arousable, even by painful stimulation. The ability to independently maintain ventilatory function is often impaired. Patients often require assistance in maintaining a patent airway, and positive pressure ventilation may be required because of depressed spontaneous ventilation or drug-induced depression of neuromuscular function. Cardiovascular function may be impaired.*

Because sedation is a continuum, it is not always possible to predict how an individual patient will respond. Hence, practitioners intending to produce a given level of sedation should be able to rescue patients whose level of sedation becomes deeper than initially intended. Individuals administering **Moderate Sedation/Analgesia ("Conscious Sedation")** *should be able to rescue patients who enter a state of* **Deep Sedation/Analgesia***, while those administering* **Deep Sedation/Analgesia** *should be able to rescue patients who enter a state of general anesthesia.*
Reflex withdrawal from a painful stimulus is NOT considered a purposeful response.

exclude it. Examples of **Minimal Sedation** include peripheral nerve blocks, local or topical anesthesia and either (1) less than 50% N_2O in O_2 with no other sedative or analgesic medications by any route, or (2) a single, oral sedative or analgesic medication administered in doses appropriate for the unsupervised treatment of insomnia, anxiety or pain. The guidelines also exclude patients who are not undergoing a diagnostic or therapeutic procedure (e.g., postoperative analgesia, sedation for treatment of insomnia). Finally, the guidelines do not apply to patients receiving general or major conduction anesthesia (e.g., spinal or epidural/caudal block), whose care should be provided, medically directed, or supervised by an anesthesiologist, the operating practitioner, or another licensed physician with specific training in sedation, anesthesia, and rescue techniques appropriate to the type of sedation or anesthesia being provided.

C. Purpose

The purpose of these guidelines is to allow clinicians to provide their patients with the benefits of sedation/analgesia while minimizing the associated risks. Sedation/analgesia provides two general types of benefit: First, sedation/analgesia allows patients to tolerate unpleasant procedures by relieving anxiety, discomfort, or pain. Second, in children and uncooperative adults, sedation/analgesia may expedite the conduct of procedures which are not particularly uncomfortable but which require that the patient not move. At times these sedation practices may result in cardiac or respiratory depression which must be rapidly recognized and appropriately managed to avoid the risk of hypoxic brain damage, cardiac arrest, or death. Conversely, inadequate sedation/analgesia may result in undue patient discomfort or patient injury because of lack of cooperation or adverse physiological or psychological response to stress.

D. Application

These guidelines are intended to be general in their application and broad in scope. The appropriate choice of agents and techniques for sedation/analgesia is dependent upon the experience and preference of the individual practitioner, requirements or constraints imposed by the patient or procedure, and the likelihood of producing a deeper level of sedation than anticipated. Because it is not always possible to predict how a specific patient will respond to sedative and analgesic medications, practitioners intending to produce a given level of sedation should be able to rescue patients whose level of sedation becomes deeper than initially intended. For moderate sedation, this implies the ability to manage a compromised airway or hypoventilation in a patient who *responds purposefully* following repeated or painful stimulation, while for deep sedation, this implies the ability to manage respiratory or cardiovascular instability in a patient who *does not respond purposefully* to painful or repeated stimulation. Levels of sedation referred to in the recommendations relate to the level of sedation intended by the practitioner. Examples are provided to illustrate airway assessment, preoperative fasting, emergency equipment, and recovery procedures. However, clinicians and their institutions have ultimate responsibility for selecting patients, procedures, medications, and equipment.

E. Task Force Members and Consultants

The ASA appointed a Task Force of 10 members to (a) review the published evidence; (b) obtain the opinion of a panel of consultants including non-anesthesiologist physicians and dentists who routinely administer sedation/analgesia as well as of anesthesiologists with a special interest in sedation/analgesia (see appendix I); and (c) build consensus within the community of practitioners likely to be affected by the guidelines. The Task Force included anesthesiologists in both private and academic practices from various geographic areas of the United States, a gastroenterologist, and methodologists from the ASA Committee on Practice Parameters.

This Practice Guideline is an update and revision of the ASA *Guidelines for Sedation and Analgesia by Non-Anesthesiologists.*[1] The Task Force revised and updated the Guidelines by means of a five-step process. First, original published research studies relevant to the revision and update were reviewed and analyzed; only articles relevant to the administration of sedation by non-anesthesiologists were evaluated. Second, the panel of expert consultants was asked to (a) participate in a survey related to the effectiveness and safety of various methods and interventions which might be used during sedation/analgesia, and (b) review and comment upon the initial draft report of the Task Force. Third, the Task Force held Open Forums at two major national meetings to solicit input on its draft recommendations. National organizations representing most of the specialties whose members typically administer sedation/analgesia were invited to send representatives. Fourth, the consultants were surveyed to assess their opinions on the feasibility and financial implications of implementing the revised and updated Guidelines. Finally, all of the available information was used by the Task Force to finalize the guidelines.

F. Availability and Strength of Evidence

Evidence-based guidelines are developed by a rigorous analytic process. To assist the reader, the Guidelines make use of several descriptive terms that are easier to understand than the technical terms and data that are used in the actual analyses. These descriptive terms are defined below.

The following terms describe the *strength* of scientific data obtained from the scientific literature:

Supportive: There is sufficient quantitative information from adequately designed studies to describe a statistically significant relationship ($P < 0.01$) between a clinical intervention and a clinical outcome, using the technique of meta-analysis.

[1]Anesthesiology 1996; 84:459-471.

Suggestive: There is enough information from case reports and descriptive studies to provide a directional assessment of the relationship between a clinical intervention and a clinical outcome. This type of qualitative information does not permit a statistical assessment of significance.

Equivocal: Qualitative data have not provided a clear direction for clinical outcomes related to a clinical intervention and (1) there is insufficient quantitative information or (2) aggregated comparative studies have found no quantitatively significant differences among groups or conditions.

The following terms describe the *lack* of available scientific evidence in the literature:

Inconclusive: Published studies are available, but they cannot be used to assess the relationship between a clinical intervention and a clinical outcome because the studies either do not meet predefined criteria for content as defined in the "Focus of the Guidelines," or do not provide a clear causal interpretation of findings due to research design or analytic concerns.

Insufficient: There are too few published studies to investigate a relationship between a clinical intervention and clinical outcome.

Silent: No studies that address a relationship of interest were found in the available published literature.

The following terms describe *survey responses* from the consultants for any specified issue. Responses were solicited on a 5-point scale; ranging from '1' (strongly disagree) to '5' (strongly agree) with a score of '3' being neutral.

Strongly Agree: Median score of '5' (At least 50% of the responses were '5')
Agree: Median score of '4' (At least 50% of the responses were '4' or '5')
Equivocal: Median score of '3' (At least 50% of the scores were 3 or less)
Disagree: Median score of '2' (At least 50% of responses were '1' or '2')
Strongly Disagree: Median score of '1' (At least 50% of responses were '1')

GUIDELINES

1. Patient Evaluation:

There is insufficient published evidence to evaluate the relationship between sedation/analgesia outcomes and the performance of a preoperative patient evaluation. There is suggestive evidence that some pre-existing medical conditions may be related to adverse outcomes in patients receiving either moderate or deep sedation/analgesia. The consultants strongly agree that appropriate pre-procedure evaluation (history, physical examination) increases the likelihood of satisfactory sedation and decreases the likelihood of adverse outcomes for both moderate and deep sedation.

Recommendations: Clinicians administering sedation/analgesia should be familiar with sedation oriented aspects of the patient's medical history and how these might alter the patient's response to sedation/analgesia. These include: (1) abnormalities of the major organ systems; (2) previous adverse experience with

Example I   AIRWAY ASSESSMENT PROCEDURES FOR SEDATION AND ANALGESIA

Positive pressure ventilation, with or without tracheal intubation, may be necessary if respiratory compromise develops during sedation/analgesia. This may be more difficult in patients with atypical airway anatomy. Also, some airway abnormalities may increase the likelihood of airway obstruction during spontaneous ventilation. Some factors which may be associated with difficulty in airway management are:

History:

Previous problems with anesthesia or sedation
Stridor, snoring, or sleep apnea
Advanced rheumatoid arthritis
Chromosomal abnormality (e.g., trisomy 21)

Physical Examination:

Habitus: Significant obesity (especially involving the neck and facial structures)
Head and Neck: Short neck, limited neck extension, decreased hyoid-mental distance (3 cm in an adult), neck mass, cervical spine disease or trauma, tracheal deviation, dysmorphic facial features (e.g., Pierre-Robin syndrome)
Mouth: Small opening (3 cm in an adult); edentulous; protruding incisors; loose or capped teeth; dental appliances; high, arched palate; macroglossia; tonsillar hypertrophy; non-visible uvula
Jaw: Micrognathia, retrognathia, trismus, significant malocclusion

---

sedation/analgesia as well as regional and general anesthesia; (3) drug allergies, current medications and potential drug interactions; (4) time and nature of last oral intake; and (5) history of tobacco, alcohol or substance use or abuse. Patients presenting for sedation/analgesia should undergo a focused physical examination including vital signs, auscultation of the heart and lungs, and evaluation of the airway. (Refer to Example I.) Preprocedure laboratory testing should be guided by the patient's underlying medical condition and the likelihood that the results will affect the management of sedation/analgesia. These evaluations should be confirmed immediately before sedation is initiated.

2. Preprocedure Preparation:

The literature is insufficient regarding the benefits of providing the patient (or her/his guardian, in the case of a child or impaired adult) with preprocedure information about sedation and analgesia. For moderate sedation the consultants agree and for deep sedation the consultants strongly agree that appropriate preprocedure counseling of patients regarding risks, benefits, and alternatives to sedation and analgesia increases patient satisfaction.

Sedatives and analgesics tend to impair airway reflexes in proportion to the degree of sedation/analgesia achieved. This dependence on level of sedation is reflected in the consultants opinion: They agree that preprocedure fasting

Example II   SUMMARY OF AMERICAN SOCIETY OF ANESTHESIOLOGISTS
PREPROCEDURE FASTING GUIDELINES[1]

Ingested Material	Minimum Fasting Period[2]
Clear liquids[3]	2h
Breast milk	4h
Infant formula	6h
Non-human milk[4]	6h
Light meal[5]	6h

[1]These recommendations apply to healthy patients who are undergoing elective procedures. They are not intended for women in labor. Following the guidelines does not guarantee a complete gastric emptying has occurred.
[2]The fasting periods noted above apply to all ages.
[3]Examples of clear liquids include water, fruit juices without pulp, carbonated beverages, clear tea, and black coffee.
[4]Since non-human milk is similar to solids in gastric emptying time, the amount ingested must be considered when determining an appropriate fasting period.
[5]A light meal typically consists of toast and clear liquids. Meals that include fried or fatty foods or meat may prolong gastric emptying time. Both the amount and type of foods ingested must be considered when determining an appropriate fasting period.

decreases risks during moderate sedation, while strongly agreeing that it decreases the risk of deep sedation. In emergency situations, when preprocedure fasting is not practical, the consultants agree that the target level of sedation should be modified (i.e., less sedation should be administered) for moderate sedation, while strongly agreeing that it should be modified for deep sedation. The literature does not provide sufficient evidence to test the hypothesis that preprocedure fasting results in a decreased incidence of adverse outcomes in patients undergoing either moderate or deep sedation.

Recommendations: Patients (or their legal guardians in the case of minors or legally incompetent adults) should be informed of and agree to the administration of sedation/analgesia including the benefits, risks, and limitations associated with this therapy, as well as possible alternatives. Patients undergoing sedation/analgesia for elective procedures should not drink fluids or eat solid foods for a sufficient period of time to allow for gastric emptying prior to their procedure, as recommended by the American Society of Anesthesiologists "Guidelines for Preoperative Fasting[2]" (Example II). In urgent, emergent, or other situations where gastric emptying is impaired, the potential for pulmonary aspiration of gastric contents must be considered in determining (1) the target level of sedation, (2) whether the procedure should be delayed or (3) whether the trachea should be protected by intubation.

[2]Anesthesiology 1999; 90:896-905.

3. Monitoring:

Level of consciousness: The response of patients to commands during procedures performed with sedation/analgesia serves as a guide to their level of consciousness. Spoken responses also provide an indication that the patients are breathing. Patients whose only response is reflex withdrawal from painful stimuli are deeply sedated, approaching a state of general anesthesia, and should be treated accordingly. The literature is silent regarding whether monitoring patients' level of consciousness improves patient outcomes or decreases risks. The consultants strongly agree that monitoring level of consciousness reduces risks for both moderate and deep sedation. The members of the Task Force believe that many of the complications associated with sedation and analgesia can be avoided if adverse drug responses are detected and treated in a timely manner (*i.e.*, prior to the development of cardiovascular decompensation, or cerebral hypoxia). Patients given sedatives and/or analgesics in unmonitored settings in anticipation of a subsequent procedure may be at increased risk of these complications.

Pulmonary ventilation: It is the opinion of the Task Force that the primary causes of morbidity associated with sedation/analgesia are drug-induced respiratory depression and airway obstruction. For both moderate and deep sedation, the literature is insufficient to evaluate the benefit of monitoring ventilatory function by observation or auscultation. However, the consultants strongly agree that monitoring of ventilatory function by observation or auscultation reduces the risk of adverse outcomes associated with sedation/analgesia. The consultants were equivocal regarding the ability of capnography to decrease risks during moderate sedation, while agreeing that it may decrease risks during deep sedation. In circumstances where patients are physically separated from the care giver, the Task Force believes that automated apnea monitoring (by detection of exhaled CO_2 or other means) may decrease risks during both moderate and deep sedation, while cautioning practitioners that impedance plethysmography may fail to detect airway obstruction. The Task Force emphasizes that because ventilation and oxygenation are separate though related physiological processes, monitoring oxygenation by pulse oximetry is not a substitute for monitoring ventilatory function.

Oxygenation: Published data suggests that oximetry effectively detects oxygen de saturation and hypoxemia in patients who are administered sedatives / analgesics. The consultants strongly agree that early detection of hypoxemia through the use of oximetry during sedation/analgesia decreases the likelihood of adverse outcomes such as cardiac arrest and death. The Task Force agrees that hypoxemia during sedation and analgesia is more likely to be detected by oximetry than by clinical assessment alone.

Hemodynamics: Although there is insufficient published data to reach a conclusion, it is the opinion of the Task Force that sedative and analgesic agents may blunt the appropriate autonomic compensation for hypovolemia and procedure-related stresses. On the other hand, if sedation and analgesia are inadequate, patients may develop potentially harmful autonomic stress responses (e.g., hypertension, tachycardia). Early detection of changes in patients' heart rate and blood pressure may enable practitioners to detect problems and intervene in a timely fashion, reducing the risk of these complications. The consultants strongly agree that regular monitoring of vital signs reduces the likelihood of adverse outcomes during both moderate and deep sedation. For both moderate and deep sedation, a majority of the consultants indicated that vital signs should be monitored at 5-minute intervals once a stable level of sedation is established. The consultants strongly agree that continuous electrocardiography reduces risks during deep sedation, while they were equivocal regarding its effect during moderate sedation. However, the Task Force believes that electrocardiographic monitoring of selected individuals (e.g., patients with significant cardiovascular disease or dysrhythmias) may decrease risks during moderate sedation.

Recommendations: Monitoring of patient response to verbal commands should be routine during moderate sedation, except in patients who are unable to respond appropriately (*e.g.,* young children, mentally impaired or uncooperative patients), or during procedures where movement could be detrimental. During deep sedation, patient responsiveness to a more profound stimulus should be sought, unless contraindicated, to ensure that the patient has not drifted into a state of general anesthesia. During procedures where a verbal response is not possible (*e.g.,* oral surgery, upper endoscopy), the ability to give a "thumbs up" or other indication of consciousness in response to verbal or tactile (light tap) stimulation suggests that the patient will be able to control his airway and take deep breaths if necessary, corresponding to a state of moderate sedation. Note that a response limited to reflex withdrawal from a painful stimulus is **not** considered a purposeful response and thus represents a state of general anesthesia.

All patients undergoing sedation/analgesia should be monitored by pulse oximetry with appropriate alarms. If available, the variable pitch "beep," which gives a continuous audible indication of the oxygen saturation reading, may be helpful. In addition, ventilatory function should be continually monitored by observation and/or auscultation. Monitoring of exhaled CO_2 should be considered for all patients receiving deep sedation and for patients whose ventilation cannot be directly observed during moderate sedation. When possible, blood pressure should be determined before sedation/analgesia is initiated. Once sedation/analgesia is established, blood pressure should be measured at 5-minute intervals during the procedure, unless such monitoring interferes with the procedure (e.g., pediatric MRI where stimulation from the BP cuff could arouse an appropriately-sedated patient). Electrocardiographic monitoring should be used in all patients undergoing deep sedation; it should also be used during moderate sedation in patients with significant cardiovascular disease or those who are undergoing procedures where dysrhythmias are anticipated.

4. Recording of Monitored Parameters:

The literature is silent regarding the benefits of contemporaneous recording of patients' level of consciousness, respiratory function or hemodynamics. Consultant opinion agrees with the use of contemporaneous recording for moderate sedation, and strongly agrees with its use for patients undergoing deep sedation. It is the consensus of the Task Force that unless technically precluded (e.g., uncooperative or combative patient) vital signs and respiratory variables should be recorded before initiating sedation/analgesia, after administration of sedative/analgesic medications, at regular intervals during the procedure, upon initiation of recovery, and immediately before discharge. It is the opinion of the Task Force that contemporaneous recording (either automatic or manual) of patient data may disclose trends which could prove critical in determining the development or cause of adverse events. Additionally, manual recording ensures that an individual caring for the patient is aware of changes in patient status in a timely fashion.

Recommendations: For both moderate and deep sedation, patients' level of consciousness, ventilatory and oxygenation status, and hemodynamic variables should be assessed and recorded at a frequency which depends upon the type and amount of medication administered, the length of the procedure, and the general condition of the patient. At a minimum, this should be: (1) before the beginning of the procedure; (2) following administration of sedative/ analgesic agents; (3) at regular intervals during the procedure, (4) during initial recovery; and (5) just before discharge. If recording is performed automatically, device alarms should be set to alert the care team to critical changes in patient status.

5. Availability of an Individual Responsible for Patient Monitoring:

Although the literature is silent on this issue, the Task Force recognizes that it may not be possible for the individual performing a procedure to be fully cognizant of the patient's condition during sedation/analgesia. For moderate sedation, the consultants agree that the availability of an individual other than the person performing the procedure to monitor the patient's status improves patient comfort and satisfaction and that risks are reduced. For deep sedation, the consultants strongly agree with these contentions. During moderate sedation, the consultants strongly agree that the individual monitoring the patient may assist the practitioner with *interruptible* ancillary tasks of short duration; during deep sedation, the consultants agree that this individual should have no other responsibilities.

Recommendation: A designated individual, other than the practitioner performing the procedure, should be present to monitor the patient throughout procedures performed with sedation/analgesia. During deep sedation, this individual should have no other responsibilities. However, during moderate sedation, this individual may assist with minor, interruptible tasks once the patient's level of sedation/analgesia and vital signs have stabilized, provided that adequate monitoring for the patient's level of sedation is maintained.

6. Training of Personnel:

Although the literature is silent regarding the effectiveness of training on patient outcomes, the consultants strongly agree that education and training in the pharmacology of agents commonly used during sedation/analgesia improves the likelihood of satisfactory sedation and reduces the risk of adverse outcomes from either moderate or deep sedation. Specific concerns may include: (1) potentiation of sedative-induced respiratory depression by concomitantly administered opioids; (2) inadequate time intervals between doses of sedative or analgesic agents resulting in a cumulative overdose; and (3) inadequate familiarity with the role of pharmacological antagonists for sedative and analgesic agents.

Because the primary complications of sedation/analgesia are related to respiratory or cardiovascular depression, it is the consensus of the Task Force that the individual responsible for monitoring the patient should be trained in the recognition of complications associated with sedation/analgesia. Because sedation/analgesia constitute a continuum, practitioners administering moderate sedation should be able to rescue patients who enter a state of deep sedation, while those intending to administer deep sedation should be able to rescue patients who enter a state of general anesthesia. Therefore, the consultants strongly agree that at least one qualified individual trained in basic life support skills (CPR, bag-valve-mask ventilation) should be present in the procedure room during both moderate and deep sedation. In addition, the consultants strongly agree with the immediate availability (1-5 minutes away) of an individual with advanced life support skills (e.g., tracheal intubation, defibrillation, use of resuscitation medications) for moderate sedation and *in the procedure room* itself for deep sedation.

Recommendations: Individuals responsible for patients receiving sedation/analgesia should understand the pharmacology of the agents that are administered, as well as the role of pharmacologic antagonists for opioids and benzodiazepines. Individuals monitoring patients receiving sedation/analgesia should be able to recognize the associated complications. At least one individual capable of establishing a patent airway and positive pressure ventilation, as well as a means for summoning additional assistance should be present whenever sedation/analgesia are administered. It is recommended that an individual with advanced life support skills be immediately available (within 5 minutes) for moderate sedation and *within the procedure room for deep sedation.*

7. Availability of Emergency Equipment:

Although the literature is silent, the consultants strongly agree that the ready availability of appropriately-sized emergency equipment reduces the risk of both moderate and deep sedation. The literature is also silent regarding the need for cardiac defibrillators during sedation/analgesia. During moderate sedation, the consultants agree that a defibrillator should be immediately available for patients with both mild (e.g., hypertension) and severe (e.g., ischemia, congestive failure) cardiovascular disease. During deep sedation, the consultants agree that a defibrillator should be immediately available for all patients.

Recommendations: Pharmacologic antagonists as well as appropriately-sized equipment for establishing a patent airway and providing positive pressure ventilation with supplemental oxygen should be present whenever sedation/analgesia is administered. Suction, advanced airway equipment, and resuscitation medications should be immediately available and in good working order (*e.g.,* Example III). A functional defibrillator should be immediately available whenever deep sedation is administered, and when moderate sedation is administered to patients with mild or severe cardiovascular disease.

8. Use of Supplemental Oxygen:

The literature supports the use of supplemental oxygen during moderate sedation, and suggests the use of supplemental oxygen during deep sedation to reduce the frequency of hypoxemia. The consultants agree that supplemental oxygen decreases patient risk during moderate sedation, while strongly agreeing with this view for deep sedation.

Recommendations: Equipment to administer supplemental oxygen should be present when sedation/analgesia is administered. Supplemental oxygen should be considered for moderate sedation and should be administered during deep sedation unless specifically contraindicated for a particular patient or procedure. If hypoxemia is anticipated or develops during sedation/analgesia, supplemental oxygen should be administered.

9. Combinations of Sedative/Analgesic Agents:

The literature suggests that combining a sedative with an opioid provides effective moderate sedation; it is equivocal regarding whether the combination of a sedative and an opioid may be more effective than a sedative or an opioid alone in providing adequate moderate sedation. For deep sedation, the literature is insufficient to compare the efficacy of sedative-opioid combinations with that of a sedative, alone. The consultants agree that combinations of sedatives and opioids provide satisfactory moderate and deep sedation. However, the published data also suggest that combinations of sedatives and opioids may increase the likelihood of adverse outcomes including ventilatory depression and hypoxemia; the consultants were equivocal on this issue for both moderate and deep sedation. It is the consensus of the Task Force that fixed combinations of sedative and analgesic agents may not allow the individual components of sedation/analgesia to be appropriately titrated to meet the individual requirements of the patient and procedure while reducing the associated risks.

Example III   EMERGENCY EQUIPMENT FOR SEDATION AND ANALGESIA

Appropriate emergency equipment should be available whenever sedative or analgesic drugs capable of causing cardiorespiratory depression are administered. The table below should be used as a guide, which should be modified depending upon the individual practice circumstances. Items in brackets are recommended when infants or children are sedated.

Intravenous Equipment:

Gloves
Tourniquets
Alcohol wipes
Sterile gauze pads
Intravenous catheters [24, 22 gauge]
Intravenous tubing [pediatric 'microdrip'--60 drops/ml]
Intravenous fluid
Assorted needles for drug aspiration, IM injection [intraosseous bone marrow needle]
Appropriately sized syringes [1 ml syringes] Tape

Basic Airway Management Equipment:

Source of compressed O_2 (tank with regulator or pipeline supply with flowmeter)
Source of suction
Suction catheters [pediatric suction catheters] Yankauer-type suction
Face masks [infant/child face masks]
Self-inflating breathing bag-valve set [pediatric bag-valve set]
Oral and nasal airways [infant/child sized airways]
Lubricant

Advanced Airway Management Equipment (for Practitioners With Intubation Skills)

Laryngeal mask airways [pediatric laryngeal mask airways]
Laryngoscope handles (tested)
Laryngoscope blades [pediatric laryngoscope blades]
Endotracheal tubes:
    Cuffed 6.0, 7.0, 8.0, mm i.d.
    [Uncuffed 2.5, 3.0, 3.5, 4.0, 4.5, 5.0, 5.5, 6.0 mm i.d.]
Stylet [appropriately sized for endotracheal tubes]

Pharmacologic Antagonists

Naloxone
Flumazenil

Emergency Medications

Epinephrine Ephedrine Vasopressin
Atropine
Nitroglycerin (tablets or spray)
Amiodarone
Lidocaine
Glucose (50%) [10% or 25% glucose]
Diphenhydramine
Hydrocortisone, methylprednisolone, or dexamethasone
Diazepam or Midazolam

Recommendations: Combinations of sedative and analgesic agents may be administered as appropriate for the procedure being performed and the condition of the patient. Ideally, each component should be administered individually to achieve the desired effect (*e.g.*, additional analgesic medication to relieve pain; additional sedative medication to decrease awareness or anxiety). The propensity for combinations of sedative and analgesic agents to cause respiratory depression and airway obstruction emphasizes the need to appropriately reduce the dose of each component as well as the need to continually monitor respiratory function.

10. Titration of Intravenous Sedative/Analgesic Medications:

The literature is insufficient to determine whether administration of small, incremental doses of intravenous sedative/analgesic drugs until the desired level of sedation and/or analgesia is achieved is preferable to a single dose based on patient size, weight, or age. The consultants strongly agree that incremental drug administration improves patient comfort and decreases risks for both moderate and deep sedation.

Recommendations: Intravenous sedative/analgesic drugs should be given in small, incremental doses which are titrated to the desired endpoints of analgesia, and sedation. Sufficient time must elapse between doses to allow the effect of each dose to be assessed before subsequent drug administration. When drugs are administered by non-intravenous routes (*e.g.*, oral, rectal, intramuscular, transmucosal), allowance should be made for the time required for drug absorption before supplementation is considered. Because absorption may be unpredictable, administration of repeat doses of oral medications to supplement sedation/analgesia is not recommended.

11. Anesthetic Induction Agents Used for Sedation/Analgesia (Propofol, Methohexital, Ketamine):

The literature suggests that when administered by non-anesthesiologists, propofol and ketamine can provide satisfactory moderate sedation, and suggests that methohexital can provide satisfactory deep sedation. The literature is insufficient to evaluate the efficacy of propofol or ketamine administered by non-anesthesiologists for deep sedation. There is insufficient literature to determine whether moderate or deep sedation with propofol is associated with a different incidence of adverse outcomes than similar levels of sedation with midazolam. The consultants are equivocal regarding whether use of these medications affects the likelihood of producing satisfactory moderate sedation, while agreeing that using them increases the likelihood of satisfactory deep sedation. However, the consultants agree that *avoiding* these medications decreases the likelihood of adverse outcomes during moderate sedation, and are equivocal regarding their effect on adverse outcomes during deep sedation.

The Task Force cautions practitioners that methohexital and propofol can produce rapid, profound decreases in level of consciousness and cardiorespiratory function, potentially culminating in a state of general anesthesia. The Task Force notes that ketamine also produces dose-related decreases in level of consciousness culminating in general anesthesia. Although it may be associated with less cardiorespiratory depression than other sedatives, airway obstruction, laryngospasm, and pulmonary aspiration may still occur with ketamine. Furthermore, because of its dissociative properties, some of the usual signs of depth of sedation may not apply (e.g., the patient's eyes may be open while in a state of deep sedation or general anesthesia). The Task Force also notes that there are no specific pharmacological antagonists for any of these medications.

Recommendations: Even if moderate sedation is intended, patients receiving propofol or methohexital by any route should receive care consistent with that required for deep sedation. Accordingly, practitioners administering these drugs should be qualified to rescue patients from any level of sedation including general anesthesia. Patients receiving ketamine should be cared for in a manner consistent with the level of sedation which is achieved.

12. Intravenous Access:

Published literature is equivocal regarding the relative efficacy of sedative/analgesic agents administered intravenously as compared to agents administered by non-intravenous routes to achieve moderate sedation; the literature is insufficient on this issue for deep sedation. The literature is equivocal regarding the comparative safety of these routes of administration for moderate sedation, and insufficient for deep sedation. The consultants strongly agree that intravenous administration of sedative and analgesic medications increases the likelihood of satisfactory sedation for both moderate and deep sedation. They also agree that it decreases the likelihood of adverse outcomes. For both moderate and deep sedation, when sedative/analgesic medications are administered intravenously, the consultants strongly agree with maintaining intravenous access until patients are no longer at risk for cardiovascular or respiratory depression, because it increases the likelihood of satisfactory sedation and decreases the likelihood of adverse outcomes. In those situations where sedation is begun by non-intravenous routes (*e.g.,* oral, rectal, intramuscular) the need for intravenous access is not sufficiently addressed in the literature. However, initiation of intravenous access after the initial sedation takes effect allows additional sedative/analgesic and resuscitation drugs to be administered if necessary.

Recommendations: In patients receiving intravenous medications for sedation/analgesia, vascular access should be maintained throughout the procedure and until the patient is no longer at risk for cardiorespiratory depression. In patients who have received sedation/analgesia by non-intravenous routes, or whose intravenous line has become dislodged or blocked, practitioners should determine the advisability of establishing or reestablishing intravenous access on a case-by-case basis. In all instances, an individual with the skills to establish intravenous access should be immediately available.

13. Reversal Agents:

Specific antagonist agents are available for the opioids (*e.g.*, naloxone) and benzodiazepines (*e.g.*, flumazenil). The literature supports the ability of naloxone to reverse opioid-induced sedation and respiratory depression. Practitioners are cautioned that acute reversal of opioid-induced analgesia may result in pain, hypertension, tachycardia, or pulmonary edema. The literature supports the ability of flumazenil to antagonize benzodiazepine-induced sedation and ventilatory depression in patients who have received benzodiazepines alone or in combination with an opioid. The consultants strongly agree that the immediate availability of reversal agents during both moderate and deep sedation is associated with decreased risk of adverse outcomes. It is the consensus of the Task Force that respiratory depression should be initially treated with supplemental oxygen and, if necessary, positive pressure ventilation by mask. The consultants disagree that the use of sedation regimens which are likely to require *routine* reversal with flumazenil or naloxone improves the quality of sedation or reduces the risk of adverse outcomes.

Recommendations: Specific antagonists should be available whenever opioid analgesics or benzodiazepines are administered for sedation/analgesia. Naloxone and/or flumazenil may be administered to improve spontaneous ventilatory efforts in patients who have received opioids or benzodiazepines, respectively. This may be especially helpful in cases where airway control and positive pressure ventilation are difficult. Prior to or concomitantly with pharmacological reversal, patients who become hypoxemic or apneic during sedation/analgesia should: (1) be encouraged or stimulated to breathe deeply; (2) receive supplemental oxygen; and (3) receive positive pressure ventilation if spontaneous ventilation is inadequate. Following pharmacological reversal, patients should be observed long enough to ensure that sedation and cardiorespiratory depression does not recur once the effect of the antagonist dissipates. The use of sedation regimens which include routine reversal of sedative or analgesic agents is discouraged.

14. Recovery Care:

Patients may continue to be at significant risk for developing complications after their procedure is completed. Decreased procedural stimulation, delayed drug absorption following nonintravenous administration, and slow drug elimination, may contribute to residual sedation and cardiorespiratory depression during the recovery period. Examples include intramuscular meperidine-promethazine-chlorpromazine mixtures and oral or rectal chloral hydrate. When sedation/analgesia is administered to outpatients, one must assume that there will be no medical supervision once the patient leaves the medical facility. Although there is not sufficient literature to examine the effects of postprocedure monitoring on patient outcomes, the consultants strongly agree that continued observation, monitoring, and predetermined discharge criteria decrease the likelihood of adverse outcomes for both moderate and deep sedation. It is the consensus of the Task Force that discharge criteria should be designed to minimize the risk for cardiorespiratory depression after patients are released from observation by trained personnel.

Recommendations: Following sedation/analgesia, patients should be observed in an appropriately staffed and equipped area until they are near their baseline level of consciousness and are no longer at increased risk for cardiorespiratory depression. Oxygenation should be monitored periodically until patients are no longer at risk for hypoxemia. Ventilation, and circulation should be monitored at regular intervals until patients are suitable for discharge. Discharge criteria should be designed to minimize the risk of central nervous system or cardiorespiratory depression following discharge from observation by trained personnel (*e.g.*, Example IV.)

15. *Special Situations:*

The literature suggests and the Task Force members concur that certain types of patients are at increased risk for developing complications related to sedation/analgesia unless special precautions are taken. In patients with significant underlying medical conditions (e.g., extremes of age; severe cardiac, pulmonary, hepatic or renal disease; pregnancy; drug or alcohol abuse) the consultants agree that preprocedure consultation with an appropriate medical specialist (e.g., cardiologist, pulmonologist) decreases the risk associated with moderate sedation and strongly agree that it decreases the risks associated with deep sedation. In patients with significant *sedation-related* risk factors (e.g., uncooperative patients, morbid obesity, potentially difficult airway, sleep apnea) the consultants are equivocal regarding whether preprocedure consultation with an anesthesiologist increases the likelihood of satisfactory moderate sedation while agreeing that it decreases adverse outcomes; the consultants strongly agree that preprocedure consultation increases the likelihood of satisfactory outcomes while decreasing the risk associated with deep sedation. The Task Force notes that in emergency situations, the benefits of awaiting pre-procedure consultations must be weighed against the risk of delaying the procedure.

For moderate sedation, the consultants are equivocal regarding whether the immediate availability of an individual with postgraduate training in anesthesiology increases the likelihood of a satisfactory outcome or decreases the associated risks. For deep sedation the consultants agree that the immediate availability of such an individual improves the likelihood of satisfactory sedation and that it will decrease the likelihood of adverse outcomes.

Recommendations: Whenever possible, appropriate medical specialists should be consulted prior to administration of sedation to patients with significant underlying conditions. The choice of specialists depends on the nature of the underlying condition and the urgency of the situation. For severely compromised or medically unstable patients (*e.g.*, anticipated difficult airway, severe

Example IV   RECOVERY AND DISCHARGE CRITERIA FOLLOWING SEDATION AND
ANALGESIA

Each patient-care facility in which sedation/analgesia is administered should
develop recovery and discharge criteria which are suitable for its specific patients
and procedures. Some of the basic principles which might be incorporated in
these criteria are enumerated below.

A. General Principles

1. Medical supervision of recovery and discharge following moderate or deep
   sedation is the responsibility of the operating practitioner or a licensed
   physician
2. The recovery area should be equipped with or have direct access to
   appropriate monitoring and resuscitation equipment
3. Patients receiving moderate or deep sedation should be monitored until
   appropriate discharge criteria are satisfied. The duration and frequency of
   monitoring should be individualized depending upon the level of sedation
   achieved, the overall condition of the patient, and the nature of the
   intervention for which sedation/analgesia was administered. Oxygenation
   should be monitored until patients are no longer at risk for respiratory
   depression.
4. Level of consciousness, vital signs and oxygenation (when indicated) should
   be recorded at regular intervals
5. A nurse or other individual trained to monitor patients and recognize
   complications should be in attendance until discharge criteria are fulfilled.
6. An individual capable of managing complications (e.g., establishing a patent
   airway and providing positive pressure ventilation) should be immediately
   available until discharge criteria are fulfilled.

B. Guidelines for Discharge

1. Patients should be alert and oriented; infants and patients whose mental
   status was initially abnormal should have returned to their baseline status.
   Practitioners and parents must be aware that pediatric patients are at risk for
   airway obstruction should the head fall forward while the child is secured in
   a car seat.
2. Vital signs should be stable and within acceptable limits.
3. Use of scoring systems may assist in documentation of fitness for discharge.
4. Sufficient time (up to 2 hours) should have elapsed following the last
   administration of reversal agents (naloxone, flumazenil) to ensure that
   patients do not become resedated after reversal effects have worn off.
5. Outpatients should be discharged in the presence of a responsible adult who
   will accompany them home and be able to report any postprocedure
   complications.
6. Outpatients and their escorts should be provided with written instructions
   regarding postprocedure diet, medications, activities, and a phone number to
   be called in case of emergency.

obstructive pulmonary disease, coronary artery disease, or congestive heart failure), or if it is likely that sedation to the point of unresponsiveness will be necessary to obtain adequate conditions, practitioners who are not trained in the administration of general anesthesia should consult an anesthesiologist.

APPENDIX: METHODS AND ANALYSES

The scientific assessment of these Guidelines was based on the following statements, or evidence linkages. These linkages represent directional statements about relationships between obstetrical anesthetic interventions and clinical outcomes.

1. A preprocedure patient evaluation, (i.e., history, physical examination, laboratory evaluation, consultation):
   a. Improves clinical efficacy (i.e., satisfactory sedation and analgesia).
   b. Reduces adverse outcomes.
2. Preprocedure preparation of the patient (e.g., counseling, fasting):
   a. Improves clinical efficacy (i.e., satisfactory sedation and analgesia).
   b. Reduces adverse outcomes.
3. Patient monitoring (i.e., level of consciousness, pulmonary ventilation (observation, auscultation), oxygenation (pulse oximetry), automated apnea monitoring (capnography), hemodynamics (ECG, BP, HR):
   a. Improves clinical efficacy (i.e., satisfactory sedation and analgesia).
   b. Reduces adverse outcomes.
4. Contemporaneous recording of monitored parameters (e.g., level of consciousness, respiratory function, hemodynamics) at regular intervals in patients receiving sedation and/or analgesia:
   a. Improves clinical efficacy (i.e., satisfactory sedation and analgesia).
   b. Reduces adverse outcomes.
5. Availability of an individual who is dedicated solely to patient monitoring and safety:
   a. Improves clinical efficacy (i.e., satisfactory sedation and analgesia).
   b. Reduces adverse outcomes.
6a. Education and training of sedation and analgesia providers in the pharmacology of sedation/analgesia agents:
   a. Improves clinical efficacy (i.e., satisfactory sedation and analgesia).
   b. Reduces adverse outcomes.
6b. The presence of an individual(s) capable of establishing a patent airway, positive pressure ventilation and resuscitation (i.e., advanced life-support skills) during a procedure:
   a. Improves clinical efficacy (i.e., satisfactory sedation and analgesia).
   b. Reduces adverse outcomes.
7. Availability of appropriately sized emergency and airway equipment (e.g., LMA, defibrillators):

a. Improves clinical efficacy (i.e., satisfactory sedation and analgesia).
b. Reduces adverse outcomes.
8. The use of supplemental oxygen during procedures performed with sedation and/or analgesia:
a. Improves clinical efficacy (i.e., satisfactory sedation and analgesia).
b. Reduces adverse outcomes.
9. Use of sedative agents combined with analgesic agents (e.g., sedative/analgesic cocktails, fixed combinations of sedatives and analgesics, titrated combinations of sedatives and analgesics):
a. Improves clinical efficacy (i.e., satisfactory sedation and analgesia).
b. Reduces adverse outcomes.
10. Titration of intravenous sedative/analgesic medications to achieve the desired effect:
a. Improves clinical efficacy (i.e., satisfactory sedation and analgesia).
b. Reduces adverse outcomes.
11. Intravenous sedation/analgesic medications specifically designed to be used for general anesthesia(i.e., methohexital, propofol and ketamine):
a. Improves clinical efficacy (ie., satisfactory sedation and analgesia).
b. Reduces adverse outcomes.
12a. Administration of sedative/analgesic agents by the intravenous route:
a. Improves clinical efficacy (i.e., satisfactory sedation and analgesia).
b. Reduces adverse outcomes.
12b. Maintaining or establishing intravenous access during sedation and/or analgesia until the patient is no longer at risk for cardiorespiratory depression:
a. Improves clinical efficacy (i.e., satisfactory sedation and analgesia).
b. Reduces adverse outcomes.
13. Availability of reversal agents *(naloxone and flumazenil only)* for the sedative and/or analgesic agents being administered:
a. Improves clinical efficacy (i.e., satisfactory sedation and analgesia).
b. Reduces adverse outcomes.
14. Post-procedural recovery observation, monitoring, and predetermined discharge criteria reduce adverse outcomes.
15. Special regimens (e.g., preprocedure consultation, specialized monitoring, *special sedatives/techniques*) for patients with special problems (e.g., uncooperative patients; extremes of age; severe cardiac, pulmonary, hepatic, renal, or central nervous system disease; morbid obesity; sleep apnea; pregnancy; drug or alcohol abuse; emergency/unprepared patients; metabolic and airway difficulties):
a. Improves clinical efficacy (i.e., satisfactory sedation and analgesia).
b. Reduces adverse outcomes.

Scientific evidence was derived from aggregated research literature, and from surveys, open presentations and other consensus-oriented activities. For purposes of literature aggregation, potentially relevant clinical studies were identified via electronic and manual searches of the literature. The electronic search covered a 36-year period from 1966 through 2001. The manual search covered a 44-year period of time from 1958 through 2001. Over 3000 citations were initially identified, yielding a total of 1876 non-overlapping articles that addressed topics related to the 15 evidence linkages. Following review of the articles, 1519 studies did not provide direct evidence, and were subsequently eliminated. A total of 357 articles contained direct linkage-related evidence.

A directional result for each study was initially determined by a literature count, classifying each outcome as either supporting a linkage, refuting a linkage, or neutral. The results were then summarized to obtain a directional assessment of support for each linkage. Literature pertaining to three evidence linkages contained enough studies with well-defined experimental designs and statistical information to conduct formal meta-analyses. These three linkages were: linkage 8 [supplemental oxygen], linkage 9 [benzodiazepines combined with opioids versus benzodiazepines alone], linkage 13 [naloxone for antagonism of opioids, flumazenil for antagonism of benzodiazepines, and flumazenil for antagonism of benzodiazepine-opioid combinations].

Combined probability tests were applied to continuous data, and an odds-ratio procedure was applied to dichotomous study results. Two combined probability tests were employed as follows: (1) The Fisher Combined Test, producing chi-square values based on logarithmic transformations of the reported p-values from the independent studies, and (2) the Stouffer Combined Test, providing weighted representation of the studies by weighting each of the standard normal deviates by the size of the sample. An odds-ratio procedure based on the Mantel-Haenszel method for combining study results using 2×2 tables was used with outcome frequency information. An acceptable significance level was set at $p < 0.01$ (one-tailed) and effect size estimates were calculated. Interobserver agreement was established through assessment of interrater reliability testing. Tests for heterogeneity of the independent samples were conducted to assure consistency among the study results. To assess potential publishing bias, a "fail-safe N" value was calculated for each combined probability test. No search for unpublished studies was conducted, and no reliability tests for locating research results were done.

Meta-analytic results are reported in Table 2. The following outcomes were found to be significant for combined probability tests: (1) *oxygen saturation*—linkage 8 [supplemental oxygen]; (2) *sedation recovery*—linkage 13 [naloxone for antagonism of opioids and flumazenil for antagonism of benzodiazepine-opioid combinations]; (3) *psychomotor recovery*—linkage 13 [flumazenil for antagonism of benzodiazepines], and (4) *respiratory/ventilatory recovery* -linkage 13 [naloxone for antagonism of opioids, flumazenil for antagonism of benzodiazepines, and flumazenil for antagonism of benzodiazepine-opioid combinations]. To be considered acceptable findings of significance, both the Fisher and weighted Stouffer combined test results must agree. Weighted effect size values for these link-ages ranged from r = 0.19 to r = 0.80, representing moderate to high effect size estimates.

Mantel-Haenszel odds ratios were significant for the following outcomes: (1) *hypoxemia*—linkage 8 [supplemental oxygen] and linkage 9 [benzodiazepine-opioid combinations versus benzodiazepines alone]; (2) *sedation recovery* -linkage 13 [flumazenil for antagonism of benzodiazepines], and (3) *recall of procedure*—linkage 9 [benzodiazepine-opioid combinations]. To be considered acceptable findings of significance, Mantel-Haenszel odds-ratios must agree with combined test results when both types of data are assessed.

Interobserver agreement among Task Force members and two methodolo-gists was established by interrater reliability testing. Agreement levels using a Kappa statistic for two-rater agreement pairs were as follows: (1) type of study design, k = 0.25 to 0.64; (2) type of analysis, k = 0.36 to 0.83; (3) evidence linkage assignment, k = 0.78 to 0.89; and (4) literature inclusion for database, k = 0.71 to 1.00. Three-rater chance-corrected agreement values were: (1) study design, Sav = 0.45, Var (Sav) = 0.012; (2) type of analysis, Sav = 0.51, Var (Sav) = 0.015; (3) linkage assignment, Sav = 0.81 Var (Sav) = 0.006; (4) literature database inclusion, Sav = 0.84 Var (Sav) = 0.046. These values represent moderate to high levels of agreement.

The findings of the literature analyses were supplemented by the opinions of Task Force members as well as by surveys of the opinions of a panel of Con-sultants, as described in the text of the Guidelines. The rate of return for this Consultant survey was 78% (N = 51/65). Median agreement scores from the Consultants regarding each linkage are reported in Table 3.

For moderate sedation, Consultants were supportive of all of the linkages with the following exceptions: linkage 3 (electrocardiogram monitoring and capnog-raphy), linkage 9 (sedatives combined with analgesics for reducing adverse out-comes), linkage 11 (avoiding general anesthesia sedatives for improving satisfactory sedation), linkage 13b (routine administration of naloxone), linkage 13c (routine administration of flumazenil), and linkage 15b (anesthesiologist consultation for patients with medical conditions to provide satisfactory moder-ate sedation). In addition, Consultants were equivocal regarding whether postgraduate training in anesthesiology improves moderate sedation or reduces adverse outcomes.

For deep sedation, Consultants were supportive of all of the linkages with the following exceptions: linkage 9 (sedatives combined with analgesics for reduc-ing adverse outcomes), linkage 11 (avoiding general anesthesia sedatives), linkage 13b (routine administration of naloxone), and linkage 13c (routine administration of flumazenil).

The Consultants were asked to indicate which, if any, of the evidence link-ages would change their clinical practices if the updated Guidelines were insti-tuted. The rate of return was 57% (N = 37/65). The percent of responding Consultants expecting *no change* associated with each linkage were as follows:

Table 2 | Meta-Analysis Summary

Linkages	No. Studies	Fisher X^2	p	Weighted Stouffer Zc	p	Effect Size	Mantel-Haenszel X^2	p	Odds Ratio	Heterogeneity Significance	Effect Size
8. Supplemental Oxygen											
Oxygen Saturation[1]	5	71.40	<0.001	5.44	<0.001	0.40	*	*	*	>0.90 (NS)	>0.50 (NS)
Hypoxemia[1]	7	*	*	*	*	*	44.15	<0.001	0.20	*	>0.50 (NS)
9a. Sedatives/Opioids Combined: Benzodiazepines + Opioids											
Sedation Efficacy	7	*	*	*	*	*	3.79	>0.05 (NS)	1.47	*	<0.01
Recall of Procedure	6	*	*	*	*	*	18.47	<0.001	2.57	*	<0.01
Hypoxemia	5	*	*	*	*	*	11.78	<0.001	2.37	*	>0.05 (NS)
13a. Reversal Agents: Naloxone for opioids											
Sedation Recovery											
At 5 *minutes*[1,2,3]	5	38.36	<0.001	3.13	<0.001	0.23	*	*	*	>0.30 (NS)	>0.02 (NS)
Respiratory Ventilation[1,2,3]	5	38.72	<0.001	3.97	<0.001	0.33	*	*	*	>0.10 (NS)	<0.001

13b. Reversal Agents: Flumazenil for benzodiazepines

Sedation Recovery											
At 5 minutes	6	*	*	*	*	*	104.76	<0.001	8.15	*	>0.10 (NS)
Psychomotor Recovery											
At 15 minutes	5	41.80	<0.001	1.69	.0455 (NS)	0.20	*	*	*	>0.70 (NS)	>0.50 (NS)
At 30 minutes	5	43.02	<0.001	3.36	<0.001	0.19	*	*	*	>0.90 (NS)	>0.50 (NS)
Respiration/Ventilation[2,3]	6	53.25	<0.001	5.03	<0.001	0.80	*	*	*	<0.01	<0.001

13c. Reversal Agents: Flumazenil for benzodiazepine-opioid combinations

Sedation Recovery											
At 5 minutes	5	72.12	<0.001	6.76	<0.001	0.37	*	*	*	<0.001	<0.001
Respiration/Ventilation[2,3]	6	55.06	<0.001	5.11	<0.001	0.25	*	*	*	>0.10 (NS)	<0.001
Nausea/Vomiting	5	*	*	*	*	*	0.28	>0.80 (NS)	1.22	*	>0.70 (NS)

[1] Non-randomized comparative studies are included.

[2] Studies in which anesthesiologist administered benzodiazepines, opioids or reversal agents are included.

[3] Studies in which subjects consist of ICU, postoperative patients or volunteers with no procedures are included.

Table 3 | **Consultant Survey Summary**

Linkage/Intervention	Outcome	Moderate Sedation		Deep Sedation	
		N	Median* or Percent	N	Median* or Percent
1. Preprocedure patient evaluation	Satisfactory sedation	51	5	51	5
	Adverse outcomes	51	5	51	5
2. Preprocedure fasting	Satisfactory sedation	51	4	51	5
	Adverse outcomes	51	4	51	5
3. Monitoring					
a. Level of consciousness	Satisfactory sedation	51	5	49	5
	Adverse outcomes	51	5	50	5
b. Breathing (observation/auscultation)	Satisfactory sedation	51	5	49	5
	Adverse outcomes	51	5	50	5
c. Pulse oximetry	Satisfactory sedation	51	5	50	5
	Adverse outcomes	51	5	50	5
d. Blood pressure/heart rate	Satisfactory sedation	50	4	49	5
	Adverse outcomes	50	5	49	5
e. Electrocardiogram	Satisfactory sedation	51	3	50	4
	Adverse outcomes	51	3	49	5
f. Capnography	Satisfactory sedation	50	3	48	4
	Adverse outcomes	50	3	49	4
4. Contemporaneous recording	Satisfactory sedation	51	4	50	5
	Adverse outcomes	51	4	50	5
5. Individual for patient monitoring	Satisfactory sedation	49	4	48	5
	Adverse outcomes	49	4	48	5

6a. Education and training	Satisfactory sedation	50	5	49	5
	Adverse outcomes	50	5	49	5
6b. Individual with basic life support skills present in room		50	5	49	5
6c. Availability of ALS skills					
In the procedure room		2	4.2%	39	79.6%
Immediate vicinity (1-5 minutes)		27	56.2%	8	16.3%
Same building (5-10 minutes)		14	29.2%	2	4.1%
Outside provider		5	10.4%	0	0.0%
7. Emergency IV and airway equipment	Adverse outcomes	51	5	49	5
8. Supplemental oxygen	Adverse outcomes	50	4	49	5
9. Sedatives combined with analgesics	Satisfactory sedation	50	4	49	4
	Adverse outcomes	50	3	49	3
10. Titration	Satisfactory sedation	51	5	50	5
	Adverse outcomes	51	5	50	5
11. Avoiding GA sedatives	Satisfactory sedation	50	3	49	2
	Adverse outcomes	50	4	49	3
12a. IV sedatives	Satisfactory sedation	51	5	50	5
	Adverse outcomes	51	4	50	4
12b. IV access	Satisfactory sedation	50	4	49	5
	Adverse outcomes	50	5	49	5
13a. Immediate availability of naloxone or flumazenil	Adverse outcomes	51	5	51	5
13b. Routine administration of naloxone	Satisfactory sedation	37	2	37	2
	Adverse outcomes	37	2	37	2
13c. Routine administration of flumazenil	Satisfactory sedation	37	1	37	2
	Adverse outcomes	37	2	37	2

Table 3 | **Consultant Survey Summary—cont'd**

Linkage/Intervention	Outcome	Moderate Sedation		Deep Sedation	
		N	Median* or Percent	N	Median* or Percent
14. Observation, monitoring & D/C criteria	Adverse outcomes	50	5	49	5
15a. Med specialist consult, med conditions	Satisfactory sedation	50	4	49	5
	Adverse outcomes	50	4	49	5
15b. Anesthesiologist consultation, patients with underlying medical conditions	Satisfactory sedation	51	3	50	4
	Adverse outcomes	51	4	50	5
15c. Anesthesiologist consultation, patients with significant sedation risk factors	Satisfactory sedation	51	4	50	5
	Adverse outcomes	51	4	50	5
16. Postgraduate training in anesthesiology	Satisfactory sedation	51	3	50	4
	Adverse outcomes	51	3	50	4
17. In emergency situations, sedate patients less deeply		51	4	51	5

From Anesthesiology 96: 1004-1017, 2002 @ 2002 American Society of Anesthesiologists Lippincott, Williams & Wilkins, Inc.

* Strongly Agree: Median score of '5' (At least 50% of the responses were '5')
Agree: Median score of '4' (At least 50% of the responses were '4' or '5')
Equivocal: Median score of '3' (At least 50% of the scores were '3' or less)
Disagree: Median score of '2' (At least 50% of responses were '1' or '2')
Strongly Disagree: Median score of '1' (At least 50% of responses were '1')

preprocedure patient evaluation—94%; preprocedure patient preparation—91%; patient monitoring 80%; contemporaneous recording of monitored parameters—91%; availability of individual dedicated solely to patient monitoring and safety—91%; education and training of sedation/analgesia providers in pharmacology—89%; presence of an individual(s) capable of establishing a patent airway—91%; availability of appropriately sized emergency and airway equipment—94%, use of supplemental oxygen during procedures—100%, use of sedative agents combined with analgesic agents—91%, titration of sedatives/analgesics—97%, intravenous sedation/analgesia with agents designed *for* general anesthesia 77%, administration of sedative/analgesic agents by the intravenous route—94%, maintaining or establishing intravenous access—97%, availability/use of flumazenil—94%, availability/use of naloxone—94%, observation and monitoring during recovery—89%, special care *for* patients with underlying medical problems—91%, and special care *for* uncooperative patients—94%. Seventy-four percent of the respondents indicated that the Guidelines would have *no effect* on the amount of time spent on a typical case. Nine respondents (26%) indicated that there would be an increase in the amount of time they would spend on a typical case with the implementation of these Guidelines. The amount of increased time anticipated by these respondents ranged from 1-60 minutes.

Appendix E

American Association of Nurse Anesthetists' Position Statement: Qualified Providers of Sedation and Analgesia; Considerations for Policy Guidelines for Registered Nurses Engaged in the Administration of Sedation and Analgesia

Wednesday, May 19, 2004
American Association of Nurse Anesthetists
Qualified Providers of Sedation and Analgesia
No. 2.2

The AANA believes the safest administration of sedation and analgesia is provided by a professional, educated in the specialty of anesthesia and skilled in the administration of sedation, monitored anesthesia care, regional and general anesthesia, providing his or her sole attention to the patient.

Sedation combined with analgesia may easily become deep sedation or loss of consciousness because of the agents used as well as the physical status and drug sensitivities of the patient. The administration of sedation requires continuous monitoring of the patient and the ability to respond immediately to any adverse reaction or complication. Sedation should only be provided by an individual who is qualified to select and administer the appropriate agents and who is capable of managing all anesthetic levels and potential complications including airway management, intubation and resuscitation.

Registered nurses have become increasingly involved in assisting physicians in providing sedation. The American Association of Nurse Anesthetists has developed *AANA Considerations for Policy Guidelines for the Registered Nurse Engaged in the Administration of Sedation and Analgesia*, to provide guidance for policy development and to promote the quality and safety of patient care when sedation is administered by persons who are not qualified anesthesia providers.

Adopted by AANA Board of Directors May 1988 Revised April 1991
Revised June 1996
Revised June 2003
http://www.aana.com/practice/qualified.asp
5/19/04
CRNA Practice
Wednesday, May 19, 2004
American Association of Nurse Anesthetists

CONSIDERATIONS FOR POLICY GUIDELINES FOR REGISTERED NURSES ENGAGED IN THE ADMINISTRATION OF SEDATION AND ANALGESIA

Introduction

Although the safest care for the patient receiving sedation and analgesia is provided by a qualified anesthesia provider, a large number of registered nurses are involved in the administration of sedation and analgesia. To promote safe care during sedation and analgesia and to address questions which have been raised by nursing organizations and healthcare institutions with respect to the necessary qualifications of registered nurses involved in this care, the American Association of Nurse Anesthetists suggests the following policy considerations. These considerations do not supersede or give the effect to more restrictive relevant laws, regulations, judicial and administrative decisions and interpretations, accepted standards and scopes of practice established by professional nursing organizations, or institutional policies applicable to registered nurses, which should be reviewed prior to the development of any sedation and analgesia policy.

Definition

Sedation and analgesia describes a medically controlled state of depressed consciousness that allows protective reflexes to be maintained. The patient retains the ability to independently maintain his or her airway and to respond purposefully to verbal commands and/or tactile stimulation. The American Society of Anesthesiologists (ASA) Task Force on Sedation and Analgesia has developed Practice Guidelines for Sedation and Analgesia by NonAnesthesiologists which states "sedation and analgesia describes a state that allows patients to tolerate unpleasant procedures while maintaining adequate cardio respiratory function and the ability to respond purposefully to verbal command and tactile stimulation. The Task Force decided that the term sedation and analgesia more accurately defines this therapeutic goal than does the more commonly used but imprecise term of 'conscious sedation.' Those patients whose only response is reflex withdrawal from a painful stimulus are sedated to a greater degree than encompassed by sedation/analgesia."

The Joint Commission on Accreditation for Healthcare Organizations has introduced to their standards definitions for four levels of sedation and anesthesia. *Minimal sedation* where the patient responds normally; *moderate seda-*

tion/analgesia (conscious sedation), where an airway and cardiovascular function is maintained; *deep sedation/analgesia,* in which the patient is not easily aroused; and, *anesthesia,* in which patients require assisted ventilation. Sedation and analgesia may easily be converted to deep sedation and the loss of consciousness because of the agents used and the physical status and drug sensitivities of the individual patient. The administration of sedation and analgesia requires constant monitoring of the patient and ability of the administrator to respond immediately to any adverse reaction or complication. Vigilance of the administrator and the ability to recognize and intervene in the event complications or undesired outcomes arise are essential requirements for individuals administering sedation and analgesia.

A. Qualifications

1. The registered nurse is allowed by state law and institutional policy to administer sedation and analgesia.
2. The health care facility shall have in place an educational/credentialing mechanism which includes a process for evaluating and documenting the individual's competency relating to the management of patients receiving sedation and analgesia. Evaluation and documentation occur on a periodic basis.
3. The registered nurse managing and monitoring the care of patients receiving sedation and analgesia is able to:
   a. Demonstrate the acquired knowledge of anatomy, physiology, pharmacology, cardiac arrhythmia recognition and complications related to sedation and analgesia sedation and medications.
   b. Assess the total patient care requirements before and during the administration of sedation and analgesia, including the recovery phase.
   c. Understand the principles of oxygen delivery, transport and uptake, respiratory physiology, as well as understand and use oxygen delivery devices.
   d. Recognize potential complications of sedation and analgesia sedation for each type of agent being administered.
   e. Posses the competency to assess, diagnose, and intervene in the event of complications and institute appropriate interventions in compliance with orders or institutional protocols.
   f. Demonstrate competency, through AClS or PClS, in airway management and resuscitation appropriate to the age of the patient.
   g. The registered nurse administering sedation and analgesia understands the legal ramifications of providing this care and maintains appropriate liability insurance.

B. Management and Monitoring

Registered nurses who are not qualified anesthesia providers may be authorized to manage and monitor sedation and analgesia during therapeutic, diagnostic or surgical procedures if the following criteria are met. These criteria should be interpreted in a manner consistent with the remainder of this document.

1. Guidelines for patient monitoring, drug administration, and protocols for dealing with potential complications or emergency situations, developed in accordance with accepted standards of anesthesia practice, are available.
2. A qualified anesthesia provider or attending physician selects and orders the agents to achieve sedation and analgesia.
3. Registered nurses who are not qualified anesthesia providers should not administer agents classified as anesthetics, including but not limited to Ketamine, Propofol, Etomidate, Sodium Thiopental, Methohexital, Nitrous oxide and muscle relaxants.
4. The registered nurse managing and monitoring the patient receiving and analgesia sedation shall have no other responsibilities during the procedure.
5. Venous access shall be maintained for all patients having sedation and analgesia.
6. Supplemental oxygen shall be available for any patient receiving sedation and analgesia, and where appropriate in the post procedure period.
7. Documentation and monitoring of physiologic measurements including but not limited to blood pressure, respiratory rate, oxygen saturation, cardiac rate and rhythm, and level of consciousness should be recorded at least every 5 minutes.
8. An emergency cart must be immediately accessible to every location where and analgesia sedation is administered. This cart must include emergency resuscitative drugs, airway and ventilatory adjunct equipment, defibrillator, and a source for administration of 100% oxygen. A positive pressure breathing device, oxygen, suction and appropriate airways must be placed in each room where and analgesia sedation is administered.
9. Back-up personnel who are experts in airway management, emergency intubations, and advanced cardiopulmonary resuscitation must be available.
10. A qualified professional capable of managing complications is present in the facility and remains in the facility until the patient is stable.
11. A qualified professional authorized under institutional guidelines to discharge the patient remains in the facility to discharge the patient in accordance with established criteria of the facility.

Adopted By AANA Board of Directors, June 1996 Revised June 2003

BIBLIOGRAPHY

American Academy of Pediatrics Guidelines for Monitoring and Management of Pediatric Patients During and After Sedation for Diagnostic and Therapeutic Procedures. Pediatrics. 1992;89:6 1110-1114.

Barr J, Donner A: Optimal Intravenous Dosing Strategies for Sedatives and Analgesics in the Intensive Care Unit. Critical Care Clinics. 1995;11:4:827-847.

Finnie G: Conscious sedation and plastic surgery. Specialty Nursing Forum. 1990;2:8.

Gunn IP: The many issues regarding IV conscious sedation. Specialty Nursing Forum. 1990;2:2.

Harvard minimal monitoring standards. JAMA. 1986;256:8.

Holzman RS, Cullen DJ, Eichhorn JK Philip JH: Guidelines for Sedation by Nonanes-thesiologists during Diagnostic and Therapeutic Procedures. Journal of Clinical Anesthesia. 1994;6

Joint Commission on Accreditation of Healthcare Organizations. Care of Patients-Examples for Use of Anesthesia and Conscious Sedation. JCAHO Accreditation Manual for Hospitals. 1996; 194-201 .

Joint Commission on Accreditation of Healthcare Organizations. Comprehensive Accreditation Manual for Hospitals, The Official Handbook. 2000;

Kallar SK- Conscious sedation for outpatient surgery. Wellcome Trends in Anesthesiol-ogy. 1991;9:3-5, 8-9.

Kingsbury JA: IV Conscious sedation: JCAHO and hospital issues. Specialty Nursing Forum. 1990;2:7-8.

Nemiroff MS: IV Conscious Sedation: Essential Techniques of Monitoring. Trends in Health Care, Law & Ethics. 1993;8-1:87-94

Nursing Care of the Patient Receiving Conscious Sedation in the Gastrointestinal Endoscopy Setting. Society of Gastroenterology Nurses and Associates, Inc. Rochester, New York. 1991.

Practice Guidelines for Sedation and Analgesia by Non-Anesthesiologists. Anesthesiol-ogy. 1996; 84;459-71.

Qualified Providers of Conscious Sedation. American Association of Nurse Anesthetists Position Statement. Park Ridge, IL: American Association of Nurse Anesthetists. 1996;2.2

Position Statement on the Role of the Registered Nurse (RN) in the Management of Patients Receiving IV Conscious Sedation for Short-Term Therapeutic, Diagnostic, or Surgical Procedures. ANA Collaborative Statement. Washington, DC. American Nurses Association. 1991.

Spry CC: Perioperative nurses should keep monitoring within their specialty. AORN Journal. 1990;51:1071-1072.

Watson DS: Recommended practices for monitoring and administering IV conscious sedation. Specialty Nursing Forum. 1990;2:3.

Council for Public Interest in Anesthesia

See the state-by-state regulations governing RNs in regards to administering sedation and analgesia: http://www.ncsbn.ora/news/stateupdates state sedation.asp

http://www.aana.com/practice/qualified.asp

Appendix F

AORN Recommended Practices for Managing the Patient Receiving Moderate Sedation/Analgesia*

The following recommended practices were developed by the AORN Recommended Practices Committee and have been approved by the AORN Board of Directors. They were presented as proposed recommended practices for comments by members and others. They are effective Jan 1, 2002.

These recommended practices are intended as achievable recommendations representing what is believed to be an optimal level of practice. Policies and procedures will reflect variations in practice settings and/or clinical situations that determine the degree to which the recommended practices can be implemented.

AORN recognizes the numerous types of settings in which perioperative nurses practice. These recommended practices are intended as guidelines adaptable to various practice settings. These practice settings include traditional ORs, ambulatory surgery units, physicians' offices, cardiac catheterization suites. endoscopy suites, radiology departments, and all other areas where operative and other invasive procedures may be performed.

Purpose: The use of moderate sedation/analgesia allows patients to tolerate unpleasant procedures while maintaining adequate cardiorespiratory function, protective reflexes, and the ability to respond purposefully to verbal and/or tactile stimulation.[1]

Moderate sedation/analgesia is a specific level or depth of sedation in the continuum of sedation (Table 1). It is not always possible to gauge how a patient may respond to sedation: therefore the health care professional intending to produce moderate sedation/analgesia should be able to rescue patients whose level of consciousness progresses to deep sedation. The possibility that the patient may enter a deeper state, such as general anesthesia, must be considered, and rescue measures by credentialed anesthesia care providers must be available.[2]

These recommended practices provide guidelines for RNs who manage the care of patients receiving moderate sedation/analgesia. Patient selection for moderate sedation/analgesia should be based on established criteria developed

*From AORN Journal, March 2002. VOL 75. No. 3; pgs 642-652.

Table 1 | **Continuum of Depth of Sedation**

	Minimal sedation	Moderate sedation/ analgesia	Deep sedation/ analgesia	General anesthesia
Responsiveness	Normal response to verbal stimulation	Purposeful response to verbal or tactile stimulation*	Purposeful response following repeated or painful stimulation*	Unarousable even with painful stimulus
Airway	Unaffected	No intervention required	Intervention may be required	Intervention often required
Spontaneous ventilation	Unaffected	Adequate	Intervention may be inadequate	Frequently inadequate
Cardiovascular function	Unaffected	Usually maintained	Usually maintained	

Reflex withdrawal from a painful stimulus in not considered a purposeful response.

through interdisciplinary collaboration by health care professionals. The type of monitoring used with patients who receive moderate sedation/analgesia, the medications selected, and the interventions taken must be within the legally defined scope of practice for perioperative RNs.[3]

Certain patients are not candidates for moderate sedation/analgesia monitored by RNs. Such patients may require more extensive sedation and should be identified, monitored, and managed by credentialed anesthesia care providers, surgeons, or other physicians.[4]

RECOMMENDED PRACTICE I

Registered nurses should understand the goals and objectives of moderate sedation/analgesia.

1. The primary goal of moderate sedation/analgesia is to reduce the patient's anxiety and discomfort. Moderate sedation/analgesia also can facilitate cooperation between the patient and caregivers.[5] Moderate sedation/analgesia produces a condition in which the patient exhibits a depressed level of consciousness and an altered perception of pain but retains the ability to respond appropriately to verbal and/or tactile stimulation and maintains protective reflexes.
2. The RN should be knowledgeable about the following desired outcomes when moderate sedation/analgesia medications are administered:

- alteration of mood;
- enhanced cooperation;
- alteration in perception of pain;
- maintenance of consciousness:
- maintenance of intact protective reflexes;
- minimal variation of vital signs;
- some degree of amnesia: and
- a rapid, safe return to activities of daily living[6]

3. The RN may be responsible for administering ordered medications based on the patient's response and according to established protocols and defined scope of practice. Adequate preoperative patient preparation and verbal reassurances from the RN facilitate the desired effects of moderate sedation/analgesia and may allow for a decrease in the dosages of opioids and sedatives.[7]

RECOMMENDED PRACTICE II

The RN managing the nursing care of the patient receiving moderate sedation/analgesia should have no other responsibilities that would require leaving the patient unattended or compromising continuous patient monitoring during the procedure.

1. There should be an additional RN serving as the circulating nurse during any procedure in which a patient receives moderate sedation/analgesia. Continuous monitoring of the patient's physiological and psychological status by a competent RN leads to early detection of potential complications and increases the likelihood of positive outcomes.[8]

RECOMMENDED PRACTICE III

The RN should be clinically competent, possessing the skills necessary to manage the nursing care of the patient receiving moderate sedation/analgesia.

1. Health care facilities should provide or make available competency-based education programs for all RNs who manage the care of patients receiving moderate sedation/analgesia. These programs should include a competency-validation process for evaluating and documenting RNs' demonstration or relevant knowledge, skills, and abilities. Standardized competency-based programs establish baseline educational requirements and ensure comparable training throughout a facility. Evaluation and documentation of competence should occur on a periodic basis according to the health care facility's policies and procedures and according to regulatory requirements.[9]

2. At a minimum, any RN monitoring the patient receiving moderate sedation/analgesia should be competent in basic life support. Additional skills for the RN should be defined by the health care facility's policies and

procedures and may include advanced cardiac life support (ACLS) certification. Health care professionals with ACLS skills should be readily available during all procedures involving moderate sedation/analgesia. The RN monitoring the patient should demonstrate the following skills and knowledge of

- proper patient selection and screening;
- anatomy and physiology;
- total patient care parameters. including, but not limited to, respiratory rate, oxygen saturation, blood pressure, cardiac rate, and level of consciousness:
- pharmacology of medications used to induce and reverse sedation/analgesia;
- respiratory physiology, airway management, and the use of oxygen delivery devices;
- the function and use of monitoring equipment;
- cardiac dysrhythmia interpretation;
- possible complications and contraindications related to the use of moderate sedation/analgesia medications; and
- age-appropriate needs and responses of patients.[10]

3. For patient safety, it is essential that the RN monitoring the patient receiving moderate sedation/ analgesia understands how to operate monitoring equipment.

Recommended Practice IV

Each patient receiving moderate sedation/analgesia should be assessed physiologically and psychologically before the procedure. The assessment should be documented in the patient's record.

1. A preoperative assessment helps determine a patient's suitability for RN-monitored moderate sedation/analgesia by identifying potential factors for undesirable outcomes. The monitoring RN should conduct the assessment and include data from numerous sources, such as chart review, patient physical assessment and interview, and consultation with other health care providers as appropriate.[11] The preoperative patient assessment should include, but not be limited to,

- chief complaint;
- level of consciousness;
- potential airway problems;
- orientation and cognitive state;
- emotional state;
- communication ability;
- patient's perception and understanding of the
- procedure and moderate sedation/analgesia:

- history and physical examination:
- current laboratory values;
- current medications, including alternative and/or complementary preparations;
- medication allergies/sensitivities;
- current medical problems;
- surgical history;
- tobacco use and substance abuse history; and
- baseline information, including vital signs,
- height, weight and age.

2. Indication of the patient's appropriateness for the procedure also should include the American Society of Anesthesiologists (ASA) physical status classification. Patients classified as P1 or P2 are considered appropriate for RN-monitored moderate sedation/analgesia. Patients with a classification of P3 may be appropriate and should be evaluated on an individual basis. Any ASA physical status classification higher than P3 is considered inappropriate for RN monitoring during moderate sedation/analgesia.[12] The ASA physical status classification is described in Table 2.

3. After analysis of assessment data and verification of written consent for the procedure and planned sedation/analgesia, the monitoring RN should develop an individualized care plan for the patient. The assessment findings and care plan should be documented in the patient's record.

Table 2 | Physical Status Classification

Definition of patient status*	Example
P1-Normal healthy patient	No physical or psychological disturbances
P2-Potient with a mild systemic disease	Asthma, obesity, diabetes mellitus
P3-Patient with a severe systemic disease	Cardiovascular disease that limits activity; severe diabetes with systemic complications
P4-Potient with o severe systemic disease that is a constant threat to life	Severe cardiac, pulmonary, renal, hepatic, or endocrine dysfunction
P5-Moribund patient who is not expected to survive without surgical intervention	Surgery is a resuscitative effort major multisystem trauma
P6-Declared brain dead patient whose organs are being removed for donor purposes	Organ donor being maintained by life support equipment

NOTE

*The PSA physical status classification system, N American Society of Anesthesiologists, http://INWN.osohq.org/ProftnfolPhysicalStatus.html (accessed 27 Sept 2001).

RECOMMENDED PRACTICE V

The RN managing the nursing care of the patient receiving moderate sedation/analgesia should be proficient in equipment selection and use and should ensure that the necessary equipment is available and working properly

1. Monitoring equipment provides the RN with patient data to identify risks and/or complications during a procedure. Airway management devices provide the needed safety equipment to decrease the risk of adverse outcomes that potentially can occur during moderate sedation/analgesia. The following equipment should be present and ready for use in the room in which moderate sedation/analgesia is administered;
   - oxygen and delivery devices,
   - suction apparatus,
   - noninvasive blood pressure device,
   - electrocardiograph,
   - pulse oximeter, and
   - narcotic and sedative reversal agents.[13]
2. Before moderate sedation/analgesia medications are administered, an oxygen delivery device should be in place or immediately available, an IV access line should be established, and appropriate hemodynamic monitoring devices should be in place.[14] The type of IV access chosen will vary depending on health care facilities' policies and procedures and physicians' preferences. Continuous IV access provides a means for administering medications used for moderate sedation/analgesia and for implementing emergency medications and fluids to counteract adverse medication effects.[15]
3. An emergency cart with resuscitative medications including narcotic and sedative reversal medications; resuscitative equipment, such as a defibrillator, suction, and airways; and a positive pressure breathing device should be immediately available in every location in which moderate sedation/analgesia is being administered.[16] Medication overdoses or adverse reactions may cause respiratory depression, hypotension, or impaired cardiovascular function requiring immediate intervention and/or cardiopulmonary resuscitation.

RECOMMENDED PRACTICE VI

Each patient who receives moderate sedation/analgesia should be monitored for adverse reactions to medications and for physiological and psychological changes.

1. Observing the patient for desired therapeutic medication reactions, preventing avoidable medication reactions, detecting and managing unexplained adverse reactions early, and accurately documenting the patient's response are integral components of the monitoring process. The RN monitoring the patient should monitor the following parameters:

- respiratory rate and effort,
- oxygen saturation,
- blood pressure,
- cardiac rate and rhythm,
- level of consciousness,
- comfort level/tolerance to procedure, and
- skin condition.[17]

2. The RN should understand the pharmacology of moderate sedation/analgesia medications and reversal agents, including the following factors:
   - indications and dosages,
   - contraindications,
   - adverse reactions and emergency management techniques,
   - interactions with other medications,
   - onset and duration of action, and
   - desired effects.[18]

3. Patient anxiety and medications used for moderate sedation/analgesia may cause rapid. adverse physiological responses in the patient. Early detection of such responses allows for rapid intervention and treatment. Desirable effects of moderate sedation/analgesia include, but are not limited to,
   - intact protective reflexes,
   - relaxation.
   - comfort,
   - cooperation,
   - appropriate level of verbal communication,
   - patent airway with adequate exchange, and
   - easy arousal from sleep.[19]

4. Sedatives may cause somnolence, confusion, diminished reflexes, depressed respiratory and cardiovascular functions, and coma. Opioids may cause respiratory depression, hypotension, nausea, and vomiting. Oversedation and adverse reactions may occur any time during the procedure and may be reversible. Any undesirable changes in patient condition should be reported immediately to the physician. Undesirable effects of moderate sedation/analgesia include. but are not limited to,
   - aspiration,
   - severely slurred speech,
   - unarousable sleep,
   - hypotension or hypertension,
   - agitation,
   - combativeness.
   - respiratory depression,
   - airway obstruction, and
   - apnea.[20]

RECOMMENDED PRACTICE VII

Documentation of the patient's care during moderate sedation/analgesia should be consistent with AORN's "Recommended practices for documentation of perioperative nursing care."[21]

1. Documentation should include a patient assessment, prioritized nursing diagnoses, identification of desired outcomes, planned interventions, and patient responses. Perioperative RNs use the nursing process to manage the care of the patient receiving moderate sedation/analgesia.

2. Documentation of nursing interventions promotes continuity of patient care and improves communication among health care team members. It provides a mechanism for comparing actual versus expected patient outcomes.[22] Perioperative documentation should include
   - preoperative assessment:
   - actual and potential nursing diagnoses, such as
     - anxiety related to the unfamiliar environment and procedure,
     - ineffective breathing patterns or impaired gas exchange related to altered level of consciousness or airway obstruction,
     - knowledge deficit related to poor recall secondary to medication effects,
     - increased or decreased cardiac output related to medication effects on the myocardium,
     - injury related to altered level of consciousness, and
   - nursing interventions and the patient's responses, including
     - dosage, route, time, and effects of all medication and fluids used;
     - IV site location, type and amount of fluids administered, including blood and blood products, monitoring devices, and equipment used;
     - physiological data from continuous monitoring at 5- to 15-minute intervals and upon significant events;
     - level of consciousness;
     - untoward significant patient reactions and their resolution; and
     - postoperative evaluation based on preoperative assessment data.

3. The Perioperative Nursing Data Set (PNDS) should be used to document the patient's care during moderate sedation/analgesia. This standardized nursing vocabulary developed by AORN can be used to improve clinical documentation and communication between clinicians and practice settings. The PNDS includes nursing diagnoses, nursing interventions, and nurse-sensitive patient outcomes. This data set has received official recognition by the American Nurses Association.[23]

RECOMMENDED PRACTICE VIII

Patients who receive moderate sedation/analgesia should be monitored post-operatively, receive verbal and written discharge instructions, and meet specified criteria before discharge.

1. Postoperative patient care, monitoring, and discharge criteria should be consistent for all patients. Recovery time will depend on the type and amount of sedation/analgesia given, procedure performed, and facility policy. Postoperative monitoring should include respiratory rate, cardiac rate and rhythm, level or consciousness, oxygen saturation, and blood pressure. The wound/dressing condition, patency of any lines or drainage tubes, and the pain level of the patient also should be monitored postoperatively.[24]

2. Discharge criteria should be developed by representatives from nursing, medicine/surgery, and anesthesia services. These are specifically for assessing and determining the patient's readiness for discharge and home care. They should reflect indications that the patient has returned to a safe physiological level. These discharge criteria should include, but are not limited to,
   - adequate respiratory function,
   - stability of vital signs,
   - preoperative level of consciousness,
   - intact protective reflexes,
   - return of motor/sensory control,
   - absence of protracted nausea,
   - adequate state of hydration,
   - skin color and condition,
   - wound/dressing condition, and
   - reasonable pain management[25]

3. Patients and/or significant others should receive verbal and written discharge instructions and be able to verbalize an understanding of the instructions to the RN. Written preoperative and postoperative instructions, as well as verbalization of understanding, is encouraged because medications used for moderate sedation/analgesia may cause significant amnesia that directly affects recall ability. A copy of the instructions should be given to the patient and a copy should be placed in the patient's medical record.[26]

RECOMMENDED PRACTICE IX

Policies and procedures for managing patients who receive moderate sedation/ analgesia should be written, reviewed periodically, and readily available within the practice setting.

1. Policies and procedures are operational guidelines that are used to minimize patient risk factors, standardize practice, direct staff members, and establish guidelines for continuous performance improvement activities. Policies and. procedures should establish authority, responsibility, and accountability.[27] Policies and procedures for managing patients receiving moderate sedation/analgesia should include, but are not limited to.
   - patient selection criteria,
   - extent of and responsibility for monitoring,

- necessary monitoring equipment,
- medications that may be administered by the RN,
- documentation of patient care, and
- discharge criteria

GLOSSARY

American Society of Anesthesiologist physical status classification:
An anesthesia risk evaluation using predetermined criteria defined by the American Society of Anesthesiologists. This system ranks patient physical status on a scale of one to six to determine appropriate patient selection for anesthesia.

Deep sedation/analgesia:
A medication induced depression of consciousness that allows patients to respond purposefully after repeated or painful stimulation. The patient cannot be aroused easily and the ability to independently maintain a patent airway maybe impaired with spontaneous ventilation possibly inadequate. Cardiovascular function usually is adequate and maintained.

General anesthesia:
Patients cannot be aroused, even by painful stimulation, during this medication induced loss of consciousness. Patients usually require assistance in airway maintenance and often requires positive pressure ventilation due to depressed spontaneous ventilation or depression of neuromuscular function. Cardiovascular function also may be impaired.

Minimal sedation:

A medication-induced state that allows patients to respond normally to verbal commands. Cognitive function and coordination may be impaired but ventilatory and cardiovascular functions remain unaffected.

Moderate sedation/analgesia:
A minimally depressed level of consciousness that allows a surgical patient to retain the ability to independently and continuously maintain a patient airway and respond appropriately to verbal commands and physical stimulation.

Monitoring:
Clinical observation that is individualized to patient needs based on data obtained from preoperative patient assessments. The objective of monitoring patients who receive moderate sedation/analgesia is to improve patient outcomes. Monitoring includes the use of mechanical devices and direct observation.

Opioid:
Pharmacological agent that produces varying degrees of analgesia and sedation and relieves pain. Fentanyl, morphine, and hydromorphone are opioid analgesic medications that may be used for moderate sedation/analgesia.

Sedative:

Pharmacological agent that reduces anxiety and may induce some degree of short-term amnesia. Diazepam and midazolam are two benzodiazepines commonly used for sedation.

NOTES

1. American Society of Anesthesiologists, Inc, "Practice guidelines for sedation and analgesia bv non-anesthesiologists," Anesthesiology 84 (February 1996) 459-471; Joint Commission on Accreditation of Healthcare Organizations, "Standards, intent statements, and examples for sedation and anesthesia care," in Comprehensive Accreditation "Manual for Hospitals, Update 3, August 2000 (Oakbrook Terrace, Ill: Joint Commission on Accreditation of Healthcare Organizations, 1999) TX15-TX19.
2. L L Yaney, "Intravenous conscious sedation: Physiologic, pharmacologic, and legal implications for nurses," Journal of Intravenous Nursing 21 (January/February 1998) 9-19; Joint Commission on Accreditation of Healthcare Organizations, "Standards, intent statements, and examples for sedation and anesthesia care," TX15-TX19.
3. "Endorsement of position statement an the role of the registered nurse (RN) in the management of patients receiving IV conscious sedation for short-term therapeutic, diagnostic, or surgical procedures," American Nurses Association, http://www.ana.org/readroom/position/joint/jtsedate.htm (accessed 27 Sept 2001); J Odom, "Conscious sedation in the ambulatory setting," Critical Care Nursing Clinics of North America 9 (September 1997) 361-370.
4. Odom. "Conscious sedation in the ambulatory setting:' 361-370; D Dlugose. "Risk management considerations in conscious sedation:' Critical Care Nursing Clinics of North America 9 (September 1997) 429-440; L Landrum, "A nursing guide to conscious sedation: Classification of current practice issues." (Critical Care Nursing Clinics of North America 9 (September 1997) 411-418; D S Watson, Conscious Sedation/Analgesia (St Louis: Mosby Year Book, Inc, 1998) 15-16.
5. American Society of Anesthesiologists. Inc. "Practice guidelines for sedation and analgesia by non-Anesthesiologists." 459-471; J D Waegerle. "Practical considerations of intravenous sedation for the perioperative nurse." Seminars in Perioperative Nursing 7 (January 1998) 21-28.
6. Watson. Conscious Sedation/Analgesia, 15-16; Landrum, " 'A nursing guide to conscious sedation: Clarification of current practice issues," 411-418.
7. Yaney. "Intravenous conscious sedation: Physiologic, pharmacologic, and legal implications for nurses,'. 9-19: Watson: Conscious Sedation/Analgesia, 15-16: Dlugose. "'Risk management considerations in conscious sedation:' 429-440.
8. "Endorsement of position statement on the role of the registered nurse (RN) in the management of patients receiving IV conscious sedation for short-term therapeutic, diagnostic, or surgical procedures": Joint Commission on Accreditation of Healthcare Organizations. "Standards, Intent statements, and examples for sedation and anesthesia care." TX16-TX19: Waegerle, "Practical considerations of intravenous

sedation for the perioperative nurse," 21-28: D L Janikowski, C A Rockefeller, "Awake and talking: Ambulatory surgery and conscious sedation," Nursing Economics 16 (January/February I 998) 37-43: M Kost. "Conscious sedation: Guarding your patient against complications." Nursing 99 (April 1999) 34-39: Dlugose'. "Risk management considerations in conscious sedation," 429-440; Odom. "Conscious sedation in the ambulatory setting:' 361-370; Watson: Conscious Sedation/Analgesia, 28. 74: American Society of Anesthesiologists. Inc, "Practice guidelines for sedation and analgesia by non-anesthesiologists," 459-471.

9. Joint Commission on Accreditation of Healthcare Organizations, "Standards, intent statements, and examples for sedation and anesthesia care." TX15-TX19: Waegerle. "Practical considerations of intravenous sedation fix the perioperative nurse," 21-28: Janikowski. Rockefeller. "Awake and talking: Ambulatory surgery and conscious sedation." 37-43.

10. "Endorsement of position statement on the role of the registered nurse (RN) in the management of patients receiving IV conscious sedation for short-term therapeutic, diagnostic or surgical procedures"; American Society of Anesthesiologists, lnc, "Practice guidelines for sedation and analgesia by nonanesthesiologists." 459-471; Landrum. "A nursing guide to conscious sedation: Clarification of Current practice issues," 411-418; Watson, Conscious Sedation/Analgesia, 72-74; Waegerle. 'Practical considerations of intravenous sedation for the perioperative nurse." 21-28.

11. American Society of Anesthesiologists. Inc. "Practice guidelines for sedation and analgesia by non-anesthesiologists:' 459-471; Joint Commission on Accreditation of Healthcare Organizations, "Standards, intent statements, and examples for sedation and anesthesia care," TX15-TX19; Dlugose, "Risk management considerations in conscious sedation:' 429-440: Kost. "Conscious sedation: Guarding your patient against complications," 34-39; R Bryan. "Administering conscious sedation: Operational guidelines,." Critical Care Nursing Clinics of North America 9 (September 1997) 289-300.

12. Watson. Conscious Sedation/Analgesia, 20; Odom, "Conscious sedation in the ambulatory setting". 361-370: Dlugose. "Risk management considerations in Conscious sedation:" 429-440.

13. Dlugose. "Risk management considerations in conscious sedation:" 429-440; American Society of Anesthesiologists, Inc. "Practice guidelines for sedation and analgesia by non-anesthesiologists," 459-471; Joint Commission on Accreditation of Healthcare Organizations, "Standards. Intent statements. and examples for sedation and anesthesia care:" TX15-TX19; "Endorsement of position statement on the role of the registered nurse (RN) in the management of patients receiving IV conscious sedation for short-term therapeutic, diagnostic. or surgical procedures"; Watson: Conscious Sedation/Analgesia, 27-38.

14. "Endorsement of position statement on the role of the registered nurse (RN) in the management of patients; receiving IV conscious sedation for short-term therapeutic, diagnostic, or surgical procedures"; Kost. "Conscious sedation: Guarding your patient against complications:' 34-39; Dlugose. "Risk management considerations in conscious sedation." 429-440: American Society of Anesthesiologists, Inc. "Practice guidelines for sedation and analgesia by non-anesthesiologists," 459-471.

15. "Endorsement of position statement on the role of the registered nurse (RN) in the management of patients receiving IV conscious sedation for short-term therapeutic, diagnostic, or surgical procedures"; American Society of Anesthesiologists. Inc. "Practice guidelines for sedation and analgesia bv nonanesthesiologists." 459-471:' Odom, "Conscious sedation in the ambulatory setting," 361-370.

16. "Endorsement of position statement on the role of the registered nurse (RN) in the management of patients receiving IV conscious sedation for short-term therapeutic, diagnostic, or surgical procedures": Odom. "Conscious sedation in the ambulatory setting," 361-370; Landrum, "A nursing guide to conscious sedation: Clarification of current practice issues, "411.418; Yaney, "Intravenous conscious sedation: Physiologic, pharmacologic and legal implications for nurses." 9-19; American Society of Anesthesiologists, Inc. "Practice guidelines for sedation and analgesia by nonanesthesiologists," 459-471.

17. "Endorsement of position statement on the role of the registered nurse (RN\) in the management of patients receiving IV conscious sedation for short-term therapeutic, diagnostic or surgical procedures"; Odom, "Conscious sedation in the ambulatory setting," 361-370; Yaney, "Intravenous conscious sedation: Physiologic, pharmacologic, and legal implications for nurses," 9-19; ,American Society of Anesthesiologists, Inc, "Practice guidelines for sedation and analgesia by non-anesthesiologists," 459-471; Watson, Conscious Sedation/Analgesia. 27-38.

18. Odom, "Conscious sedation in the ambulatory setting," 361-370; Yaney, "Intravenous conscious sedation: Physiologic, pharmacologic, and legal implications for nurses," 9-19; Waegerle, "Practical considerations of intravenous conscious sedation for the perioperative nurse." 21-28; Dlugose, "Risk management considerations in conscious sedation," 429-440.

19. Landrum. " A nursing guide to conscious sedation: Clarification of current practice issues," 411-418; American Society of Anesthesiologists, Inc, "Practice guidelines for sedation and analgesia by nonanesthesiologist.s," 459-471; Kost, "Conscious sedation: Guarding your patient against complications," 34-39: Watson. Conscious Sedation/ Analgesia, 14.

20. Kost. "Conscious sedation: Guarding your patient against complications," 34-39; Bryan, "Administering conscious sedation: Operational guidelines," 289-300; Watson, Conscious Sedation/Analgesia, 14; Yaney. "Intravenous conscious sedation: Physiologic, pharmacologic, and legal implications for nurses," 9-19.

21. "Recommended practices for documentation of perioperative nursing care, in Standards, Recommended Practices, and Guidelines (Denver: AORN. Inc, 2001) 199-201.

22. J C Rothrock. "(Generic care planning: AORN patient outcome standards," in Perioperative Nursing Care Planning, second ed, J C Rothrock ed (St. Louis: Mosby-Year Book, Inc, 1996) 91.

23. S Beyea, ed. Perioperative Nursing Data Set (Denver: AORN, Inc., 2000) 5, 17-18.

24. American Society of Anesthesiologists, Inc. "Practice guidelines for sedation and analgesia bv non-anesthesiologists." 459-471; Bryan, "Administering conscious sedation: Operational guidelines." 289-300; Watson. Conscious Sedation/Analgesia, 98-100.

25. American Society of Anesthesiologists, Inc, "Practice guidelines for sedation and analgesia by non-anesthesiologists," 459-471; Bryan, "Administering conscious sedation: Operational guidelines" 289-300; Watson, Conscious Sedation/Analgesia. 101-103: Odom, "Conscious sedation in the ambulatory setting." 361-370; Joint Commission on Accreditation of Healthcare Organizations, "Standards, intent statements, and examples for sedation and anesthesia care," TX15-TX19.

26. Odom. "Conscious sedation in the ambulatory setting," 361-370; Watson, Conscious Sedation Analgesia, 103.

27. Joint Commission on Accreditation of Healthcare Organizations, "Standards, intent statements, and examples for sedation and anesthesia care," TX15-TX19.

RESOURCES

"Endorsement of position statement on the role of the registered nurse (RN) in the management of patients receiving TV conscious sedation for short-term therapeutic, diagnostic, or surgical procedures," American Nurses Association, http://www.ana.org/readroom/position/joint/jtsedate.htm (accessed 26 Sept 2001).

Foster, F. "Conscious sedation: Coming to a unit near you." Nursing Management (April 2000) 45-51.

Hayes, J S. et al. "Oral meperidine, atropine, and pentobarbital for pediatric conscious sedation."

Pediatric Nursing 26 (September/October 2000) 500-504,

Poe, S, et al. "Ensuring safety of patients receiving sedation for procedures: Evaluation of clinical practice guidelines." Journal on Quality Improvement 27 (January 2001) 28-41.

"Policy statement: Guidelines for monitoring and management of pediatric patients during and after sedation for diagnostic and therapeutic procedures (RE9252)," American Academy of Pediatrics, http://www .aap.org/policy/04789.html (accessed 27 Sept 2001).

"Revisions to anesthesia care standards," Joint Commission on Accreditation of Healthcare Organizations. http://www.jcaho.org/standard/aneshap.html (accessed 26 Sept 2001).

Shields. R E. "A comprehensive review of sedative and analgesic agents," Critical Care Nursing Clinics of North America 9 (September 1997) 281-288.

Appendix G

Pediatric Sedation Standards
2002-2004

CHILDREN'S HOSPITAL BOSTON, MASSACHUSETTS

The language for these standards has been adopted in part from: "Practice Guidelines for Sedation and Analgesia by Non-Anesthesiologists." Anesthesiology 96:1004-1017, 2002; the American Academy of Pediatrics, Pediatrics 89: 1110-1115, 1992; American College of Emergency Physicians (1995) Guidelines for Pediatric Sedation; and the Model Guidelines for Sedation by Non-Anesthesiologists During Diagnostic and Therapeutic Procedures as approved by the Risk Management Committee Departments of Anesthesia, Harvard Medical School, Boston, MA 1992.

Revised 2001, 2002, 2003. Approved by Sedation Committee November 2003.

PURPOSE

The purpose of these Standards is to provide patients with the benefits of sedation/analgesia while minimizing the associated risks.

* Sedation/analgesia provides two primary benefits: (1) During uncomfortable procedures, sedation and analgesia minimizes anxiety and discomfort, while also reducing undesirable autonomic responses to painful stimuli, and (2) sedation may also help the patient through a procedure that is not uncomfortable but requires that they remain still for an extended period of time.
* Excessive sedation/analgesia may result in respiratory or cardiac depression that must be rapidly recognized and appropriately managed to avoid the risk of hypoxia and/or cardiac arrest.
* Inadequate sedation/ analgesia may result in inaccurate/incomplete test results and/or patient injury.

The level of sedation/analgesia necessary to ensure patient comfort through a procedure is highly variable and dependent upon the actual or perceived invasiveness of a procedure, the developmental level of the infant/child, the patient's history of interacting with personally challenging environments, and patient's evolving capacity to tolerate stress.

To achieve comfort in infants and children during procedures three levels of *Sedation and Analgesia* are described:

- Sedation: Describes a state that allows a patient to tolerate unpleasant procedures while maintaining adequate cardiorespiratory function and the ability to respond purposefully to verbal and/or tactile stimulation.
- Deep Sedation: Describes a state that allows a patient to tolerate unpleasant procedures while maintaining adequate cardiorespiratory function BUT not the ability to respond purposefully to verbal and/or nonpainful tactile stimulation; airway reflexes remain intact and the patient continues to withdraw from painful stimulation.
- Anesthesia: Describes a state of controlled unconsciousness accompanied by a loss of protective reflexes, including the ability to maintain an airway independently and respond purposefully to painful stimulation.

These standards apply to sedated and deeply sedated patients undergoing a diagnostic or therapeutic procedure; they do not apply to otherwise healthy patients receiving peripheral nerve blocks, local or topical anesthesia, or to patients receiving up to 50% nitrous oxide, provided no other systemic sedatives or analgesics are administered. In situations where patients require anesthesia, an anesthesiologist must be involved. These standards do not apply to intensive care and perioperative areas where the patient vigilance is continuously monitored.

SEDATION PLAN

Prior to a diagnostic or therapeutic procedure, an individualized sedation plan is developed for a patient. The sedation plan includes: (1) the intended level of sedation and (2) the strategy to achieve the intended level of sedation given the individual capacities of the patient. The level of sedation and analgesia necessary to accomplish the diagnostic or therapeutic procedure is identified by the practitioner performing the procedure and communicated to members of the care team. A clinical sedation score is used to enhance communication and assessment of the end-point of therapy (see Table 1):

In addition to medication, the use of complementary alternative therapy (CAM) is encouraged. CAM includes but is not limited to the therapeutic use of parents, distraction, guided imagery, acupuncture, and therapeutic touch. Topical agents, specifically EMLA cream, may be used when time and indications permit.

FACILITIES FOR SEDATION AND ANALGESIA

A. Responsibility

The practitioner who utilizes any type of medication for sedation must assure that the proper personnel and equipment are immediately available to manage any emergency situation. Practitioner: Refers to a:

Table 1 | **Clinical Sedation Score**

Clinical Score	Level of Sedation	Patient Characteristics
1		Anxious, agitated or restless
2	Sedation	Cooperative, orientated, or tranquil
3	Sedation	Asleep, brisk response to a light stroke to the cheek
4	Sedation	Asleep, sluggish response to a light stroke to the cheek
5	Deep Sedation	No response to a light stroke to the cheek but responds to a painful stimulus (i.e. nail bed pressure)
6	Anesthesia	No response to a painful stimulus (i.e. nail bed pressure) **Consult with Department of Anesthesia**

Modified from Ramsey MAE, Savege TM, Simpson BRJ, Goodwin R. (1974). Controlled sedation with Alphaxalone-alphadolone. British Medical Journal, 2, 656-659.

- Member of the active medical/dental staff as defined in the Hospital's Bylaws (i.e. a licensed physician or dentist who is granted privileges to attend patients at Children's Hospital and its clinics), that has been credentialed.
- Nurse Practitioner privileged to prescribe schedule II-V drugs and credentialed to administer sedation.

B. Personnel

All personnel caring for the sedated patient must be able to manage a sudden deterioration in clinical status with an emphasis on acute airway management. Thus, all personnel must be certified in basic life support and knowledgeable regarding the resources available to summon emergency services.

C. Back-up Emergency Services

Back-up emergency services include the Anesthesia STAT beeper and/or the Code Blue Team in the event of a potential life-threatening situation. It must be recognized that when an anesthesiologist arrives to care for the patient, (s)he assumes responsibility for the patient care and the decision whether or not to proceed with the sedation for the diagnostic or therapeutic procedure.

D. Equipment

1. A pulse oximeter for non-invasive monitoring of heart rate and oxygen saturation is required.
2. An appropriate sized bag—mask—valve system (i.e., Ambu, Mapelson) capable of administering greater than 90% oxygen at a 15 L/min flow for at least 60 minutes must be immediately available.
3. An appropriate suction apparatus, including catheters, must be immediately available.

4. A standard emergency cart must be readily accessible.
5. Reversal agents, flumazenil and naloxone, are immediately available if benzodiazepines and opioids are being administered.

CANDIDATES FOR SEDATION

While all patients are potential candidates for sedation, those that have significant comorbidities very often need special attention. Sedative and analgesic medications may cause significant respiratory and cardiovascular depression; doses may need to be reduced in patients with pre-existing pulmonary or cardiac disease. Patients with hepatic or renal abnormalities may have impaired drug metabolism and excretion, thus causing sedation duration to be longer than expected. Patients on anticonvulsant therapy may require higher doses of sedatives per kilogram of body weight.

Infant Standard for Procedural Sedation with Routine Monitoring is as follows:

1. Four weeks post-conceptual age for full term infants (>37 weeks gestation) without a history of apnea/bradycardia or respiratory distress.
2. Sixty weeks post-conceptual age for premature infants (<37 weeks gestation) and/or history of apnea/bradycardia or respiratory distress, with no residual apnea and bradycardia.

Infant Standard for Procedural Sedation with Overnight Observation with an Apnea Monitoring is as follows:

1. Full term infants (<37 weeks gestation) that are < 4 weeks post-conceptual age.
2. Premature infants (<37 weeks gestation) that are < 60 weeks post-conceptual age.
3. Infants with a history of apnea/bradycardia or respiratory distress >60 weeks post-conceptual age with residual apnea and/or bradycardia.
4. Siblings (under 12 months) of SIDS patients.

Clinicians should consult with members of the Department of Anesthesia regarding any concerns about the use of procedural sedation with specific patients.

INFORMED CONSENT AND COMMUNICATION

A. Informed Consent

Separate consent forms are required for the procedure and for the sedation. In all instances, the sedation plan shall be outlined to the patient and/or legal guardian. Each family shall be informed of risks and benefits related to sedation. This discussion must be documented in the Medical Record on the Sedation Consent Form (See Figure 1). Congruent with existing policy, one initial consent for sedation for multiple procedures within a therapeutic regimen will suffice provided that the patient's medical condition has not changed. Informed consent is obtained by the responsible practitioner or registered nurse who has sufficient expertise to communicate relevant information (alternatives, risks and benefits)

CONSENT FOR SEDATION AND ANALGESIA

Children's Hospital Patient Stamp
300 Longwood Avenue
Boston, Massachusetts 02115

TO THE PARENT/GUARDIAN AND/OR PATIENT: This consent form is designed to confirm the discussion of the proposed sedation and analgesia you/your child will receive during you/your child's proposed diagnostic or therapeutic procedure(s).

Name _____ has explained to me and/or my child that a fully licensed practitioner from the Department of _____ will be responsible for the administration of sedation and analgesia appropriate to my/my child's condition and will monitor vital bodily functions during the procedure(s). I understand that sedation and analgesia involve risks in addition to the risks of the procedure itself. These include, but are not limited to, such things as respiratory (breathing) problems, allergic or other unexpected drug reactions, irritability, vomiting, prolonged drowsiness, unsteadiness, minor pain and discomfort, failure to achieve adequate sedation and/or possible awareness or memory of the procedure. Severe drug reactions may occur but are rare.

I also realize that the following additional sedation and analgesia related risks may occur in conjunction with the particular procedure(s) proposed for me/my child:

_____
_____

Additional comments or observations:

_____
_____

This information has been explained to me and I understand it. I voluntarily give my authorization and consent to the administration of sedation and analgesia.

Date: _____   Signed: _____
                                          ◇
                                          (Parent or Guardian necessary if Patient is under
                                          18 years of Age)

Witnessed: _____   Signed: _____
                                          ◇
© Children's Hospital   (Telephone Consents)   Patient (if 12 years or older and Physician
Boston 2003.   determines signature is appropriate)

Figure 1

and to answer questions so that understanding and agreement occur between the medical team and the patient/legal guardian.

B. Supervising Physician or Dentist

The name and beeper number of the credentialed supervising physician responsible for the procedure and sedation must be recorded on the sedation monitoring form.

C. Outpatient Procedures

All patients sedated as outpatients must be accompanied to and from the hospital by a responsible adult, who shall be required to remain on-site for the entire duration of treatment. Patients and the responsible adult will be provided with post sedation written instructions. Instructions shall include the explanation of potential or anticipated post sedation behavior and problems, any limitations of activities that are recommended, and the 24-hour contact number of an available practitioner.

PRE-SEDATION ASSESSMENT

A. Dietary guidelines are outlined in Table 2.

Table 2 | NPO Guidelines

Patients undergoing sedation/analgesia for elective diagnostic or therapeutic procedures should not drink fluids or eat solid foods for a sufficient period of time to allow for gastric emptying before the procedure (see below). In urgent, emergent, or other situations when gastric emptying is impaired, the potential for pulmonary aspiration of gastric contents must be considered in determining the timing of the intervention and the degree of sedation/analgesia.

Gastric emptying may be influenced by many factors, including anxiety, pain, abnormal autonomic function (e.g., diabetes), pregnancy, and mechanical obstruction. Therefore, the suggestions listed do not guarantee that complete gastric emptying has occurred. Unless contraindicated, pediatric patients should be offered clear liquids until 2-3 hours before sedation to minimize the risk of dehydration. Critical oral medications are excluded from NPO guidelines.

	Solids and Nonclear Liquids*	Clear Liquids**
>16 years	none after midnight	2-3 h
>36 months	6-8 h	2-3 h
6-36 months	6 h	2-3 h
<6 months	4-6 h	2 h

*This includes milk, formula (high fat content may delay gastric emptying).
**Breast milk is considered a clear liquid.
© Children's Hospital Boston 2003.

B. Pre-procedure health evaluation prior to the administration of sedating drugs: an evaluation of the patient shall be performed by the credentialed physician, dentist, or registered nurse, and verified by the practitioner prescribing the sedation. Signature of the prescribing practitioner implies that the pre-sedation assessment review and verification has occurred.

Such health evaluation must include the patient:

1. Weight in kilograms, measured within one week of the sedation. The age of the patient.
2. Allergies and previous allergic reactions.*
3. Concurrent medications, herbs, dietary supplement including name, dose, route of administration.*
4. Time of last oral intake.
5. History of tobacco, alcohol use or substance abuse.*
6. History of other co-morbidities, disorders, hospitalizations.*
7. History of sedation/anesthesia and problems that have been experienced by the patient.*
8. Family history of problems relating to anesthesia and or sedation.*
9. Established coping mechanisms, for example, meditation techniques.
10. Review of systems with specific statement describing the airway assessment.
11. Baseline vital signs including blood pressure, heart rate, respiratory rate, and level of consciousness.
12. Physical exam to include an examination of airway, pulmonary and cardiac status.

Pre-procedure laboratory testing are guided by the patient's underlying medical condition and the likelihood that the results will effect the management of sedation/analgesia (e.g., current hospital policy for pregnancy testing of female patients). Pre-Sedation assessment is documented on the Sedation Monitoring Form (see Box 1).

* Inpatient areas may cross-reference to existing documentation in the Medical Record.

PRESCRIPTION AND ADMINISTRATION OF AGENTS

A. Prescribing Medications

The practitioner responsible for the treatment of the patient and/or administration of the drugs for sedation shall be educated in sedation practices and credentialed. A signed and dated written order including dose, route and frequency of administration is required. The practitioner's signature on the sedation monitoring record (See Box 1) will meet this requirement.

B. Administration of Medication

Medications for sedation may only be administered by a credentialed physician, dentist, nurse practitioner or registered nurse.

Box 1 DOCUMENTATION GUIDELINE

PURPOSE: To provide a concise, current, factual, and legal record of pediatric patients receiving sedation for diagnostic or therapeutic procedures.

DEMOGRAPHIC DATA: The monitoring tool is stamped with the patient addressograph. Date, age, weight, location of procedure, diagnosis, procedure to be performed, and current medications are included in this section. For inpatients, the medication administration record can be referenced.

INFORMED CONSENT: Risks and benefits are to be outlined to the patient and/or legal guardian. Informed consent is to be obtained by the responsible practitioner or registered nurse who has sufficient expertise to communicate relevant information (alternatives, risks, and benefits) and to answer all questions so that understanding and agreement occur. Informed consent may be obtained for multiple procedures for patients on protocol and designated as such on the informed consent. The parent/legal guardian must remain in the hospital during the procedural sedation.

DIETARY HISTORY: This section should include date and time of last solid and clear intake.

PAST HISTORY: A check in the box would indicate usage of tobacco products, alcohol, or substances. If a check is indicated, type and amount should be listed. A recent infectious exposure would warrant a check. A check would also indicate allergies. Allergies may be cross-referenced to the patient's medical record. Diseases, disorders, past hospitalizations pertinent to the administration of sedation should be documented. A prior history of personal or family problems with sedation/anesthesia should be documented. Established coping strategies such as imagery, meditation, relaxation, use of pacifiers and favorite toys should be listed.

REVIEW OF SYSTEMS: A check in each section would indicate a normal assessment. Absence of a check would indicate an aberrance and should be documented in the comment section.

SEDATION PLAN: Prior to a diagnostic or therapeutic procedure, an individualized sedation plan should be developed for the patient. The sedation plan includes (1) the intended level of sedation and (2) the strategy to achieve the intended level of sedation. A clinical sedation score is used to communicate the desired endpoint of therapy. **The sedation strategy is the order for sedation**. The sedation strategy and practitioner's signature meet the standard for the physician's order, that is, no separate order sheet is necessary. The practitioner will note the time of anticipated peak drug effect. The practitioner responsible for sedation will have a contact number in the allotted space. Drug administration is noted in the far right hand column under monitoring.

EQUIPMENT CHECK: A check indicates the presence of functional equipment.

BASELINE VITAL SIGNS: The time and initial vital signs is documented. A Glasgow Coma Scale quantifies baseline assessment. A Glasgow Coma Score of 15 is considered normal.

Box 1   DOCUMENTATION GUIDELINE—cont'd

TIME PROCEDURE STARTED: Time procedure started is documented in military time.

TIME PROCEDURE STARTED/ENDED: Time procedure ended is documented in military time.

MONITORING: The flow sheet begins with time. The level of sedation utilizing the sedation score is documented in the second column. The Glasgow Coma scale quantifies the patient's level of consciousness during the procedure. Pulse oximeter readings are documented in columns 4 and 5. Tidal volume is a subjective assessment of the patient's respiratory effort. A check would indicate adequate respiratory effort. An absence of a check would indicate otherwise. Pulse, respiratory rate, and blood pressure are documented in the last three columns. The extra space provided is used to document medication administration and any other pertinent observation. Frequency and documentation of vital signs are outlined in the Hospital Sedation Standards.

TIME RETURN TO BASELINE LEVEL OF MONITORING: A check would indicate the vital signs are stable and with in the patient baseline. A check would indicate the level of consciousness and function are back to baseline and more than two hours have elapsed if a reversal agent was used. A check indicates the parents/guardians/adults were given written instructions. A contact person should be provided to the parents/guardian/patient should any concerns arise. Discharge location and person accompanying patient is noted.

DEPARTMENTAL MONITORING: This section is provided to track any adverse effects or untoward outcomes as a result of sedation. Either the yes or no box should be checked. Definition of adverse effects are noted on the back side of the Sedation Monitoring form as a reference.

© Children's Hospital Boston 2003.

C. Selection and Dose of Sedatives/Analgesics

Clinical areas will develop practice guidelines on the selection and dosage of sedatives used within their department. The guidelines should reflect the special needs of their patient population, the most common procedures performed within the department, and the desired level of sedation to safely accomplish a routine procedure. In addition, Home Care Instructions After Sedation (see Box 2) provides general recommendations for home care after sedation.

Clinical areas are encouraged to adopt unique strategies to ensure the comfort of their patient population but are required to have these strategies approved by the Sedation Committee prior to implementation. An evaluation plan must accompany all proposals.

PERSONNEL

Administration of sedation/analgesia and/or deep sedation requires that a minimum of two credentialed individuals be immediately available. The operator who performs a procedure and a registered nurse with the responsibility of monitoring the patient. The documentation of physical parameters may be accomplished using automated devices and may be delegated to a clinical assistant/technician, however, interpretation of the physical parameters and clinical decisions requires the clinical judgment of the registered nurse, nurse practitioner or a member of the medical/dental staff.

MONITORING

A. General

Whenever a patient is sedated a credentialed individual shall monitor the patient until the desired level of sedation and peak drug effect has been achieved. Those patients who are deeply sedated must be continuously monitored by a registered nurse, nurse practitioner or a member of the medical/dental staff.

B. Prior to the Procedure

Level of sedation/analgesia is assessed frequently (1-minute intervals) during the onset of sedation hallmarked by a change in the level of consciousness. Once the desired level of sedation is achieved, the patient may be aroused less frequently to avoid interfering with the diagnostic or therapeutic procedure.

C. During the Procedure

1. The patient's heart rate and oxygen saturation are continuously monitored using a pulse oximeter. The heart rate and saturation derived from the pulse oximeter are recorded at least every five minutes.
2. The patient's head position, airway, and chest excursion are continuously monitored. The patient is repositioned as necessary to ensure adequate spontaneous tidal volume. Respiratory rate is documented at least every 5 minutes. In cases where a sedated patient cannot be continuously observed (e.g., during a MRI) continuous SpO2 monitoring will serve as an acceptable proxy for adequate ventilation.
3. Patients with a history of cardiovascular instability must have continuous EKG monitoring; blood pressure monitored and recorded at least every five minutes.
4. Patients receiving medication therapy for hypertension should have their blood pressure monitored and recorded at least every five minutes.
5. The use of a Sedation Monitoring Form is required in all patient care areas (see Box 1).

D. After the Procedure

1. The duration of monitoring after a procedure is individualized depending upon the level of sedation achieved, overall condition of the patient and the nature of the intervention for which sedation/analgesia was administered.
2. The practitioner shall be responsible for assuring that the patient is appropriately monitored after the procedure. Monitoring shall continue until the patient is no longer at risk for respiratory or cardiac depression; specifically, until sufficient time has lapsed from drug administration through peak drug effect.
3. During the recovery period, pulse oximetry monitoring continues. The patient heart rate and oxygen saturation, respiratory rate, blood pressure, motor activity, level of consciousness/sedation score, are monitored and recorded at least once every fifteen minutes.
4. Sedated patients may need to be transported between care areas. The appropriate level of care and monitoring will continue during transport. Sedated patients are to be transported in a crib/bed with a pulse oximeter, oxygen, and registered nurse, nurse practitioner or medical/dental staff.
5. The decision to discontinue monitoring may be made by a registered nurse, nurse practitioner or medical/dental staff. Patients are discharged after a post procedure assessment by a qualified practitioner or according to criteria approved by the Medical Staff Executive Committee.
6. Guidelines for discharge:
   a. Prior to discharge, the patient level of cognition/function should be returned/progressing toward baseline.
   b. Vital signs should be stable and within the patient baseline.
   c. Sufficient time (up to 2 hours) should have elapsed after the last administration of reversal agents (naloxone, flumazenil) if used.
   d. The patient should be tolerating fluids. Prior to discharge the patient and/or their legal guardians will be provided with post procedure written instructions (see Box 2).
   e. *Discharge Score Sheet* (see Table 3).

QUALITY MONITORING

Each department is responsible for the implementation of these Standards within their department and/or clinical program. This includes, but is not necessarily limited to:

1. Assurance that practitioners are appropriately credentialed to prescribe, administer, and/or monitor sedation within their clinical area (see Box 3).
2. Adherence to standards for the safe administration of sedation.
3. Identification and monitoring of indicators (see Box 4).
4. Discussion and follow-up within specific departments and the Sedation Committee of all untoward complications.

Box 2   HOME CARE INSTRUCTIONS AFTER SEDATION

Your child received medicine today for sedation during a test or treatment. Medicine used for sedation helps relieve anxiety and decrease discomfort. This sheet gives you information on caring for your child after he or she has received sedation.

Safety

Some effects of the medication may linger on. Plan to watch your child closely for the next 24 hours especially during the ride home.

When traveling in the car, tilt the car seat slightly back. Your child's head should stay upright and tilted back. If the head falls forward, your child could have trouble breathing.

Activity

Your child may be slightly dizzy and groggy for up to 24 hours. Plan quiet activities, such as videos, TV, and quiet music.

Your child should not do anything that requires concentration or coordination. Some examples of activities not to do include bike riding, rollerblading, swimming, or studying.

Older patients should not drive a car or operate machinery for at least 24 hours.

Diet

Give clear liquids for the first few hours at home. Some examples are water, apple juice, ginger ale, Popsicles®, Jello®, broth, and tea. Advance the diet slowly as tolerated.

For infants who are breastfed, you may go back to breastfeeding after the test.

For infants who take formula, give one feeding of water or Pedialyte® before giving formula.

Do not give your child a heavy meal for the next few hours. Some children may have an upset stomach or vomit once or twice.

Older patients should not drink alcohol for at least 24 hours after sedation.

Sleeping

If your child naps or goes to bed for the night within 2 hours after leaving the hospital, you will need to check him or her once more after they go to sleep. Two hours after he or she has fallen asleep, awaken your child briefly and check the breathing pattern and skin color.

When to Call the Doctor or Nurse

Get emergency help if:

breathing appears difficult, shallow, slow, or different than usual; skin color has become extremely pale or gray.

Call _____ at _____ if:

it is very difficult to wake your child from sleeping;
your child vomits more than twice; or
you have any questions or concerns.

© Children's Hospital Boston 2003.

Table 3 | **Procedural Sedation Discharge Score**

Motor Activity

Active voluntary motion on command................................... = 2

Weak voluntary motion on command or any
nonpurposeful motion.. = 1

No motion... = 0

Respiration

Coughing on command or crying.............................. = 2

Maintaining good airway... = 1

Airway requires maintenance.................................... = 0

Blood Pressure (Systolic)

BP +/−20 mm Hg of preprocedure level
(or normal for age).. = 2

BP +/−20-50 mm Hg of preprocedure level............................. = 1

BP +/−50 mmHg of preprocedure level.................................... = 0

Consciousness

Fully awake or fully arousable on calling...................................... = 2

Responding to stimuli and intact
protective reflexes.. = 1

Not responding or absence of
protective reflexes.. = 0

Room Air Saturation

100-98%.. = 2

97-95%.. = 1

<95%.. = 0

Discharge Observation Criteria

Ready for discharge... ≥9

Re-evaluation in 30 minutes.. 7-8

Continuous monitoring until stable................................ ≤6

© Children's Hospital Boston 2003.

Box 3 DEPARTMENTAL GUIDELINES FOR CREDENTIALING

All persons caring for sedated patients must be able to manage a sudden deterioration in the patient's clinical status, with an emphasis on airway management. Thus, all persons must be certified in basic life support and know how to summon emergency services. Pediatric Advanced Life Support is suggested.

Practitioner: Individuals responsible for ordering sedatives, analgesics, or reversal agents must be familiar with the clinical pharmacology of the medications, their potential interactions, and side effects. Practitioner credentialing includes successful completion the scenario-based sedation pharmacology exam with a minimal score of 90%. The Department of Anesthesia will monitor practitioner practice. Credentialed practitioners who perform less than 5 procedural sedations annually are required to take the scenario based pharmacology exam on a yearly basis. A credentialed practitioner who has successfully completed the scenario-based pharmacology exam and who performs at least 5 procedural sedations annually without level 3 or 4 adverse events is required to maintain records of evidence.

Registered Nurse: Individuals responsible for administering sedatives, analgesics, or reversal agents must be familiar with the clinical pharmacology of the medications, their potential interactions, and side effects. Individuals responsible for using their clinical judgment when caring for sedated patients must be able to accurately assess an infants/child's level of sedation, be familiar with the clinical signs of hypoventilation, and be able to rapidly detect abnormal vital signs. RN credentialing includes successful completion the sedation monitoring exam with a minimal score of 90%. Credentialed practitioners who perform less than 5 procedural sedations annually are required to take the scenario based pharmacology exam on a yearly basis. A credentialed practitioner who has successfully completed the scenario-based pharmacology exam and who performs at least 5 procedural sedations annually without level 3 or 4 adverse events is required to maintain records of evidence. Departments may elect to participate in the credentialing process or use the sedation consulting service. The sedation consulting service is available 24 hours/day by beeper and utilizes Room 20 in the operating room for procedural sedation.

© Children's Hospital Boston 2003.

5. Yearly review and updating of departmental practices.

The Department of Anesthesia through the Sedation Committee is responsible for reviewing these standards on a yearly basis and for institutional quality monitoring. This includes, but is not necessarily limited to:

1. Credentialing practitioners (Fellow-MD level and above, Nurse Practitioners, Registered Nurses) in the safe prescription of sedation.
2. Approving all departmental specific practices regarding sedation.

> **Box 4**   DEPARTMENTAL GUIDELINE FOR QUALITY MONITORING
>
> **Patient Sedation Information**
>
> Sedation Monitoring forms are sent to the Department of Quality Improvement immediately after the procedure is completed. The Department will log the case into a data file and review the form for adverse events. The Sedation Committee will formally review all adverse events on a monthly basis. Each adverse event will be rated for level and severity of event.
>
> *Level:*
>
> 1. Expected
> 2. Unexpected and no identifiable opportunity to improve care.
> 3. Unexpected and potentially avoidable with an opportunity to improve care.
> 4. Unexpected and definitely avoidable with an opportunity to improve care.
>
> Severity:
>
> a. No sustained problem.
> b. Sustained problem, resolved before discharge
> c. Sustained problem, expected to resolve before discharge
> d. Permanent or semi-permanent complication
> e. Death
>
> The Sedation Committee will provide individual and departmental follow-up on all adverse events rated above level 3b within one month of notification. **Note: Practitioners should notify Risk Management immediately of all serious events.** Risk Management will then notify the Sedation Committee Chairs. A complete analysis of a single month's data will be performed yearly to assess for evolving trends and departmental compliance with the established standard of care.
>
> © Children's Hospital Boston 2003.

3. Oversee quality monitoring of Level 3-4 adverse events including:
   - providing feedback to all practitioners
   - reporting adverse events to department chiefs and nursing directors
   - contributing data to hospital profiling system.
4. Reviewing and updating hospital-wide sedation standards when appropriate (see Box 5).

© Children's Hospital Boston 2003.

Box 5 SEDATION COMMITTEE CHILDREN'S HOSPITAL BOSTON

Request for Sedation Strategy Which Differs from Hospital Guidelines

To ensure that all patients receive optimal care, the Sedation Committee has implemented hospital-wide standards of care for procedural sedation. While these standards include drug selection guidelines, the committee does not limit any department from the introduction of a new sedation strategy that may improve the quality of care provided to a particular patient population. However, in order to implement the administration of a drug strategy not specified by the current guidelines, a written request must be formally submitted to the Sedation Committee. The following criteria must be included in a department's formal request:

– Location of the practice change
– Supervising physician
– Strategy including drug, dosage, route, and frequency of administration
– Procedures in which the new strategy will be used
– Patient inclusion/exclusion criteria
– Desired level of sedation
– A list of practitioners who will prescribe the drug
– Education plan for staff responsible for drug administration
– Desired outcome and monitoring plan

I. Aim: What are you trying to accomplish?—Purpose statement, including pertinent background information. Please be specific, narrow in scope, and quantify if possible (i.e., Adverse events are occurring because of the use of multiple drug agents. We will reduce the use of multiple drugs by 20%)

II. How will you know a change is an improvement?

a. Include a summary of baseline measures that will be used to determine the effectiveness of the changes (i.e. a chart review of x patients will be done monthly).
b. Specify the desired goal(s) and outcome(s). (i.e. 85% of our patients will be sedated using a single drug).

III. Results: Data must be presented to the Committee 6 months following implementation.

All aspects of the current standard of care will apply unless a specific change in practice is outlined within the request. The Sedation Committee will review the request at its monthly meeting (4th Thursday of the month) then notify the department/requesting Practitioner of the Committee's decision in writing. All requests will be approved for a 6-month pilot period. After 6 months, pilot results must be presented to the Committee for final review and approval.

© Children's Hospital Boston 2003.

Index

A

AAAASF. *See* American Association for Accreditation of Ambulatory Surgery Facilities (AAAASF)

AANA. *See* American Association of Nurse Anesthetists (AANA)

AAP. *See* American Academy of Pediatrics (AAP) guidelines

ACLS. *See* Advanced cardiac life support (ACLS)

Adolescents developmental approaches, 169

Adult respiratory distress syndrome (ARDS), 188

Advanced cardiac life support (ACLS), 231
  metanalyses, 287t

AGA. *See* American Gastroenterological Association (AGA)

Agency for Healthcare Research and Quality (AHRQ), 8-9

Age specific competency, 184-185, 185t

Aging physiologic changes, 180-183

Agitation, 187, 188, 195, 196, 206
  causes of, 194b
  medications for, 201t-202t
  pathophysiologic mechanisms of, 189-196

AHRQ. *See* Agency for Healthcare Research and Quality (AHRQ)

Airway
  assessment of, 84-85, 165-166
  ASA guidelines, 276
  of children, 161-162
  management competencies, 151, 151t

Alabama state board of nursing information, 243

Alaska state board of nursing information, 243

Alcohol withdrawal, 195-196

Allergic reactions, 102-103

Alphabet boards in mechanically ventilated patient, 214

Alprazolam (Xanax), 206

American Academy of Pediatrics (AAP) guidelines, 157-158, 158b

American Association for Accreditation of Ambulatory Surgery Facilities (AAAASF), 11

American Association of Nurse Anesthetists (AANA), 11, 12b

American Association of Oral and Maxillofacial Surgeons guidelines, 10

American College of Chest Physicians, 198

American Dental Society of Anesthesiology guidelines, 10

American Gastroenterological Association (AGA), 11

American Nurses Association (ANA)
  moderate sedation monitoring, 38t
  NAPS, 12b
  nursing practice standards, 6, 7b

American Society of Anesthesiologists (ASA)
  fasting guidelines, 277
  guidelines, 157-158
    airway assessment procedures, 276
    anesthetic induction used for sedation, 273
    combination agents, 272
    deep sedation, 277-279
    discharge criteria, 279

Note: Page numbers followed by "f" refer to illustrations; page numbers followed by "t" refer to tables; page numbers followed by "b" refer to boxes.

American Society of Anesthesiologists
(ASA) *(Continued)*
emergency equipment, 271, 278
general anesthesia, 280
intravenous access, 273-274
medication titration, 272-273
minimal sedation, 277
moderate sedation, 277
monitoring, 267-268
individuals responsible for,
270
patient evaluation, 266
personnel training, 270-271
preprocedure preparation, 266-267
recording monitored parameters,
269
recovery care, 275, 279
reversal agents, 274-275
special situations, 275-280
supplemental oxygen, 271-272
MAC, 3-4
moderate sedation monitoring, 38t
NAPS, 11
patient classification status, 85-86
physical status classification, 36t,
124t-131t, 304
practice guidelines, 9
preprocedure fasting guidelines, 34t,
40b-41b
sedation continuum, 140t
Task Force on Sedation and Analgesia
by NonAnesthesiologists, 261-289
American Society of Hospital
Pharmacists, 198
American Society of PeriAnesthesia
Nurses (ASPAN)
moderate sedation monitoring, 38t
standards, 110
Amiodarone interactions, 27t
Amnesia, 17, 159
ANA. *See* American Nurses Association
(ANA)
Analgesia, 262

Analgesics, 199-205
Anaphylaxis, 102-103, 103t
Anesthesia and sedation instructions,
117f
Anesthesia monitoring standards, 238-
241
body temperature, 240-241
circulation, 240
oxygenation, 239
personnel, 238-239
ventilation, 239-240
Anesthetic agents, 234-236
Angiotensin converting enzymes
interactions, 27t
Antagonists, 208-209
Antiarrhythmics interactions, 27t
Anticoagulants interactions, 27t
Anxiety, 213
with blood pressure measurement, 45
mechanically ventilated patient, 214
medications for, 199t
spectrum of control, 54f
Anxiolysis. *See* Minimal sedation
Anxiolytics, 205-208
Anxious patients, 187
Aphrodisiac, 207
Apprehension, 191, 193
APRN. *See* Association of Perioperative
Registered Nurses (APRN)
ARDS. *See* Adult respiratory distress
syndrome (ARDS)
Arizona state board of nursing
information, 243
Arkansas state board of nursing
information, 244
ASA. *See* American Society of
Anesthesiologists (ASA)
ASPAN. *See* American Society of
PeriAnesthesia Nurses (ASPAN)
Aspiration, 96-98, 97t
Association of Perioperative Registered
Nurses (APRN)
moderate sedation monitoring, 38t

Association of Perioperative Registered Nurses (APRN) *(Continued)*
patient discharge, 107
recommended practices, 10
Asthma, 25, 161
children, 88
Ativan. *See* Lorazepam (Ativan)
Auscultatory gap with blood pressure measurement, 45

B

Bacteremia, 207
Bag valve mask device, 94
Barbiturates, 103
Basic life support (BLS), 231
Behavior, 159
Benzodiazepine, 3, 56-63, 88, 198
causing respiratory depression, 90
clinical uses, 57
mechanism of action, 56
metanalyses, 284t
pharmacokinetics, 56
pharmacology, 56
rapid withdrawal of, 223
Benzodiazepine antagonists, 63-65
Beth Israel Deaconess Medical Center (BIDMC) sedation manual, 132f-139f
Bispectral Index (BIS), 218
monitor, 219f
range guidelines, 220f
Black cohosh, 30t
Blood pressure
assessment of, 45-46
metanalyses, 286t
Blood urea nitrogen (BUN), 195
BLS. *See* Basic life support (BLS)
Body temperature with anesthesia monitoring, 240-241
Bolus doses, 198
Brain function, 192b, 193
Breach of duty, 228
Breathing metanalyses, 286t
Bronchodilators for children, 88

Bronchospasm, 96
BUN. *See* Blood urea nitrogen (BUN)
Butorphanol (Stadol), 66, 66t, 74-76

C

CAD. *See* Coronary artery disease (CAD)
California state board of nursing information, 244
CAM. *See* Complementary and alternative medication (CAM)
CAM ICU scale. *See* Confusion assessment method for ICU (CAM ICU scale)
Capnography, 42, 43f
metanalyses, 286t
Cardiac dysrhythmias, 101-102
Cardiovascular problems
history of, 24-25
NPPE, 98-99
Cardiovascular system in elderly, 180-182
Cards, mechanically ventilated patient, 214
Catapres. *See* Clonidine (Catapres)
Causation, 228
Centers for Disease Control and Prevention, 10
Central nervous system in elderly, 182
Certified respiratory nurse anesthetists (CRNA), 290-293
Chest pain, 189
Children
airway assessment of, 161-162
asthma, 88
bronchodilators, 88
communication guidelines, 156b
developmental approaches to, 167
fainting history, 162
heart rates, 167t
ICP, 88
intramuscular sedation, 171
intravenous administration, 171-172
midazolam, 170

Children (Continued)
  nursing care of, 163b-164f
  oral sedation, 170-171
  pain assessment, 162
  physical examination of, 161
  preoperative assessment, 162t
  rectal sedation, 171
  respiration rates, 167t
  respiratory distress
    signs of, 166t
Chloral hydrate, 175t
Chlorpromazine hydrochloride
  (Thorazine), 209
Chronic obstructive pulmonary disease
  (COPD), 87
Chronic renal failure (CRF), 88
Circulation
  anesthesia monitoring standards, 240
  assessment of, 42-45
Clinical sedation score, 311t
Clonidine (Catapres), 210-211
  side effects of, 202t
Coffee withdrawal, 195-196
Cognition, 35
Colorado state board of nursing
  information, 244
Combination therapy, 211-213
  metanalyses, 284t
Combined probability tests, 282, 283
Communication, 141
  with children, 156b
  with mechanically ventilated patient,
    214
  moderate sedation, 232
Competence, 146-153
  determining appropriate, 147-148
  moderate sedation, 230-231, 230b,
    297-298
  program implementation, 152
  sedation specific, 148-152
Competencies
  age specific, 184-185, 185t
  airway management, 151, 151t
  with core practice areas, 150t

Competency outcomes and performance
  (COPA) model, 149f
Competency statement, 150t
Complementary and alternative
  medication (CAM), 26, 310
Complications, 82-103
  management, 89-103
  trends, 82-83
Confusion, 195
  causes of, 194b
  mechanically ventilated patient, 214
Confusion assessment method for ICU
  (CAM ICU scale), 189, 190-191
Connecticut state board of nursing
  information, 244
Consciousness
  assessing level of, 46-48
Conscious sedation
  complications, 82-103
  depth continuum, 15t
  drug dosage, 124t-125t
  history of, 1-18
    nursing perspective, 3-4
  intraprocedure record, 128t
  levels of, 13-16
  nursing diagnosis, 131t
  objectives of, 16-17
  patient selection for, 17-18
  position statements, 8
  post procedure recovery, 130t
  practice guidelines, 8-10
  procedure record, 126t-128t
  recommended practices, 10-11
  vital signs record, 129t
Contin. See Morphine (MS Contin)
Cooperation, 16
Coordination, 191
COPA. See Competency outcomes and
  performance (COPA) model
COPD. See Chronic obstructive
  pulmonary disease (COPD)
Core practice, 149t
Core practice area competencies,
  150t

Coronary artery disease (CAD), 87
CRF. *See* Chronic renal failure
  (CRF)
Critical care guidelines for sedation,
  224f
Critically ill, 187
  family crisis, 213
CRNA. *See* Certified respiratory nurse
  anesthetists (CRNA)

D

Damages, 229
Deep sedation, 14, 15, 15t, 140t, 263t,
  304
  ASA guidelines, 277-279
  defined, 156
Delaware state board of nursing
  information, 245
Delirium, 189, 209, 223
  medications for, 201t-202t
  pathophysiologic mechanisms of, 189-
  196
Demerol. *See* Meperidine (Demerol)
Demerol, 65
Dexmedetomidine (Precedex), 211
  side effects of, 202t
Diabetes, 89
Diagnostic assessment, 36
Diazemuls. *See* Diazepam (Valium)
Diazepam (Valium), 3, 56, 57-59, 57t,
  173t, 199t, 205-206
  side effects of, 201t
Difficult airway management
  physical examination findings
  associated with, 86t
Dilaudid, 199t
  side effects of, 202t
Dilaudid (hydromorphone), 205
Diprivan. *See* Propofol (Diprivan)
Discharge criteria
  ASA guidelines, 279
  moderate sedation, 303
Discomfort, 191, 198
  medications for, 199t

District of Columbia state board of
  nursing information, 245
Diuretics
  interactions, 27t
Documentation, 49-50
  guidelines for, 316-317
  moderate sedation, 233, 302
Drug addiction, 88
Drug interactions, 27t-28t
Drug solubility, 55t
Drug tolerance, mechanically ventilated
  patient, 221-222
Duty, 228
Dyspnea, 188, 191
Dysrhythmia, 101-102
  recognition and management, 151

E

Echinacea, 30t
Education and competence, moderate
  sedation, 230-231
Education and training, metanalyses,
  287t
Elderly, 88
  cardiovascular system in, 180-182
Elderly surgical patients, improving care
  for, 180t
Electrocardiogram, 45-46, 46f
  metanalyses, 286t
Emergency
  cart, 300
  equipment, 48, 89-90
    ASA guidelines, 271, 278
  management, 152
  moderate sedation, 232, 300
  services, 311
EMLA. *See* Eutectic mixture of local
  anesthetics (EMLA)
Emphysema, 25
Ephedra, 30t
Equipment, 135f, 311-312
  moderate sedation, 300
Eutectic mixture of local anesthetics
  (EMLA), 171-172

Extended elimination half lives, 212-213

F

Facilities, 158-161
Fainting history, children, 162
Family crisis, critically ill, 213
Fasting, 29
    guidelines for, 165f
        ASA, 277
Fentanyl, 54, 65, 199t, 200
    activity sites, 66t
    side effects of, 201t
Fentanyl (Sublimaze), 71-73, 88, 204
Feverfew, 30t
Fibrinolytic drug interactions, 28t
Fisher Combined Test, 282
Florida state board of nursing
        information, 245
Flumazenil (Romazicon), 57, 63-65, 95,
        176t, 208-209
    metanalyses, 285t

G

Garlic, 30t
Gastric motility, 200
Gastroesophageal reflux, 161
Gastrointestinal system in elderly,
        183
General anesthesia, 15t, 140t, 263t,
        304
    ASA guidelines, 280
Genitourinary system in elderly, 183
Georgia state board of nursing
        information, 246
Geriatric sedation, 179-185
    patient care, 184
    patient selection for, 183-184
Ginger, 32t-33t
Ginkgo biloba, 32t-33t
Ginseng, 32t-33t
Glasgow Scale, 218
Glucuronide conjugation, 56

H

Haloperidol (Haldol), 199t, 209-210
    side effects of, 201t
Hawaii state board of nursing
        information, 246
Head tilt chin lift procedure, 92f
Heart rates
    children, 167t
    metanalyses, 286t
Hemodynamics, 268
Heparin interactions, 27t
Hepatic dysfunction, 89
Herbs, 30t-34t
High risk patients, 86-89
Home care instructions, 320
Hydromorphone. See Dilaudid
        (hydromorphone)
Hyperactive delirium, 190
Hypercapnia, 89, 90
Hyperthyroidism, 26, 89
Hypnotics, 205-208
Hypoactive delirium, 190
Hypoglycemia, 195
Hypoglycemic agent interactions, 28t
Hypotension, 99-101, 195
    algorithm, 100f
Hypothyroidism, 26, 89
Hypoventilation, 89
Hypoxia, 89, 90, 193

I

ICP. See Intracranial pressure (ICP)
ICU. See Intensive care unit (ICU)
Idaho state board of nursing
        information, 246
Illinois state board of nursing
        information, 246
Indiana state board of nursing
        information, 246
Infants, developmental approaches to,
        168
Informed consent, 37, 136f, 312-313
Injuries, 229

Institution policy and guideline
    development for standard of care,
    120-144
Instructions for local anesthesia and
    sedation, 117f
Insulin interactions, 28t
Integumentary system in elderly, 183
Intensive care unit (ICU), 187
    psychosis, 189
    route of administration, 197
    visiting hours, 213
Interdisciplinary conscious sedation use
    documentation review, 142f-144f
Intracranial pressure (ICP) in children,
    88
Intramuscular sedation for children,
    171
Intraprocedural care and
    documentation, 140-141
Intraprocedural monitoring, 37-48
Intravenous (IV)
    access ASA guidelines, 273-274
    administration, 53-56, 197
        children, 171-172
    benzodiazepines, 57t
    conscious sedation, 258
    continuous infusion, 55-56
    push, 54
    titration, 55
Intubation, recommended equipment
    for, 94t
Ionization, 55t
Iowa state board of nursing
    information, 246
IV. See Intravenous (IV)

J

Jaw thrust maneuver, 92f
Joint Commission on Accreditation of
    Healthcare Organizations
    (JCAHO), 10
    moderate sedation monitoring, 38t
    patient discharge, 111-115

Joint Commission on Accreditation of
    Healthcare Organizations (JCAHO)
    (Continued)
    patient identification, 21
    sedation protocols, 38-39

K

Kansas state board of nursing
    information, 247
Kava, 32t-33t
Kentucky state board of nursing
    information, 247
Ketamine (Ketalar), 79-80, 175t
    ASA guidelines, 273
Ketorolac tromethamine (Toradol), 200
    side effects of, 201t

L

Laryngospasm, 95-96
Learning needs, 36-37
Legal issues, 227-236
Level of consciousness metanalyses,
    286t
Liability causes, 229b
Lidocaine, 102
Lipid solubility, 55t
Liver disease, 25
Local anesthesia and sedation
    instructions, 117f
Lorazepam (Ativan), 56, 57t, 59-61, 174t,
    199t, 206, 212
    side effects of, 201t
Louisiana state board of nursing
    information, 247
Luer Scale, 216t

M

MAC. See Monitored anesthesia care
    (MAC)
Maine state board of nursing
    information, 248
Mallampati technique, 23, 24f, 125t
Malpractice, 228-229

Mantel Haenszel odds ratio, 283
Manual, BIDMC, 132f-139f
MAO. *See* Monoamine oxidase (MAO)
    inhibitor interactions
Maryland state board of nursing
    information, 248-249
MASS. *See* Motor Activity Assessment
    Scale (MAAS)
Massachusetts state board of nursing
    information, 249
Mechanically ventilated patient
    communication, 214
    daily wake up, 219-221
    drug tolerance, 221-222
    nonpharmacologic measures, 213-214
    pharmacologic measures, 196-208
    sedation, 187-225
    sedation scale, 214-219
    weaning, 221
    withdrawal symptoms, 222
Medicare, MAC, 3
Medication, 173t-176t
    administration of, 149, 315
        pediatric sedation, 169-172
    allergy, 26
    prescribing, 315
Meperidine (Demerol), 3, 70-71, 200
Metabolic acidosis, 195
Metabolic disturbances, 193-195
Metanalyses, 283, 284t-287t
Methohexital, 173t
    ASA guidelines, 273
Michigan state board of nursing
    information, 249
Microstream capnography, 157
Midacolam, 174t-175t
Midazolam (Versed), 56, 57t, 61-63,
    199t, 207
    children, 170
    pharmacokinetics, 56
    side effects of, 201t
Minimal sedation, 14, 15t, 140t, 263t,
    304
    ASA guidelines, 277

Minnesota state board of nursing
    information, 249
Mississippi state board of nursing
    information, 249
Missouri state board of nursing
    information, 250
Mixed delirium, 190
Moderate sedation, 14, 15t, 140t, 263t,
    304. *See also* Conscious sedation
    anesthetic agent administration, 234-
        236
    ASA guidelines, 277
    communication, 232
    competence, 230-231, 230b, 297-298
    discharge criteria, 303
    documentation, 233, 302
    education, 230-231
    emergencies, 232
    equipment, 300
    goals and objectives of, 296-297
    medication administration, 231-232
    monitoring, 38t, 300-301
    patient assessment, 298-299
    patient monitoring, 232
    policies and procedures, 230, 303-
        304
    postoperative monitoring, 302-303
    practice issues, 229-230
    preoperative assessment, 298-299
    preprocedural care, 231
    recommended practices, 295-308
    risk management, 229-236
    wrong site surgery, 233, 233f
Modified PostAnesthesia Discharge
    Scoring System, 111b
Monitored anesthesia care (MAC)
    reimbursement, 3
Monitoring, 137f-138f, 304, 318-319
    ASA guidelines, 267-268
    individuals responsible for, 270
    metanalyses, 286t
    moderate sedation, 300-301
Monoamine oxidase (MAO) inhibitor
    interactions, 28t

Montana state board of nursing information, 250
Mood, 16
Morphine (MS Contin), 65, 67-70, 199t, 200, 203-204
    activity sites, 66t
    side effects of, 202t
Motor activity, 187
Motor Activity Assessment Scale (MAAS), 218
MS Contin. See Morphine (MS Contin)

N

Nalbuphine (Nubain), 66, 67, 73-74
    activity sites, 66t
Naloxone (Narcan), 76-77, 95, 208, 274
    metanalyses, 284t
NAPS. See Nurse administered propofol sedation (NAPS)
Narcan. See Naloxone (Narcan)
Nasopharyngeal artificial airway, 91, 93f
National Guideline Clearinghouse (NGC), 8-9, 9b
Nausea, 213
Nebraska state board of nursing information, 250
Neck assessment, 84-85
Negative pressure pulmonary edema (NPPE), 98-101
    physiology of, 99f
    risk factors for, 98t
Neuroleptics, 209-211
Neuromalignant syndrome, 209-210
Nevada state board of nursing information, 250
New Hampshire state board of nursing information, 251
New Jersey state board of nursing information, 251
New Mexico state board of nursing information, 252
New York state board of nursing information, 252

NGC. See National Guideline Clearinghouse (NGC)
Nonanesthesia providers, 1
    practice guidelines, 261-289
    scope of practice, 4-13
Nonanesthesia registered nurses, 1
    procedures performed by, 2b
    standard of care, 4
    standards of practice, 5-10
Nonclear liquids, 314
Nonsteroidal antiinflammatory drugs (NSAID), 103
    interactions, 27t
Norepinephrine, 193
North Carolina state board of nursing information, 252
North Dakota state board of nursing information, 252
Nothing by mouth (NPO)
    guidelines, 314-315
    status, 84
NPPE. See Negative pressure pulmonary edema (NPPE)
NSAID. See Nonsteroidal antiinflammatory drugs (NSAID)
Nubain. See Nalbuphine (Nubain)
Nurse administered propofol sedation (NAPS), 11
Nursing practice standards, ANA, 6, 7b

O

Obesity, 87
    with blood pressure measurement, 45
Occupational Safety and Health Administration (OSHA), 10
Ohio state board of nursing information, 253
Oklahoma state board of nursing information, 253
Opiates, 198
    rapid withdrawal of, 223
Opioid agonist-antagonists, 73-76
Opioid agonists, 65-73
Opioid antagonists, 76-77

Opioids, 304
   activity sites, 66t
   adverse effects, 301
   causing respiratory depression, 90
   metanalyses, 284t
Oral hypoglycemic agent interactions,
   28t
Oral sedation, children, 170-171
Oregon state board of nursing
   information, 253
Oropharyngeal airway, 92, 93f
OSHA. *See* Occupational Safety and
   Health Administration (OSHA)
Outcomes evaluation, 141-144
Outpatient procedures, 314
Oxygenation, 268
   anesthesia monitoring standards, 239
Oxygen saturation, 39, 283
   elderly, 184
Oxyhemoglobin dissociation curve, 41f

P

PACU. *See* Postanesthesia care unit
   (PACU)
PADSS. *See* PostAnesthesia Discharge
   Scoring System (PADSS)
Pain, 158, 188, 191, 193, 213
   assessment in children, 162, 163b-
      164f
   history of, 29
   spectrum of control, 54f
   threshold, 16
PAR. *See* Postanesthetic Recovery (PAR)
   Score for Outpatient's Street
   Fitness
Parkinson's disease, 210
Patient
   ASA evaluation guidelines, 266
   assessment, 29
      position, 23
      for sedation, 17-18, 159, 298-299
   discharge, 107-118, 159
      guidelines for, 116b
      phase II, 114b-115b

Patient *(Continued)*
      phase II unit goals, 113b
      planning, 141
      postprocedure assessment, 109-110
      postprocedure phone call, 116-118
      report, 107-108
      teaching and instructions, 115-116
   education, 36-37
   identification, 21-22
   information, 323
   monitoring, 37-39
      moderate sedation, 232
   risk factors, 84-89
   safety, 21-22, 158
Peak airway pressure, 188, 195
Pediatric sedation, 155-172
   intraprocedure assessment, 165-166
   medication administration, 169-172
   postprocedure assessment, 166-169
   preprocedure assessment, 161-165
Pennsylvania state board of nursing
   information, 254
Pentobarbital, 173t
Perioperative Nursing Data Set (PNDS),
   302
Personality disorders, 191
Personnel, 133f-134f, 158-161, 311,
   318
   privileging of, 134f-135f
   standards for, 238-239
   training of, 134f-135f
Personnel training, ASA guidelines,
   270-271
pH, 55t
Pharmacology, 53-80
Phencyclidine derivative, 79-80
Phlebitis, 206
Physical evaluation, 21-22, 22t-23t
Physical status classification, 299t
   ASA, 124t-131t
Physicians, children, 160
Piercings, 29
PNDS. *See* Perioperative Nursing Data
   Set (PNDS)

Pneumothorax, 188
Policies and procedures for moderate
    sedation, 303-304
PONV. *See* Postoperative nausea and
    vomiting (PONV)
Position statements
    conscious sedation, 8
    on role of RN, 258-270
Postanesthesia care unit (PACU), 107
PostAnesthesia Discharge Scoring
    System (PADSS), 109, 110b,
    111b
Postanesthetic Recovery (PAR) Score for
    Outpatient's Street Fitness, 109,
    112b
Postoperative monitoring for moderate
    sedation, 302-303
Postoperative nausea and vomiting
    (PONV), 11, 96-97
Postprocedure assessment, 48-49
    patient discharge, 109-110
Postprocedure patient care and
    discharge planning, 138f-139f
Postprocedure phone call for patient
    discharge, 116-118
Practice guidelines
    ASA, 9
    conscious sedation, 8-10
    nonanesthesia providers, 261-289
Practitioners, 322
Precedex. *See* Dexmedetomidine
    (Precedex)
Premature ventricular contractions
    (PVC), 102
Preoperative assessment for moderate
    sedation, 298-299
Preprocedure assessment, 20-24
    and documentation, 136f-137f
    metanalyses, 286t
Preprocedure fasting
    guidelines, 34t
    metanalyses, 286t
Preprocedure preparation, ASA
    guidelines, 266-267

Preschool children
    developmental approaches to, 168-169
Presedation assessment, 314-315
Presedation history, 21-22, 22t-23t
Private insurers, MAC, 3
Procedural documentation, 49b
Procedural Sedation Discharge Score,
    321t
Professional negligence, 228-229
Professional performance standards,
    ANA, 7b
Propofol (Diprivan), 11-12, 77-78, 103,
    176t, 199t, 207-208, 212, 222
    ASA guidelines, 273
    side effects of, 201t
Protective reflexes, 16
Protein binding, 55t
Psychomotor recovery, 283
Psychosocial assessment, 35
Pulmonary ventilation, 267-268
Pulse
    assessment of, 42-43, 44t
        quality, 44
        rate, 43-44
        rhythm, 44
    oximetry, 39-42, 157
        metanalyses, 286t
PVC. *See* Premature ventricular
    contractions (PVC)

Q

QT interval, 210
Quality monitoring, 319-320

R

Ramsay sedation scale, 47, 47b, 215,
    216t
Rapid recovery from conscious sedation,
    17
Receptor side effects, 65t
Recommended practices
    conscious sedation, 10-11
Recording monitored parameters, ASA
    guidelines, 269

Recovery care, ASA guidelines, 275, 279
Rectal sedation, children, 171
Registered nurses (RN), 322
    liability causes of, 229b
    management and monitoring by, 292-293
    moderate sedation, 296-305
    policy guidelines for, 291-293
    position statement on role of, 258-270
    qualifications of, 292
Renal disease, 25
Renal system in elderly, 183
Report for patient discharge, 107-108
Respiration rates for children, 167t
Respiratory complications, 90-98
Respiratory depression, 90, 206
    management of, 91t
Respiratory distress, signs in children, 166t
Respiratory system in elderly, 182
Reversal agents
    ASA guidelines, 274-275
    metanalyses, 284t, 285t
Rhode Island state board of nursing information, 254
Riker Sedation Agitation Scale, 217t, 218
Risk analysis, 227
Risk evaluation, 227
Risk identification, 227
Risk management, 227-236
    moderate sedation, 229-236
RN. See Nonanesthesia registered nurses; Registered nurses (RN)
Romazicon. See Flumazenil (Romazicon)
Roxanol. See Morphine (MS Contin)

S

SAS. See Sedation Agitation Scale (SAS)
Saw palmetto, 32t-33t
School age children, developmental approaches to, 169

Scope of practice, nonanesthesia providers, 4-13
Sedation
    candidates for, 312
    complications, 296t
    continuum of, 83f, 156, 263t
    critical care guidelines for, 224f
    defined, 262
    mechanically ventilated patient, 187-225
    standards, 309-324
    strategy differing from hospital guidelines, 324
Sedation Agitation Scale (SAS), 217t, 218
Sedation instructions, 117f
Sedation protocols, JCAHO, 38-39
Sedation rating scale, 125t, 133f
Sedation recovery, 283
Sedation related risk factors, 183-184
Sedation scales, 48b, 222
    comparison of, 216t-217t
    mechanically ventilated patient, 214-219
Sedatives, 305
    adverse effects, 301
    dosage of, 317
    metanalyses, 284t
    selection of, 317
Seizure, history, 24
Sensory input, emotional response to, 193
Sensory system in elderly, 183-184
SGNA. See Society of Gastroenterology Nurses and Associates (SGNA)
Shelly Scale, 216t-217t
Short term memory deficit, 191
Sleep apnea, 85t
Smoking, 89
Society of Critical Care Medicine, 198
Society of Gastroenterology Nurses and Associates (SGNA), moderate sedation monitoring, 38t

Solids, 314
South Carolina state board of nursing
    information, 254
South Dakota state board of nursing
    information, 254
St. John's Wort, 32t-33t
Stadol. *See* Butorphanol (Stadol)
Standard of care
    development of, 12-13, 121-144
    institution policy and guideline
        development, 120-144
    nationally endorsed guidelines
        evaluation, 122-123
    nonanesthesia providers, 4
    policy format, 123, 140
    team member selection, 121-122
Standards of practice
    nonanesthesia registered nurses (RN),
        5-10
    sedation, 309-324
State boards of nursing, 5, 242-247
    moderate sedation monitoring,
        38t
    NAPS, 11
Stouffer Combined Test, 282
Streptokinase interactions, 28t
Sublimaze. *See* Fentanyl (Sublimaze)
Substance abuse, 26
Supervising dentist, 314
Supervising physician, 314
Supplemental oxygen
    ASA guidelines, 271-272
    metanalyses, 284t
Sympathetic inhibiting agents, 209-211

T

Teaching and instructions, patient
    discharge, 115-116
Tennessee state board of nursing
    information, 254
Texas state board of nursing
    information, 254
Thiopental, 173t

Third party payers, MAC, 3
Thorazine. *See* Chlorpromazine
    hydrochloride (Thorazine)
Thyroid disorders, 25-26
Tilt chin lift maneuver, 91
Tissue drug uptake, 55t
Tissue mass, 55t
Toddlers, developmental approaches to,
    168
Tolerance, 212-213
Tongue piercings, 29
Toradol. *See* Ketorolac tromethamine
    (Toradol)
TPA interactions, 28t

U

Urokinase interactions, 28t
Utah state board of nursing
    information, 255

V

Valerian, 34t-35t
Valium. *See* Diazepam (Valium)
Valrelease. *See* Diazepam (Valium)
VAS. *See* Visual analog scale (VAS)
Ventilation, anesthesia monitoring
    standards, 239-240
Ventilatory function, 39-42
Vermont state board of nursing
    information, 255
Versed. *See* Midazolam (Versed)
Virginia state board of nursing
    information, 255
Visiting hours, ICU, 213
Visual analog scale (VAS), 68f, 69f
Vital signs, 16
Vivol. *See* Diazepam (Valium)
Vomiting, 213

W

Warfarin interactions, 27t
Washington state board of nursing
    information, 255

Weaning mechanically ventilated patient, 221
West Virginia state board of nursing information, 256
Wisconsin state board of nursing information, 256
Wrong site surgery, moderate sedation, 233, 233f

Wyoming state board of nursing information, 256

X

Xanax. *See* Alprazolam (Xanax)

Z

Zetran. *See* Diazepam (Valium)

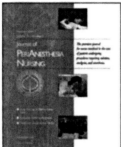